Problems of Veterinary Education, Science and Profession

Problems of Veterinary Education, Science and Profession

Guest Editor

Joanna Wojtacka

MDPI • Basel • Beijing • Wuhan • Barcelona • Belgrade • Novi Sad • Cluj • Manchester

Guest Editor
Joanna Wojtacka
Faculty of Veterinary Medicine
University of Warmia and Mazury in Olsztyn
Olsztyn
Poland

Editorial Office
MDPI AG
Grosspeteranlage 5
4052 Basel, Switzerland

This is a reprint of the Special Issue, published open access by the journal *Animals* (ISSN 2076-2615), freely accessible at: https://www.mdpi.com/journal/animals/special_issues/N9PCVS45UP.

For citation purposes, cite each article independently as indicated on the article page online and as indicated below:

Lastname, A.A.; Lastname, B.B. Article Title. *Journal Name* **Year**, *Volume Number*, Page Range.

ISBN 978-3-7258-8251-9 (Hbk)
ISBN 978-3-7258-8252-6 (PDF)
https://doi.org/10.3390/books978-3-7258-8252-6

Contents

About the Editor

Joanna Wojtacka

Joanna Wojtacka is an associate professor at the Department of Veterinary Public Health, Faculty of Veterinary Medicine, University of Warmia and Mazury in Olsztyn. She has been involved in the didactic process for future and post-graduate veterinarians across various One Health subjects. She specializes in the hygiene of animal origin products, and has a special interest in bee products, their chemical composition and the biological hazards posed by anaerobic microflora. She has expertise in food law and problems related to work of veterinarians in all fields of the public health sector, particularly in relation to veterinary food inspectors.

animals

MDPI

Article

Veterinary Expert: Legal Nature and Responsibility

Andrzej Dzikowski

Department of Food Hygiene and Public Health Protection, Warsaw University of Life Sciences, 159 Nowoursynowska St., 02-787 Warsaw, Poland; andrzej_dzikowski@sggw.edu.pl

Simple Summary: The issuing of expert opinions is rarely found as a topic of discussion in veterinary colleges as one of the forms of veterinary practice. At the same time, it has a significant social, legal, and economic impact. This article examines veterinary experts and expertise from an interdisciplinary ethical and comparative legal perspective, regarding different definitions and underlying basic assumptions concerning the meaning of veterinary expertise. Analysis reveals how the terminology used changes the perception of the examined institution. Legally relevant factors of an expert opinion are identified: direct connection with the law and the intended, applied use of this opinion in a legal context. A variety of sources of legal and ethical duties and the related liability of the veterinary expert are revealed, both as a proficient and as a member of a public trust profession. Different theoretical and practical suggestions are made to clarify and facilitate expertise in various contexts of veterinary professional practice.

Abstract: Veterinary professional practice can be performed in many forms, including expert activity. The importance of veterinary expertise is, however, often underrated and limited to only one of its areas. Nonetheless, veterinary expert opinions have significant social, legal, and economic impacts. This study investigates veterinary expertise from an interdisciplinary, comparative perspective. Ethical and legal analysis and interpretation are performed. Essential concepts and relevant aspects of veterinary expertise are analysed. Legally relevant factors of an expert opinion are identified. The relationship between the law, the language, and the understanding of the role and duties of a veterinary proficient is demonstrated. A variety of possible expert opinions and the multiplicity of veterinary scopes of such activity is presented. It is argued that the ranges of forensic veterinary medicine and of veterinary expertise are broader than is predominantly assumed. Veterinary forensic medicine is a crucial part of veterinary specialisation. Ethical and legal basics, and the scope of veterinary expert's liability, are revealed and discussed. The conclusion is that the duties and responsibilities of expert veterinarians are particularly great due to the exercise of the public trust profession, with large importance for the whole society. Their observance is, however, crucial to ensure the highest quality of expert opinions issued by veterinarians.

Keywords: veterinary ethics; veterinary forensic medicine; veterinary law; expertise; expert opinion; civil law; penal law; legal procedure

1. Introduction

Among the forms of veterinary professional practice, the issuing of decisions, predicates, certificates, reports, and opinions of various kinds can be indicated [1,2]. Not only decisions on the state of health of an animal, which are the everyday work of general practitioners, but also expert opinions belong to this sphere of professional activity.

The general definition of an expert is based on the special skills or knowledge of a certain person [3–13]. Similarly, the definition of "expertise" could refer simply to a specific skill or type of knowledge [12]. These are abstract and globally consistent definitions. They are independent of a given jurisdiction and its specific, detailed legal regulations, or local traditions. Moreover, they are uniform and unanimous throughout science. This common, universal basis allows for the current analysis.

Any veterinary professional is, and should be, in fact, professional par excellence, and thus an expert in veterinary medicine [14–16]. He or she could specialise, with expertise in a particular scope of study, knowledge, and skills. Every veterinary surgeon is—or could be—an expert.

Therefore, a fundamental question may be asked about whether an expert includes

- any veterinary surgeon;
- a specialist, in the sense that a veterinarian deals with a given, specific problem area and has knowledge and skills in this respect;
- a specialist, in the sense of an officially recognised title, such as veterinary surgeon; or
- the legal function of a proficient?

The goal of the author is to analyse, prove, and present universal and essential features developed by science, professional ethics, and law worldwide, regardless of the jurisdiction. Such a general and universal type of study is possible due to the fundamental homogeneity of the considered problem, the essential identity of legal solutions on a global scale, and the uniformity of veterinary sciences.

The inevitability of interdisciplinary knowledge used in all types of veterinary practice, including expertise in all its meanings, is indicated [14,17]. Therefore, the current analysis has an interdisciplinary and comparative veterinary, legal, linguistic, and ethical nature.

A comparative legal analysis of the concept of the veterinary expert is carried out. Nevertheless, it is decided to reduce the number of citations of legal acts to a minimum, selecting only the most representative ones. An etymological and linguistic analysis of the legal vocabulary also sheds light on the definitions accepted and adopted, and the background of the terms used. Functional and teleological paths of legal interpretation are also used.

2. Expert and Expertise

The definitions of "expert" and "expertise" are comprehensive and have existed since, at least, the second half of the 19th century [12], although the institution of expert veterinarians is much older [18]. It should be noted that the definitions of the discussed concepts are sometimes subject to logical fallacy, being defined as *idem per idem* (i.e., a vicious circle) [19].

Additional characteristics of an expert are emphasised, however, in the literature. According to the established opinions of the scientific community, a veterinary expert is a person qualified in veterinary medicine in terms of not only knowledge and skills but also his or her education, experience, training, and thus—personal cognizance [10,20–22]. The roles of long-term and ongoing practice, the current work at the time that the expert opinion is issued, experience in researching a given issue, and experience in issuing opinions are especially appreciated [9,19,21,22].

It should be noted that this covers not only any specific field of veterinary science or practice, but also a general veterinary medical cognizance, which laymen do not possess [1,6,10,12,16]. The point of reference is the state of the general, common knowledge of a typical citizen with an average education and no particular interests.

2.1. When a Veterinary Expertise Is Not Possible

It should be noted that veterinary peer courts, as a rule, should not commission expert opinions in veterinary sciences. As persons who possess special knowledge, the judges of such courts should assess the case investigated by themselves. According to the author, this is a specific variant of the *iura novit curia* (the court knows the laws) rule.

The only exception should be considered for highly specialised and rare aspects of veterinary medicine. Such a statement is an effect of the extensive teleological interpretation of the legal provisions, analogous to the possibility of admitting evidence from an expert opinion on international law before a court of justice [11].

On the other hand, if there was a judge in a civil or criminal court, who is a veterinary surgeon, he/she cannot use his/her personal veterinary knowledge and should order an expert opinion [11]. The accumulation of different procedural roles by the judge would violate the adversarial, contradictory nature of the court proceedings and would undermine the constitutional guarantees for the parties.

This conclusion does not apply only to exceptional situations in which the legislator has provided for the possibility of veterinarians acting as experts and arbitrators [23–25], and private arbitration at the request of the parties, where the veterinarian acts simultaneously as an expert and as a *iudex privatus* (private judge).

2.2. Scope and Impact of Veterinary Expertise

The veterinarian's expert opinion can apply to all matters related to animals, as well as nature protection, environmental and ecosystem protection, interspecies interactions, public health protection, food safety, fodder, drugs, etc. [7,8,20,26–28].

A specific, underestimated type of veterinary experts is those who can be described as "scientific experts". They could work on behalf of public authorities, government, non-governmental organisations, or industry, providing scientific veterinary expertise in biosecurity, food safety and public health, animal production and productivity, agriculture, etc. [12,15,16,28–30]. This includes expert opinions issued within state veterinary authorities, both carried out purely in the laboratory and as a result of "field work" with the principle of "learning by doing", e.g., in the eradication of transmissible diseases [12,16,28,29]. This type of expertise may have an impact on society via the implementation and application of the scientific work and veterinary knowledge [12,28].

Another impact that veterinary expertise could have is its incorporation into the law-making process, at the local, national, and international levels (e.g., food safety laws, infectious disease combat and prevention, animal welfare, statutes regulating the economic use of animals and their productivity). As with the introduction of interdisciplinary elements of other sciences, including technical and ethics, into veterinary expertise [2,17,30], it is also possible and desirable to introduce elements of veterinary medicine, through expert opinions, into other technical sciences, humanities, and the law.

A very important area of expertise is the assessment of veterinary malpractice in civil and disciplinary proceedings [11,31].

3. Terminology Used and the Understanding of the Position and Duties of an Expert

In addition to the mentioned considerations, it is necessary to examine how the terminology used affects the (in)correct understanding of the legal institution, position, and duties of the veterinary expert.

3.1. Who Is an Expert?

The word "expert" is derived from the Latin *expertus*, *ex-peritus*. It is a designation of a person who is skilful or who is experienced in something. The word *experior*, likewise, means to try, to test, to put to the test, to make trial of a person or thing, to find out, to prove [32–34].

As already indicated, any veterinarian could be an expert in a legal sense [4,15]. Every veterinarian, including general practitioners, is a specialist in his field and is recognised as such by the law. As has been stated above, all veterinary knowledge is a special factor that laymen do not possess [15,16].

Veterinarians could practice issuing "opinions", even unknowingly or unaware [8], but this does not imply that every aspect of veterinary practice is expertise. The factors that make a given activity an expert opinion will be presented in the following part of the analysis.

The conducted research allowed the conclusion that the term "expert witness" is widely abused [35–38]. The nomenclature "expert witness" greatly (and faultily) influences the perceptions of experts in the Anglophone world. It should be observed that linguistic issues overlap in this respect with the legal regulations of the common law.

Many authors, as well as professional legislators, seem to be trapped in their linguistic imaginings, and—despite noticing and demonstrating fundamental differences—still place the expert opinion on par with evidence given by a factual witness [1,4,10,13,36,37,39].

There should be no doubt that the duties, powers, and the entirety of the legal institution of a veterinary expert differ significantly and fundamentally from cases in which a veterinary surgeon is called as a witness of a fact in a case. A veterinary expert's opinion differs from factual evidence to the same extent. Indeed, these differences are so profound that they can be indicated without any doubt [10,13,36,37], so it was decided not to repeat these arguments in the current work.

3.1.1. Professional Witness

Problematic, however, are the so-called "professional expert opinions", as some [1,3], but not all [13], researchers refer to cases in which a veterinarian testifies before a court or other authority about information obtained in the course of his/her professional work. The equivalent term "professional witness' evidence" is also used [1,3,10,35]. The activities of such a witness could include not only providing facts but also collecting evidence [9].

Notions are presented [1,9,10] according to which the "professional expert opinion" or "professional witness' evidence" is a legal institution that lies between an expert opinion and a witness' testimony. Supporters of this theory maintain that it is a specific form of a "*de facto* expert", due to his/her professional qualifications.

This position is not only fundamentally errant but also internally contradictory. There should be no doubt that this is *nec plus ultra* the testimony of a factual witness (nothing further beyond). No particular knowledge is used directly in this testimony, and it is not the subject of evidence. The fact that the veterinary surgeon will use, in his testimony as a witness, the knowledge he/she has gained from education, practice, and experience is irrelevant. As with other witnesses, everyone has a certain degree of knowledge, background, and life experience. In the discussed case, the veterinarian is to provide only factual information. His/her profession has no particular legal relevance and is merely accidental.

3.1.2. Professional Secrecy

Nevertheless, the witness testimony of a veterinary surgeon regarding any information obtained in the course of professional work is a very complex issue. It relates to one of the most important ethical and deontological obligations of a veterinarian, as a representative of a profession of public trust, namely professional secrecy [10,20,27,40,41].

This is one of the oldest duties of professional medical ethics, included in the Hippocratic oath [13,42]. It should be noted that professional secrecy applies to *all* information obtained during the work of a veterinarian. It applies to *all* facts, not merely the animal itself or its state of health or the animal's owner. Moreover, it is not limited to clinical practice only and includes also official veterinarians and veterinary scientists.

A veterinarian may testify about the facts that he/she has gained as information in the course of his professional work only if he is released by an authorised body, such as the court, in the appropriate procedure. Alternatively, the person to whom the information relates may release the veterinary surgeon from confidentiality.

3.2. Further Terminology

A veterinary expert can also be named, particularly in the judicial context, a proficient. The word "proficient" is also derived from Latin, referring to somebody acting on behalf of somebody else [32–34].

It is the expert veterinary who conducts the examination, issues a decision, draws up a report, and presents it. He or she works for the layman, such as the judge. Expert opinion allows laymen to understand complex, specialised issues and problems. It is a particular form of assistance [1,4,6,10,19,22,26,31], and advice [1,4,6,14,15,32,43].

It has been found that in the veterinary scientific literature, the use of the aforementioned *terminus technicus* is extremely rare. The author hereby proposes the more frequent use of this term and the discontinuation of the usage of the ambiguous term "expert witness".

Other terms used in a related sense include "connoisseur" (and "connoisseurship"), borrowed from French and used predominantly in relation to cuisine, music, and the fine arts, as well as the Italian term "cognoscente", derived from Latin. Similar is the Yiddish-based "maven". Etymologically, they all refer to someone who has specialised, above-average knowledge in a particular field [32–34]. A different, yet related, meaning is attributed to the word "doyen" (f. "doyenne"), meaning the oldest, and therefore the most experienced, individual [33]. Unlike the term "proficient", their use in a veterinary context is not recommended.

As has been shown, most of the terminology is derived from Latin. A similar situation can be observed in most of the European languages. In other languages, particular terms referring to the expert carry the following semantic loads: knowledgeable, professionally competent, reasonable appraiser (e.g., German *Sachverständiger*), proper estimator, evaluator, adjudicator, adviser (e.g., German *Gutachter*), or somebody fluent and eloquent (e.g., Polish *biegły*).

3.3. Specialisation and Expertise

A "specialist" is a person devoted to a particular, specialised branch of science or a profession, particularly a medical one, such as a branch of veterinary medicine. The initial use of this term in English was in a medical context, similarly in French. Becoming specialised is a result of differentiation, adopting a specific area of study and practice, e.g., veterinary surgery, canine diseases, cariology, or neurology [44]. It should be noted that in most jurisdictions, there is no separate postgraduate specialisation in forensic veterinary medicine or forensic veterinary pathology [1,21,36,43].

Such specialised, above-average (compared to other veterinarians) knowledge and skills are the basis for being an expert—and, moreover, being one in an effective and correct way. They, however, do not in themselves make a given veterinarian legally proficient.

Synonymous terms "specialisation" and "expertise" are both used with different meanings, depending on the context [10,27], i.a., the specialised knowledge itself, the possession of such knowledge, the actual specialisation, the title of specialist, the administrative duties, and the performance of an expert opinion. The expert opinion itself can be also referred to as "expertise".

Specialisation, or expertise, in a given field of veterinary medicine, e.g., in neurology, proves deepened professionalisation. It has a significantly positive impact on the cognizance of a given veterinarian [4,14] and increases their likelihood of examining a given type of case. The same must be said both for actual expertise in a certain field of veterinary medicine and for the officially recognised title of the specialised DVM.

On the other hand, it should be observed that specialisation in such a narrow sense is not a prerequisite and *sine qua non* condition for becoming a forensic veterinary expert [21]. As has been already mentioned, the reference point is the average level of a layman. The exact subject and complexity of the case are also important.

Doctoral and professor titles, as well as various training courses and scientific conferences, should be treated in a manner analogous to what was stated above for the legally recognised specialisation.

Indeed, the vast majority of veterinary experts are academics or specialised practitioners [1,21]. There are very few "experts by profession" who are devoted solely to examining cases and producing reports [1,21].

Nevertheless, a certain doctrinal consensus can be observed: actual skills and knowledge tested in practice are far more important than the title itself [7,9,19,45]. Such a certified title helps in obtaining a court order or a civil contract [1] and helps the expert to demonstrate his/her proficiency and professionalism [7]. Each diploma can be used as a credential, a certification of quality, and a justification of the competencies that one possesses in a tangible way [7,9,46].

In the case of a court expert, it is the court (the judge) who assesses the proficiency and decides and grants the status to the given veterinarian [7,11].

As has been revealed, above-average knowledge and skills are not, by themselves, enough. Being an expert in light of the law is also not tantamount to having the title of a specialist or actually specialising in a given branch of veterinary medicine.

3.4. Legally Relevant Factors

The above-mentioned question should be reposed, but from a slightly different point of view: what factors are legally relevant for the proficient or expert in the strictest sense?

The conducted research allowed the conclusion that these factors are

- a direct connection with the law, and
- the intended, applied use of the expert opinion or report in a legal context.

Therefore, for example, clinical examinations performed as part of the diagnostics and therapy of animals, post-slaughter examinations of meat, administrative examinations of district veterinary officers, or state veterinary hygienists and scientific tests do not provide an expert opinion *per se*. The listed factual and legal cases lack the simultaneous, cumulative occurrence of the two mentioned *sine qua non* prerequisites. In particular, administrative decisions regarding the suitability of meat for consumption, or designating an outbreak of an infectious animal disease, are not expert opinions. Such decisions are classified differently, due to being the fulfilment of administrative obligations imposed by the law.

3.5. Veterinary Expert and Veterinary Forensic Medicine

The term "veterinary forensic medicine" should also be understood similarly to the definition of the veterinary proficient. It covers any usage of veterinary medicine for the purpose of the law [1,36].

The author, however, strongly rejects the limitation of the legal institution of an expert to judiciary proceedings or to forensic pathology. Such a limitation would be contradicted by the arguments of both historical and current legal provisions on a global, comparative scale. One of the reasons for such a false, narrow understanding of the analysed issues is, as has already been shown, the abuse of the term "expert witness".

Different types of expert opinions [4,11,17,36,39], together with the differentiation criteria, are presented in Table 1.

Table 1. Types of expert opinions.

<table>
<tr><th>Criteria</th><th colspan="2">Types of Opinions</th></tr>
<tr><td rowspan="6">Commissioning entity</td><td rowspan="4">Court</td><td>Prepared by registered experts</td></tr>
<tr><td>Prepared by experts appointed ad hoc or ad casum</td></tr>
<tr><td>Commissioned ex officio/motu proprio</td></tr>
<tr><td>Commissioned at the request of the party to the proceedings</td></tr>
<tr><td colspan="2">Official (ordered by the police, procurature, public authority)</td></tr>
<tr><td colspan="2">Private, extrajudicial (such opinion may be used in the court as a substantive support, source of arguments, source of further evidence requests, motion or request for an evidence, private document evidence, basis for a supplementary opinion of another expert, or for appointing an expert, etc.)</td></tr>
<tr><td rowspan="2">Mandatority/not</td><td colspan="2">Mandatory (required by the law)</td></tr>
<tr><td colspan="2">Facultative</td></tr>
</table>

Table 1. *Cont.*

Criteria	Types of Opinions	
Form of realisation	Independent, individual expert	
	Collective (prepared by two or more veterinary surgeons) and complex (one opinion prepared by the veterinary expert and expert(s) from another field of expertise)	
	Institutional (prepared by scientific institutions, public veterinary administrative institutions, veterinary clinics, or veterinary laboratories; form excluded in some jurisdictions, yet very useful in veterinary science, where elaborate opinions that require equipment and many specialists can be developed)	
Content of the opinion/report	*Sensu largo* (containing course of activities, examinations, and conclusions, as well as additional documents, e.g., results of laboratory tests)	
	Sensu stricto (solely conclusions, allowed predominantly in the course of purely clinical or administrative practice)	
Form of the opinion/report	Oral	
	Written	
	Mixed	
Type of material	Abstract (theoretical)	
	Examination-based	
	Based on case files	
	Based on case files and examination	
Order, task assigned, or importance	Primordial	
	Ultimate	
	Partial	Preliminary
		Provisional
		Supplementary (by the same expert as the primordial one)
		Accessory
	Counter-expertise (by another veterinary expert besides the primordial one, having the same value as evidence)	
	Super-expertise (in German: *Oberexpertise;* improperly named "consulting expertise" by some authors; by other veterinary experts besides the previous expert(s), evaluating previous opinion(s), having higher value as evidence; type present only in some jurisdictions, such as Switzerland, while in others it is explicitly excluded by the law)	
Type of expert's conclusion or justification	Categorical (unequivocal)	
	Probable (alternate)	
Content of expert's conclusion or justification	Total	
	Partial	

Henceforth, the legal context of veterinary medicine shall be broadly understood [5,36]: as court proceedings, administrative proceedings, legislation, contract conclusion, etc. Neither veterinary expertise nor veterinary forensic medicine are limited solely to court evidence or to pathology, as some hold [6,7,10,19].

Most of the veterinary literature focuses on forensic veterinary court experts in criminal proceedings [6–8,17,22,31,36,38,47–49], while other contexts of the activity of expert veterinarians are merely mentioned [1,2,5,7,26,31,44,48,50]. Animal abuse, animal welfare, animals as victims of accidents, animals causing injuries to people, and other issues related to pathomorphology provide relevant examples of veterinary expertise, but they are definitely not exhaustive.

Forensic veterinary medicine is a separate, broad, and interdisciplinary branch of science, and it is not the same as forensic veterinary pathology, which is its subdivision; a veterinary expert is not the same as a veterinary pathologist [8,14,17,36,47]. Nevertheless, according to the author, veterinary forensic medicine cannot be interpreted as synonymous with veterinary specialisation [5], the latter being a broader term.

In particular, attention should be paid to the private-law aspects of forensic veterinary medicine, and of veterinary expertise, such as animal-sales-related examinations and opinions. The author's statement is based on the legal provisions of many legal regimes [31,51] and on the practical and economical significance of such expert opinions. This crucial theme is notoriously ignored in the majority of the veterinary scientific literature discussing expert opinions.

Moreover, the author's view is supported by the linguistic interpretation, as the word "forensic" is derived from the Roman *forum* (market). Therefore, it is incorrect to claim that the extension of the meaning of forensic veterinary medicine (from forensic pathology to veterinary jurisprudence) is a trend of the recent past [1,26]. On the contrary, it is a return to the origins of the discussed discipline.

3.6. *Untrue Novelty*

It is often stated in the literature that veterinary forensic medicine is a new scientific discipline and that the activities of expert veterinarians are a "new form" of practicing the profession [1,8,47]. These are definitely erroneous and untrue statements of novelty.

The use of expert opinion in relation to veterinary medicine in its modern meaning in various normative acts dates back (at least) to the end of the 18th century. Eminent examples include expert veterinarians adjudicating on the occurrence of physical defects in animals, performing official examinations, and deciding on price reductions. Such regulations are, or have been, present in the following states: Austria, Belgium, Germany, France, Luxembourg, Poland, Spain, and Switzerland [23–25,46,52–57].

Sales-Related Expert Opinions

Bearing in mind the above examples, the author would like to return to the aforementioned sales-related veterinary examinations and issuing of sales-related expert opinions. It should be noted that the use of terms such as "vetting" or "pre-purchase examinations" [10,26,58–61] does not cover the entire scope of the issue in question.

These synonyms apply only to veterinary examinations conducted, and opinions issued, *before* concluding of the contract of the sale of an animal. Meanwhile, veterinary examinations are often carried out, and opinions issued, *after* the conclusion of the contract, *after* the animal's delivery, when a physical defect in the animal is revealed and manifested. Examinations and opinions can be carried out both intravitally [17,26,36] and post-mortem [47], including post-slaughter.

There is no substantial difference between a veterinary examination aimed at issuing expert opinions before and after the conclusion of the contract, before and after the delivery, or those ordered by the seller, by the buyer, or by the court (in the event of a dispute regarding the animal warranty). German veterinary science provides a variety of names for sales-related veterinary examinations and opinions [57–62]; nevertheless, according to the author, they should not be differentiated [51,60].

A similar legal nature is presented in opinions issued by veterinarians after examining an animal's health in relation to exhibiting it at competitions, shows, or races or allowing it to breed.

There is no doubt that the development of veterinary expertise and specialisation in the legal veterinary field has already taken place: in terms not only of the proper performance of the role of veterinary expert, and thus acting *lege artis*, but also legal obligations and professional ethics and deontology [51,57–61].

4. Characteristics of the Veterinary Expert Opinion

Unlike factual witnesses, who provide facts and information to the court, other authorities, or private persons, the expert witness provides an opinion: conclusions and interpretations of the results obtained [8,13].

It is reasonable to distinguish between a veterinary surgeon's decision—a comprehensive verdict on an animal's health status—and an expert opinion, also called a report. The first is a manifestation of the activity conducted by a clinician or pathologist, or a public veterinary officer. As has been revealed, decisions may be issued not only in the case of expert opinions.

The report/opinion is the final formulation of the results, observations, and conclusions of a proficient [51]. It should be noted that not all opinions of expert veterinarians are based on decisions on an animal's health. Both decisions and reports may be presented in oral, written, or mixed form.

An opinion/report should be balanced, clear, complete, concise, confidential, considered (taking into account all data and materials, even those that detract from the conclusion), consistent with life experience, convenient, fact-based, impartial, independent, intelligible and understandable (to the layman), integral, in relation to the matter, justified, lawful, logical, methodologically appropriate, objective, precise, prepared within a certain period of time, professional, properly appointed and in accordance with the provisions of the procedure in question, qualified, relevant, reliable, scientifically based, scrupulous, self-confident, sound, truthful, unbiased, and uninfluenced [1,3,7–11,13,19,36,43]. It is especially important that the opinion is not written in an over-intellectualised or incomprehensible manner regarding its addressee, the layman [7,8,11,12,36]. The court, the public administration, the industry, and the animal owner must understand the opinion in order to benefit from it.

Opinion-making and the preceding examinations are dependent on the personal performance of the commissioned expert [11,51]. Acting by proxy or deputy is strictly prohibited, due to the strict personal nature of this obligation. As has been shown, the personal skills, knowledge, experience, and cognizance of a given proficient are the factors of key importance.

Moreover, the opinion/report should contain appropriate reservations, regarding, i.a., aspects that go beyond the scope of questions asked to the expert; that go beyond the scope of the specialisation, knowledge, skills, and competence of the expert; that go beyond the area, scope, or range of expertise; for which a decision cannot be made on the basis of the available research material or other insufficient data; and on which discrepancies or differing opinions are presented in the scientific discourse [8–10,13,21,40,50].

Expert's Liability

Therefore, the following opinions should be considered defective: those that are incomplete, those that go beyond the subjective or the objective, or the expert's cognizance; and those that are illogical, internally contradictory, contradictory (in the case of several opinions), unscientific (contrary to current knowledge), illogical, intentionally falsified, unclear, methodologically incorrect, suggested, or biased [11].

In the case of court expert opinions, after analysing them in accordance with the principle of discretion (free assessment of evidence), the court accepts the opinion when it meets the requirements of correctness, rejects the opinion in its entirety, or partly rejects the opinion [4,19,22,48]. The court may also order a supplementary opinion (*ex officio*, or at the request of the party). The expert bears public-law liability for a faulty opinion, e.g., imprisonment or a pecuniary fine [11]. Penal liability for inappropriate behaviour in the courtroom is also possible [11]. The court expert is a public-law institution, and thus bears public-law liability of a criminal and administrative nature.

The issue of private, extra-judicial opinions is different. In the case of a defect in the opinion, the commissioning party (e.g., owner, seller, buyer of the animal) may not accept the defective opinion as a defective performance of the obligation (and, thus, a breach of contract), or they may possibly accept it. The commissioner is entitled to compensation, and, in some jurisdictions, also to a warranty for defects in the opinion. It is a civil, private-law liability [23,51–54,59,61,62], as the expertise commissioned in a civil contract has a private-law nature.

In addition, a veterinarian may be held professionally and disciplinarily liable in the case of defective opinions, both judicial and extra-judicial [51]. A veterinarian working in a scientific or state institution, or in a clinic, may also be liable as an employee [51].

Such a situation has, moreover, a significant negative effect on his/her scientific and professional reputation. His/her moral responsibility towards the whole society is, therefore, worth considering.

5. Duties of Veterinary Experts

The abstract, general, and unspecific obligations and duties of experts are well established both in legal acts—especially the codes of criminal, civil, and administrative procedures—and in judicial decisions, and the scientific literature. At the same time, these rules are the features of a proper expert opinion. Therefore, the same can be said about the duties of an expert [1]. These are interdependent and inextricably intertwined issues. Compliance with the expert's duties results in the issuance of a proper opinion. All of these aspects are established and are uniform for all types of expert opinions; hence, they will not be discussed in more detail.

Instead, the author's intention is to focus on a more complex problem: are the duties, responsibilities, and liability of a veterinary expert the same as the duties, responsibilities, and liability of proficients in other areas of expertise?

The conducted analysis allowed the conclusion that there are significant differences in the case of experts performing professions of public trust, such as veterinary medicine, and burdened with professional ethics [2,5,6,14,26,44,51,59,63,64]—in relation to experts who do not perform such professions and are not required to comply with professional ethics.

The duties of a veterinary professional and the duties of an expert overlap and complement each other. They arise from different sources and different systems of social control and result in different legal liabilities. In addition, there may be further mixing of duties derived from other sources, e.g., religion, national law, international law, labour law, civil law, scientific ethics, etc. [51]. All these conditions create a specific, individual, and uniform model of the bonds resting on a given entity [51].

Nevertheless, the premise that distinguishes the veterinary expert from other proficients is the professional ethics and deontology [13,26,51,64].

The risk of liability of the veterinary expert is, in the author's opinion, greater than in other cases. Being a representative of the profession of public trust [57,62] is an additional criterion affecting the increase in the rigor of the liability and the lowering of its threshold.

Regardless of criminal and professional liability, a veterinary expert may also bear civil responsibility. In particular, the following civilian liability can be indicated: liability for damages, for *culpa in contrahendo* (fault in conclusion of the contract, in the case of private opinions), and tort liability [57,60,62], as well as liability towards third parties, e.g., an animal buyer who does not order an expert opinion [57–60,62].

It should be noted that in some jurisdictions, it is necessary for the court to notify the veterinary professional organisation and obtain its input (but not binding consent) regarding the person to be appointed as a proficient [45].

5.1. *Secrecy and Documentation*

One of the key ethical aspects is the obligation to maintain veterinary professional secrecy and confidentiality, as mentioned in the earlier part of the current study.

In addition, an obligation for any expert to maintain confidentiality related to *any* knowledge gained in the course of examination and the issuing of an opinion should be raised. The problem of the expert's confidentiality is crucial in terms of the rule of law and is often present in normative acts, but it is considered extremely rarely in the veterinary literature [10,11,45]. According to the author, this gap in the veterinary literature may be caused by the "natural" conviction of veterinary surgeons about the need to maintain secrecy.

While the two legal obligations of secrecy overlap in the discussed area of veterinary expert opinions, in other areas of expertise, this regularity is not observed due to the lack of the ethical principle of professional secrecy. Meanwhile, the obligation of veterinary ethics is broader and more general than that of any expert. The former includes, as has already been demonstrated, *any* knowledge gained in the course of *any* professional activity of *any* veterinary surgeon, including information gained as a proficient. One should, however, bear in mind that the legal basis of these two overlapping obligations is different.

Another very important duty, associated with secrecy, to be guided by the veterinary proficient, is documentation. It concerns the entire course of the expert's study, the results of all analyses and tests conducted, as well as the report, as the final summary of the expertise. This obligation has its sources in professional law (veterinary medical documentation, possibly also concerning informed consent), in court procedural law, and in civil law (proper performance of the obligation, due diligence) [4,10,20,27,40,41,51].

5.2. *Independency and Advocacy*

It is argued that the expert veterinarian should remain independent of any influence and never assume the role of an advocate [8,9,13]. This undoubtedly applies to the parties to the court proceedings, such as the accused, defendant, or claimant [10]. Regardless of whether the expert was appointed at the request of one of the parties to the proceedings, or *ex officio* or *motu proprio*, he/she appears before the court and for the court. Furthermore, the principle of independency applies to certain influence groups, politicians, social organisations, relatives, friends, representatives of certain views, etc. The rule of objectivity includes also the deontological prohibition of issuing opinions in relation to one's own clinical cases, owned animals, or enterprises [20,27].

A provocative question could be, however, posed: does this also apply to animal advocacy?

In order to answer this question correctly, one should set aside specific legal regulations and one's own views and prejudices and try to look at the problem in a general and holistic way. The research carried out made it possible to present a functional interpretation of the discussed problem.

It is a well-known fact that animal advocacy is the highest ethical and deontological rule of the veterinary profession in many jurisdictions, especially Anglo-Saxon ones [10,13,14,40,41], but, nowise, in all. According to some regulations [20], the most important rule in the veterinary profession is to ensure the welfare of mankind, while other professional veterinary organisations do not indicate any primary rule *explicite*.

Consequently, does a veterinarian presenting an expert opinion in which, in order to maintain impartiality, independency, and objectivity, he/she evades assessment based on animal advocacy or another guiding rule and acts against the law, deontology, and ethics of a professional corporation? The answer is no. As has been shown, the primary duty of the expert is to maintain objectivity and impartiality, and the primary role of the expert is to provide independent, substantive assistance. Therefore, an expert cannot adopt any point of view that favours any side of the proceedings, on the basis of animal advocacy or the good of mankind.

Nevertheless, he/she may and should include in his/her opinion a statement that, in accordance with the prevailing rule of professional ethics, the case analysed in the opinion takes a certain rating. The aforementioned rule is also the part of specific knowledge of the expert. It is the court (or the other authority ordering the opinion) that proceeds to its comprehensive and free assessment.

The case of private veterinary opinions is slightly different; hence, the expert veterinarian is afforded greater freedom of expression but should always indicate the ethical basis for his/her claim.

Thus, another principle of veterinary professional ethics is also implemented: the exclusion and disclosure of any possible conflicts of interest [3,10,14,20,40]. As has been already mentioned, this deontological imperative applies primarily to one's own clinical cases and owned animals [27]. According to the author, such a legal and ethical provision implements the general principle of law: *nemo iudex in causa sua* (no-one is judge in his own cause).

5.3. Cognizance and Correctness

Another important aspect of the expert's duties, and of the characteristics of the opinion, which the author would like to raise, is basing the opinion on scientific grounds, methodological correctness, and the use of appropriate research methods [13]. This is the implementation of another important requirement and professional rule applicable to all veterinarians: the use of current medical knowledge [10,20,27,40,41]. This statement is related to another deontological obligation of each veterinarian, continuous self-education as a part of the *lege artis* practice [11,14,20,65]. The provision of specialised knowledge in a given field does not, however, imply the veterinary medical training of the person, or authority, that commissioned the expert's opinion [66].

A veterinary expert exceeding his/her own competences, expertise, the level of his/her own knowledge, skills, scientific competences, education, or professional experience, and the scope of the procedural competences expressed in the questions asked, will bear professional liability in the veterinary peer court [10,20,27,40,41,51].

Similarly, professional liability will be implied for malpractice and medical errors committed during the preparation of the opinion and the examination. Professional liability for malpractice is independent of the civil one (damages) [23,25,51–54,61,62].

Another eminent example of a deficiency implying professional liability is the commission of a crime by the expert, e.g., issuing a false opinion or bribery.

It should be noted that in some jurisdictions, appointing a veterinary surgeon as an expert by the court requires the veterinary professional corporation to be informed. The corporation should express its opinion (but not consent) in this matter [45].

5.4. Non-Universal Duties

Another issue worthy of deeper analysis is the collection of evidence by the veterinary expert. This part of the expert's work is often pointed out in the literature on veterinary experts written in Anglophone circles [7–9,21,22,26,36,38,48], and thus in the common law context.

The obligation to collect evidence, inspect the crime scene, conduct the chain of custody, and other resulting responsibilities [7,9,10,21,22,26,36,38,48,49,67,68], and liability for non-compliance with the law, results from the Anglo-Saxon penal law system, including the offices of a coroner or medical examiner.

In continental law, the situation is completely different. Statutory provisions explicitly or implicitly prohibit the collection of evidence and sampling by any experts, including veterinarians [11]. Under such provisions, the expert may examine only evidence (e.g., animals, animal corpses, case files, documents, laboratory test results) provided by procedural entities, such as the police, or the prosecutor.

A significant exception to this prohibition has been developed in the legal doctrine and jurisprudence. Thus, collecting additional evidence in the examined material is possible in the case of the threat of destruction of this evidence, or the impossibility of its subsequent analysis [11]. It is the result of the systemic and teleological interpretation of the law, with which the author does agree and affirm.

The discussed essential legal difference between continental and common law countries is not reported in the global veterinary literature. It has been discussed only in local analyses, focused on the legal system of the particular state, usually in non-congress languages [11,64]. In the author's opinion, therefore, this problem needs to be analysed and discussed in the current study. Hereby, significant differences in the court procedure, duties, and empowerment of the expert veterinarian in different legal systems are revealed, as well as fundamental disparities in the judicial proceedings. The issue of the contradictory nature of the trial in the common law system, and the behaviour in the courtroom related to it, should be assessed in an analogous way.

The discussed differences significantly affect the course of expertise, as well as the duties of veterinary experts.

5.5. *Veterinary Experts' Legal Knowledge*

It should be observed that legal knowledge is a legal requirement for an expert in all types of legal systems [26,31,45]. Moreover, it is also a legal and deontological obligation of every veterinarian [10,17,20,26,27,41]. It is therefore, as analysed above, a duty for veterinary experts of a double nature, double source, and broad, multifarious liability. The importance of legal awareness in this regard among veterinary surgeons is revealed, especially in the face of progressive globalisation and cases of appointing outstanding, foreign veterinarians as experts.

5.6. *Wide Range of Responsibility*

The responsibility of the veterinary expert, as a professional *par excellence* and a member of a public trust profession, to the general public can be derived from ethical codes [6,10,14,20,27,41]. The moral responsibility of all experts and of all scientists can also be assumed, but there is no way to respect it directly, unlike the morality of veterinarians, the violation of which is punishable by professional liability before peer tribunals.

Modern changes in humans and humans in relation to animals bring about changes in public morality. These are accompanied by changes in the law. Changes in the professional veterinary ethics, including the strengthening of the obligations of expert veterinarians to maintain a level of due diligence in their practice, are implied. Social implications, public expectations, and inter-systemic connections require new tasks, behaviours, and approaches from veterinarians [14,43]. The development of the professional activities of veterinarians within their expertise is associated with a rise in the level of responsibility, and liability—primarily ethical and civil.

6. Conclusions

Proficiency and expertise—the comprehensive work of an expert veterinarian—are crucial from theoretical, practical, legal, and veterinary points of view. It is a significant form of veterinary practice. It should be emphasised that veterinary forensic medicine has been found to be an important part of the complex phenomenon of veterinary specialisation.

It has been found that the role of a veterinary expert can be defined as the legal function of a proficient: a veterinary surgeon whose substantive statement (opinion/report) is based on specific veterinary knowledge and skills and meets the legally relevant criteria: a direct connection with the law and the intended, applied use of this opinion in a legal context.

It has been revealed that the diversity of terminological forms significantly affects the correct and incorrect understanding of the institution, role, tasks, and responsibilities of veterinary experts. It has been shown that limiting oneself to only one legal system, without comparative studies, significantly narrows the understanding of the discussed problem. Moreover, it has been proven that the global view allows for a uniform and consistent foundation for all veterinarians who will act as expert witnesses in the future.

It has been revealed that the problem of the responsibility of a veterinary expert for the, broadly understood, defectiveness of judgments and conclusions issued by him/her on the basis of the conducted examination is complex and multifaceted. The basis of this complexity is, above all, the multitude and complexity of the obligations imposed on the veterinarian providing the expertise. The origin of these obligations (from different, but complementary, source systems of values and obligations) is not without significance.

The development of the practice and theory of the analysed problem has had a significant impact on the development of veterinary medicine, especially in terms of research procedures and of specifying the standards of due diligence and the compliance of conduct with ethical and deontological principles.

Trends for the future in veterinary expertise are expected to gain the interest of both public and private commissioners, which corresponds to an increase in the frequency of disputes [1,43,47]. This applies to evaluating the malpractice and unethical behaviour of other veterinarians as well [43].

An increase in the importance of veterinary expertise is expected, in terms of not only legal matters but also in the further development of veterinary medicine—as a science, and as an ethical system of professional duties [14]. Thus far, the predictions have been realised [1,43]; it is, therefore, expected that these processes will continue in the future.

In particular, it may be important to intensify the use veterinary proficient opinions in legislative processes and in economic development, through the use of interdisciplinary knowledge and skills and the navigation of public discourse in animal matters.

The analysis conducted indicates that the ultimate goal of litigation, as well as of scientific research and of issuing expert opinions, is to discover the truth. This brings the court trial and the expert opinion formation process closer to the research and the publication of its results in science. Axiology and praxeology, as well as professional and social liability, are analogous and comparable in these areas of veterinary professional activity.

Funding: This research received no external funding.

Institutional Review Board Statement: Not applicable.

Informed Consent Statement: Not applicable.

Data Availability Statement: Not applicable.

Conflicts of Interest: The author declares no conflict of interest.

References

1. Cooper, J.E. What Is Forensic Veterinary Medicine? Its Relevance to the Modern Exotic Animal Practice. *Semin. Avian Exot. Pet Med.* **1998**, *7*, 161–165. [CrossRef]
2. Harris, J.M. The Role of the Practicing Veterinarian as an Expert Witness. *Semin. Avian Exot. Pet Med.* **1998**, *7*, 176–181. [CrossRef]
3. Dobson, J. Role of the expert witness and report-writing considerations. *Vet. Times* **2011**, *41*, 29–31.
4. Balkin, D.E.; Janssen, L.A.; Merck, M.D. The Legal System: The Veterinarian's Role and Responsibilities. In *Veterinary Forensics: Animal Cruelty Investigations*, 2nd ed.; Merck, M.D., Ed.; Wiley & Sons: Hoboken, NJ, USA, 2013; pp. 1–16.
5. Forbes, N. An exacting science: The veterinary surgeon as expert witness. *In Pract.* **2004**, *26*, 503–506. [CrossRef]
6. Howey, A. Criminal Liability of the Dog Owner under the Animal Welfare Act 2006. *Vet Times*, 10 November 2014. Available online: https://vettimes.co.uk/app/uploads/wp-post-to-pdf-enhanced-cache/1/criminal-liability-of-dog-owners-under-the-animal-welfare-act.pdf (accessed on 1 June 2023).
7. Munro, R. Forensic Necropsy. *Semin. Avian Exot. Pet Med.* **1998**, *7*, 201–209. [CrossRef]
8. Newbery, S.; Munro, R. Forensic veterinary medicine: 1. Investigation involving live animals. *In Pract.* **2011**, *33*, 220–227. [CrossRef]
9. Roger, P. Expert Witness. In *Bovine Medicine*, 1st ed.; Cockcroft, P.D., Ed.; Wiley & Sons: Hoboken, NJ, USA, 2015; pp. 55–60.
10. Royal College of Veterinary Surgeons, Code of Professional Conduct for Veterinary Surgeons. Available online: https://www.rcvs.org.uk/setting-standards/advice-and-guidance/code-of-professional-conduct-for-veterinary-surgeons/ (accessed on 1 June 2023).
11. Szarek, J. *Lekarz Weterynarii Jako Biegły*, 4th ed.; UWM: Olsztyn, Poland, 2003; pp. 9–177. (In Polish)
12. Woods, A. From practical men to scientific experts: British veterinary surgeons and the development of government scientific expertise, c. 1878–1919. *Hist. Sci.* **2013**, *51*, 457–480. [CrossRef]
13. Yeates, J. Dealing with possible criminal cases: Witness work. *In Pract.* **2017**, *39*, 187–189. [CrossRef]
14. De Paula Vieira, A.; Anthony, R. Recalibrating Veterinary Medicine through Animal Welfare Science and Ethics for the 2020s. *Animals* **2020**, *10*, 654. [CrossRef] [PubMed]
15. Lowe, P. Unlocking Potential. A Report on Veterinary Expertise in Food Animal Production. Available online: https://eprints.ncl.ac.uk/file_store/production/157494/88D16007-9B91-460D-A5D9-94E17A5CACCA.pdf (accessed on 1 June 2023).
16. Wenzel, J.G.W.; Nusbaum, K.E. Veterinary expertise in biosecurity and biological risk assessment. *J. Am. Vet. Med. Assoc.* **2007**, *230*, 1476–1480. [CrossRef]
17. Cooper, J.E.; Cooper, M.E. *Introduction to Veterinary and Comparative Medicine*, 1st ed.; Blackwell: Oxford, UK, 2007; pp. XI, 5, 22, 24, 37, 117–167, 285–303.

18. Shaham, R. *The Expert Witness in Islamic Courts: Medicine and Crafts in the Service of Law*, 1st ed.; University of Chicago: Chicago, IL, USA; London, UK, 2010; pp. 74–75.
19. Maxwell, Á. Expert Evidence and the Role of the Expert Witness—A practical Guide. *Fish Vet. J.* **2005**, *8*, 93–100.
20. Kodeks Etyki Lekarza Weterynarii. Uchwała 3/2008/VII Nadzwyczajnego VII Krajowego Zjazdu Lekarzy Weterynarii. Available online: https://vetpol.org.pl/dmdocuments/Kodeks%20etyki%20lekarza%20weterynarii.pdf (accessed on 1 June 2023). (In Polish).
21. Newbery, S.G.; Cooke, S.W.; Martineau, H.M. A Perspective on Veterinary Forensic Pathology and Medicine in the United Kingdom. *Vet. Pathol.* **2016**, *53*, 894–897. [CrossRef]
22. Stroud, R.K. Wildlife Forensics and the Veterinary Practitioner. *Semin. Avian Exot. Pet Med.* **1998**, *7*, 182–192. [CrossRef]
23. Code Civil des Français, Loi du 30 Ventôse an XII sur la Réunion des Lois Civiles en un Seul Corps, Sous le Titre de Code Civil des Français. Version Consolidée; Amended. Available online: https://www.legifrance.gouv.fr/codes/texte_lc/LEGITEXT000006070721/ (accessed on 1 June 2023). (In French).
24. Code Rural et de la Pêche Maritime (Nouveau). Version Consolidée; Amended. Available online: https://www.legifrance.gouv.fr/codes/texte_lc/LEGITEXT000006071367/ (accessed on 1 June 2023). (In French).
25. Dzikowski, A.; Szarek, J. Stan prawny wad głównych zwierząt w aktach normatywnych Francji, Belgii i Luksemburga. *Stud. Prawnoustroj.* 2023; *submitted*.
26. Cooper, J.E.; Cooper, M.E. Forensic veterinary medicine: A rapidly evolving discipline. *Forensic Sci. Med. Pathol.* **2008**, *4*, 75–82. [CrossRef]
27. L'Ordre National des Vétérinaires. Code de Déontologie Vétérinaire. Available online: https://www.veterinaire.fr/system/files/files/2023-03/CNO%20VETOS%20-%20Code%20deontologie%20%20V1.pdf (accessed on 1 June 2023). (In French).
28. Woods, A. The farm as clinic: Veterinary expertise and the transformation of dairy farming, 1930–1950. *Stud. Hist. Phil. Biol. Biomed. Sci.* **2007**, *38*, 462–487. [CrossRef]
29. Enticott, G. Geographies of Veterinary Experts and Expertise. In *Routledge Handbook of Biosecurity and Invasive Species*, 1st ed.; Baker, K., Francis, R.A., Eds.; Routledge: Abingdon-on-Thames, UK, 2021; pp. 63–74.
30. Enticott, G.; Donaldson, A.; Lowe, P.; Power, M.; Proctor, A.; Wilkinson, K. The changing tole of veterinary expertise in food chain. *Philos. Trans. R. Soc. Lond. B Biol. Sci.* **2011**, *366*, 1955–1965. [CrossRef]
31. Cooper, M.E. Birds, Exotic Animals, and the Law. *Semin. Avian Exot. Pet Med.* **1998**, *7*, 166–175. [CrossRef]
32. Onions, C.T.; Friedrichsen, G.W.S.; Burchfield, R.W. (Eds.) *Oxford Dictionary of English Etymology*, 1st ed.; Clarendon: Oxford, UK, 1966.
33. Oxford English Dictionary. Available online: https://www.oed.com/ (accessed on 1 June 2023).
34. Glare, P.G.W. (Ed.) *Oxford Latin Dictionary*, 2nd ed.; University Press: Oxford, UK, 2008; Volumes 1 and 2.
35. Veterinary Council of New Zealand. Code of Professional Conduct for Veterinarians. Available online: https://vetcouncil.org.nz/common/Uploaded%20files/Web/Publications/2020_01%20Code%20of%20Professional%20Conduct.pdf (accessed on 1 June 2023).
36. Touroo, R.; Brooks, J.W.; Lockwood, R.; Reisman, R. Medicolegal Investigation. In *Veterinary Forensic Pathology*, 1st ed.; Brooks, J.W., Ed.; Springer: Cham, Switzerland, 2018; Volume 1, pp. 1–8.
37. Porter, A.R.W. The veterinary surgeon as a witness. *Vet. Rec.* **1971**, *89*, 505–509. [CrossRef]
38. Rogers, E.; Stern, A.W. Expert Witness Testimony and Report Writing. In *Veterinary Forensics: Investigation, Evidence Collection, and Expert Testimony*, 1st ed.; Rogers, E., Stern, A.W., Eds.; Taylor & Francis: Boca Raton, FL, USA, 2018; pp. 389–404.
39. Frederickson, R. Demystifying the Courtroom: Everything the Veterinary Pathologist Needs to Know About Testifying in an Animal Cruelty Case. *Vet. Pathol.* **2016**, *53*, 888–893. [CrossRef]
40. American Veterinary Medical Association. Principles of Veterinary Medical Ethics. Available online: https://www.avma.org/ (accessed on 1 June 2023).
41. Canadian American Veterinary Medical Association. Principles of Veterinary Medical Ethics. Available online: https://www.canadianveterinarians.net/media/o5qjghc0/principles-of-veterinary-medical-ethics-of-the-cvma.pdf (accessed on 1 June 2023).
42. Hippocrates of Kos. *The Hippocratic Oath: Text, Translation, and Interpretation*; Edelstein, L., Ed.; Johns Hopkins Press: Baltimore, MD, USA, 1943.
43. Cooper, J.E. Future Trends in Forensic Veterinary Medicine. *Semin. Avian Exot. Pet Med.* **1998**, *7*, 210–217. [CrossRef]
44. Pugliese, M.; Voslarova, E.; Biondi, V.; Passantino, A. Clinical Practice Guidelines: An Opinion of the Legal Implication to Veterinary Medicine. *Animals* **2019**, *9*, 577. [CrossRef]
45. Rozporządzenie Ministra Sprawiedliwości z dnia 24 stycznia 2005 r. w Sprawie Biegłych Sądowych. Available online: https://isap.sejm.gov.pl/isap.nsf/download.xsp/WDU20050150133/O/D20050133.pdf (accessed on 1 June 2023). (In Polish)
46. Rozporządzenie Ministra Rolnictwa z dnia 7 października 1966 r. w Sprawie Odpowiedzialności Sprzedawców za Wady Główne Niektórych Gatunków Zwierząt. Available online: https://isap.sejm.gov.pl/isap.nsf/download.xsp/WDU19660430257/O/D19660257.pdf (accessed on 1 June 2023). (In Polish)
47. Listos, P.; Gryzinska, M.; Kowalczyk, M. Analysis of cases of forensic veterinary opinions produced in a research and teaching unit. *J. Forensic Leg. Med.* **2015**, *36*, 84–89. [CrossRef]
48. Merck, M.D. *Veterinary Forensics: Animal Cruelty Investigations*; Wiley & Sons: Chichester, UK, 2013; pp. 10, 17–36, 41.

49. Parmalee, K. Crime Scene Investigation. In *Veterinary Forensics: Investigation, Evidence Collection, and Expert Testimony*, 1st ed.; Rogers, E., Stern, A.W., Eds.; Taylor & Francis: Boca Raton, FL, USA, 2018; pp. 23–52.
50. Martin, D. Role of the expert witness. *Vet. Rec.* **2013**, *173*, 1. [CrossRef]
51. Dzikowski, A. Veterinary surgeons' legal obligations in sales-related animal health status examinations. *Med. Weter.* **2021**, *77*, 309–313. [CrossRef]
52. Allgemeines Bürgerliches Gesetzbuch für die Gesammten Deutschen Erbländer der Œsterreichischen Monarchie. Amended. Available online: https://www.ris.bka.gv.at/GeltendeFassung.wxe?Abfrage=Bundesnormen&Gesetzesnummer=10001622 (accessed on 1 June 2023). (In German).
53. Code Des Obligations/Obligationenrecht/Diritto Delle Obbligazioni, Loi Fédérale Complétant le Code Civil Suisse (Livre Cinquième: Droit Des Obligations) du 30 Mars 1911/Bundesgesetz Betreffend die Ergänzung des Schweizerischen Zivilgesetzbuches (Fünfter Teil: Obligationenrecht) vom 30. März 1911/Legge Federale di Complemento del Codice Civile Svizzero (Libro Quinto: Diritto Delle Obbligazioni) del 30 Marzo 1911. Amended. Available online: https://www.fedlex.admin.ch/en/cc/internal-law/22 (accessed on 1 June 2023). (Official Text in German, Italian, and French; English Version Available).
54. Código Civil. Real Decreto de 24 de Julio de 1889 por el que se Publica el Código Civil, Texto Consolidado. Amended. Available online: https://boe.es/buscar/act.php?id=BOE-A-1889-4763 (accessed on 1 June 2023). (In Spanish).
55. Ordonnance sur la Procédure en Matière de Garantie dans le Commerce du Bétail du 14 Novembre 1911/Verordnung Betreffend das Verfahren bei der Gewährleistung im Viehhandel vom 14. November 1911/Ordinanza sulla Procedura in Materia di Garanzia nel Commercio del Bestiame del 14 Novembre 1911. Amended. Available online: https://www.fedlex.admin.ch/eli/cc/27/877_903_899/de (accessed on 1 June 2023). (In German, Italian, and French).
56. Vaquer, A. *Contract Law in Spain*; Wolters Kluwer: Alphen aan den Rijn, The Netherlands, 2012; pp. 152, 187–190.
57. Wolkowski, B. *Die Rechtliche Behandlung der Kaufuntersuchung Beim Pferdekauf*; Dr. Kovač: Hamburg, Germany, 2010; pp. 23–28, 36, 178, 219–254. (In German)
58. Von Bardeleben, G. *Rechtliche Besonderheiten des Pferdekaufs unter Besonderer Berücksichtigung der Tierärztlichen Kaufuntersuchung*; Agricola: Hildesheim, Germany, 2013; pp. 172–179, 183–184, 187–188, 196–199. (In German)
59. Bleckwenn, E. *Die Haftung des Tierarztes im Zivilrecht*; Springer: Berlin/Heidelberg, Germany, 2014; pp. 38–39, 50–70, 327, 350, 358, 377. (In German)
60. Eichelberg, S. *Kaufuntersuchungen Beim Pferdekauf*; Dr. Kovač: Hamburg, Germany, 2018; pp. 42–45, 89–118. (In German)
61. Fink, C. *Aufklärungspflicht von Medizinalpersonen (Arzt, Zahnarzt, Tierarzt, Apotheker)*, 1st ed.; Stämpfli: St. Gallen, Switzerland, 2008; pp. 213–228. (In German)
62. Bürgerliches Gesetzbuch vom in der Fassung der Bekanntmachung vom 2. Januar 2002. Amended. Available online: https://www.gesetze-im-internet.de/bgb/BJNR001950896.html (accessed on 1 June 2023). (In German).
63. Soave, O.A. *An Introduction to Veterinary Law*; Saunders: Philadelphia, PA, USA, 1962; pp. 1–105.
64. Szarek, J.; Fabczak, J. Analiza obowiązków lekarza wetrynarii będącego biegłym. *Życie Wet.* **1992**, *67*, 208–211. (In Polish)
65. Sehn, J. Dowód z biegłych w postępowaniu sądowym. *Nowe Prawo* **1956**, *3*, 22–34. (In Polish)
66. Last, W.J. Beratung in der Nutztierpraxis. *Veterinärspiegel* **2011**, *21*, 83. (In German) [CrossRef]
67. Crime Scene Investigation: A Guide for Law Enforcement. Available online: https://www.ojp.gov/pdffiles1/nij/178280.pdf (accessed on 1 June 2023).
68. Touroo, R.; Fitch, A. Crime Scene Findings and the Identification, Collection, and Preservation of Evidence. In *Veterinary Forensic Pathology*, 1st ed.; Brooks, J.W., Ed.; Springer: Cham, Switzerland, 2018; Volume 1, pp. 9–25.

animals

MDPI

Article

Workplace Strategies to Reduce Burnout in Veterinary Nurses and Technicians: A Delphi Study

Angela J. Chapman *, Pauleen C. Bennett and Vanessa I. Rohlf

School of Psychology and Public Health, La Trobe University, Bundoora, VIC 3086, Australia; pauleen.bennett@latrobe.edu.au (P.C.B.); v.rohlf@latrobe.edu.au (V.I.R.)
* Correspondence: a.chapman@latrobe.edu.au

Simple Summary: Veterinary nurses and technicians experience burnout, which affects their mental and physical health, the likelihood of leaving their job, and their quality of work. Burnout is caused by workplace issues, and existing research has identified specific causes in veterinary nurses and technicians. But little is known about how to address these issues within veterinary clinics in ways that are both effective and feasible. To address this gap, we consulted a panel of 40 veterinary nurse and technician leadership or wellbeing experts to seek their opinions on the challenges to addressing burnout and recommended management approaches. Responses were collected via two anonymous surveys between October 2024 and January 2025. The lack of, or unclear, regulation, poor leadership knowledge, poor team culture, an unwillingness to change, and existing burnout were found to make burnout management more difficult. Thirty-nine possible solutions, with recommended actions, were developed. These focused on improving communication, progression pathways, delegation, and leadership. Panel experts rated the proposed solutions as being highly, or very highly effective. When making changes in the workplace, current workplace problems, such as poor team culture and poor leadership, need to be considered first, as these will reduce the likelihood of success.

Abstract: Veterinary nurses and technicians are at risk of burnout, which negatively impacts mental and physical health, turnover, and patient care. Workplace contributors to burnout have been identified in this population, but little is known about best practice management strategies. This study used the Delphi method to explore barriers to addressing burnout and develop expert recommendations for workplace management strategies. Forty participants with a minimum of 5 years' industry experience in leadership, or wellbeing, were recruited via purposive sampling from the USA, UK, Australia, New Zealand, and Canada. Participants completed two anonymous, online, mixed-methods surveys between October 2024 and January 2025. Qualitative survey data were analysed using content analysis to identify codes and categorise solutions. Quantitative data were analysed using descriptive statistics. Barriers to addressing burnout included industry-wide barriers, such as lack of, or unclear, regulation and lack of leadership knowledge, and clinic specific barriers, such as poor team culture, unwillingness for change, and existing burnout. Thirty-nine solutions were developed and rated as being highly, or very highly effective. These focused on themes such as improving communication, developing progression pathways, and providing leadership training and support. Existing workplace barriers must be evaluated prior to selecting strategies, to maximise effectiveness in specific contexts.

Keywords: workplace mental health; animal care professional; leadership; wellbeing; retention; workload; regulation; utilisation

1. Introduction

Veterinary team members are prone to burnout, with veterinary nurses and technicians (VN/Ts) at particular risk [1]. The existing body of evidence on burnout in veterinarians and the unique contributors to burnout in their role is growing [2,3], however, research specific to burnout in VN/Ts is lacking [4]. A recent study found that VN/Ts were twice as likely to experience high/very high levels of burnout compared to the general population, with exhaustion being a key contributor [5]. The same study identified that having a good work-life balance was the biggest predictor of low burnout levels [5]. Burnout has well documented negative physical and mental health consequences for the individual, with potential welfare implications for veterinary patients under their care. Burnout is also a known contributor to intentions to leave, thus leading to increased staff turnover and increased economic costs for veterinary practice owners [6–8]. Effective prevention and management of burnout within VN/Ts is, therefore, critical to ensuring team wellbeing, business sustainability, and patient outcomes.

Burnout is defined as a syndrome resulting from chronic workplace stress which has not been adequately managed [9] and is, therefore, considered an occupational health issue. According to the International Labour Organisation (ILO), a United Nations agency that sets international labour guidelines for its 187 member states, a safe and healthy work environment is a fundamental right for employees [10]. Furthermore, the World Health Organisation (WHO) guidelines on mental health at work, written in consultation with the ILO, state that employers have a responsibility to ensure that psychosocial risks, which can contribute to burnout, are managed within the workplace to protect employee's mental health [11]. Psychosocial risks are defined as "anything in the design or management of work that increases the risk of work-related stress" [12] (psychosocial risks section). This may include a lack of work variety, lack of job control or inflexible hours, poor communication, lack of support, and poor work-life balance [12]. A shared responsibility exists between the workplace and the employee to manage and protect the mental health and wellbeing of individuals through preventing burnout.

Burnout contributors can be divided into risk and protective factors, with protective factors describing aspects of the workplace that can help to reduce an individual's risk of experiencing burnout. Protective factors in VN/Ts have been found to include manageable workloads, teamwork and support, clear and respectful communication, appropriate staffing levels, recognition of work, and knowledge of making a difference to clients and patients [13]. Risk factors describe aspects of the workplace that increase an individual's risk of experiencing burnout. These factors may be experienced across a range of industries, for example, co-worker incivility [14], or may be unique to individuals working in animal care roles, for example, exposure to animal abuse and euthanasia [15]. In VN/Ts, risk factors have been found to include high workloads, lack of skill utilisation, negative team culture, unclear communication, poor management or leadership, lack of schedule control, poor remuneration, lack of progression opportunities, negative client interactions, and lack of appreciation [13,16]. Some of these contributors, including high job demands, low job control, lack of support, and team conflict in VN/Ts, were identified in studies published over 10 years ago and, therefore, awareness of these problems is not new [17,18]. Despite this, recent research suggests that they are still being inadequately managed [13,16]. In addition to understanding the contributors to burnout it is, therefore, necessary to identify any barriers and enablers that may prevent, or support, organisations in addressing these contributors, so as to maximise the chances of success.

Barriers are factors that impede the ability of people leaders to address burnout risk factors. These are multifactorial and may be internal to the workplace. This includes barriers related to the interventions themselves, for example, technology that is not suited for the intended use; barriers related to the process of implementation, for example a lack of planning; or barriers related to the characteristics of the team or workplace, for example opposing values within the team. Barriers may also be external to the workplace, related to industry or legislative limitations, for example a lack of standardised educational competencies for professional licensing requirements [19]. Enablers are factors that facilitate people leaders to manage burnout. These may also arise from internal workplace sources, for example clear goals that have been collaboratively developed; or external sources, for example existing research to help understand the impact of changes [19].

Burnout prevention strategies can be classified as primary and secondary interventions, which may be organisational or individual focused, and tertiary interventions, which are generally individual focused [20]. Primary interventions are aimed at addressing the antecedents of burnout and preventing the onset of signs. Secondary interventions focus on identifying signs of burnout in the early stages and preventing the development of longer-term impacts. Tertiary interventions are aimed at addressing existing burnout and minimising the long-term effects through healing and rehabilitation [20]. Implementation of primary and secondary interventions by the organisation requires an understanding of the unique contributors to burnout in VN/Ts.

Existing research exploring burnout in VN/Ts includes recommendations on strategies that can be implemented within the workplace to better support individuals. These include providing opportunities for professional development, greater control over shift pattern and length, and management training on development of positive interpersonal relationships [17,21,22]. No studies to date, however, have explored barriers to implementation. Furthermore, existing studies typically include researcher recommendations to address burnout [21–24]. While these recommendations are informed by research findings derived from VN/Ts, they have not been evaluated for their perceived effectiveness or feasibility. Gaining this information, particularly from experienced wellbeing and leadership experts in the veterinary industry, is critical to ensure best practice recommendations target the known risk and protective factors and are also evaluated as effective and feasible.

Delphi studies are a research method commonly used in the development of human healthcare recommendations, allowing researchers to gain consensus through expert opinion [25]. The Delphi technique has been used in studies to develop workplace guidelines for the prevention of mental health problems [26], as well as to rate the importance of factors in the occurrence of burnout in nurses [27], and is therefore well-suited to research in the area of VN/T burnout. The Delphi method is used to collect objective opinions from participants in geographically diverse locations, across successive iterative rounds, to develop recommendations based on collective expert views. Delphi studies are particularly useful in areas where limited research exists and consensus is absent, and the technique transforms expert opinions into group consensus to elevate the quality of research evidence [25]. The lack of existing research on barriers, enablers, and feasibility of management strategies to address burnout in VN/Ts makes this an ideal framework for developing recommendations in this area.

The aim of this study was to employ a Delphi method to develop effective and feasible organisational management strategies to address known contributors to burnout in VN/Ts. This addressed the existing literature gap by producing recommendations based on expert consensus. This was achieved by, first, identifying perceived barriers and enablers to addressing the contributors, then, second, by exploring perceived ease of implementation and effectiveness of proposed strategies in addressing burnout in the workplace.

2. Materials and Methods

The Delphi method [28] was used to conduct the study, and it is reported following the Delphi studies in social and health sciences—recommendations for an interdisciplinary standardized reporting (DELPHISTAR) guideline [29].

2.1. Research Design

The Delphi method is a structured consultation process whereby a panel of experts contribute their views on an issue via an anonymous survey. Surveys incorporate both quantitative and qualitative questions to allow experts to rate items and provide feedback on their reasoning [25]. Panel members then revise their views through multiple survey rounds based on summarised feedback and responses from other participants, until consensus is reached. Anonymity is maintained throughout the process to minimise risk of bias resulting from perceptions of dominance and group conformity [25]. The current study comprised two rounds of data collection, with additional planned rounds being cancelled due to consensus being reached. In this study, consensus was defined as at least 75% endorsement by the panel across two consecutive ratings, following guidelines from similar research [27,30]. This process can be seen in Figure 1.

2.2. Participant Recruitment

Purposive sampling was utilised to identify experts with a minimum of five years' experience in VN/T leadership, leadership consulting, or wellbeing, as utilised in similar studies [25,31]. Potential participants were identified through their involvement in, or contributions to, VN/T wellness publications, conference presentations, veterinary industry wellbeing initiatives and awards, VN/T wellbeing podcasts, LinkedIn profiles, and existing professional networks of the researchers. Potential participants were contacted via email or LinkedIn and invited to contribute to the study. The panel size in Delphi studies is recommended to be greater than 20, after taking into account attrition across survey rounds [30]. Out of 84 experts invited, 40 consented to participate in the initial round. Participant recruitment was not directed toward specific countries, however, all recruited participants belonged to nations considered as the global West and English speaking. Participants who completed each round were invited to participate in subsequent rounds.

2.3. Measures

The aim of Round 1 was to explore barriers, enablers, and proposed strategies to address risk and protective factors for burnout in VN/Ts. The survey comprised a mixture of four questions which were developed by the authors. Participants were asked to respond to the same four questions for each of 10 risk and three protective factors derived from the findings of Chapman et al. [13,16]. For the 10 risk factors, Question 1 asked participants to rate how easy, or difficult, they believe it is to address the issue. Responses were rated on a 5-point Likert scale from 'very difficult' to 'very easy'. Three open-ended questions then asked participants to identify (1) what, if any, barriers they are aware of that increase the difficulty for managers or leaders to address the issue, (2) what, if any, enablers they are aware of that support managers or leaders to address the issue, and (3) what solutions or strategies they are aware of that effectively address the issue. For the three protective factors, the same questions were asked but rephrased to reflect the protective aspect. For example, the words "to address this issue" were replaced with "to promote this factor". The final open-ended question in the protective factors section removed the word "solutions" and sought strategies to promote the protective factor only, as solutions for protective factors are not required (Supplementary Materials S1). Responses to the questions in Round 1 were analysed and informed the development of solutions to the 10 risk factors, and promotions strategies for the three protective factors, which were then reviewed in the second round of data collection.

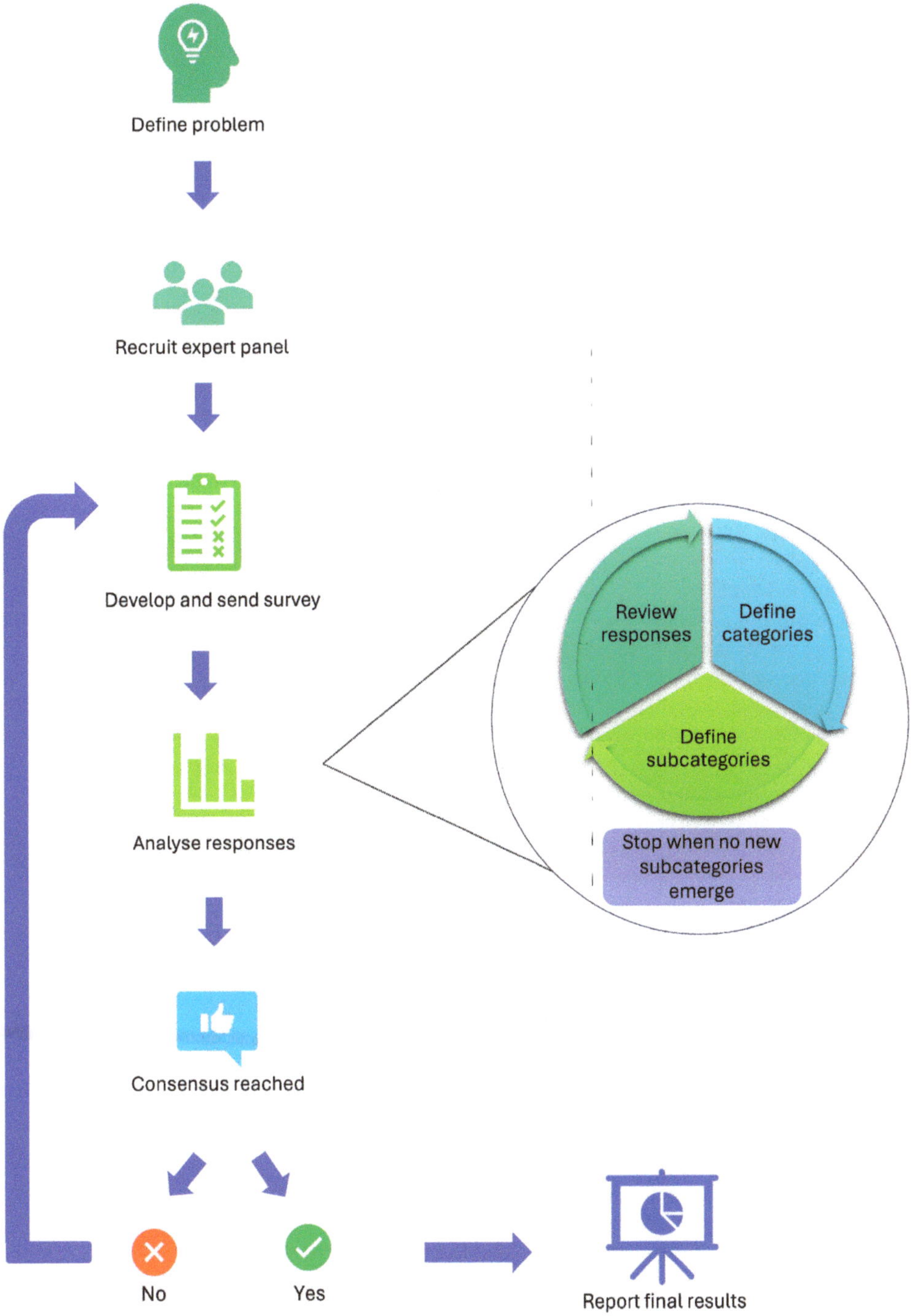

Figure 1. Delphi technique flow chart.

The aim of Round 2 was to rate the ease with which each solution or promotion strategy, developed in Round 1, could be implemented, as well as to rate the perceived effectiveness of the solutions in addressing the 10 risk factors. The survey comprised a mixture of three questions developed by the authors. Participants were asked to respond to the same three questions for each of the 10 risk factors, and two of those three questions for the three protective factors. Rating questions asked participants to rate how easy, or difficult, they believed it would be to implement each solution, for the risk factors, and each strategy, for the protective factors, as well as how effective, or ineffective, they believed the solutions for each risk factor would be. Items were measured on 5-point Likert scales ranging from 'very difficult' to 'very easy' for ease of implementation, and from 'very ineffective' to 'very effective' for effectiveness of solutions. Open-ended questions asked participants to provide feedback on proposed improvements to both solutions and strategies (Supplementary Materials S2).

2.4. Procedure

The study was conducted in accordance with the National Statement on Ethical Conduct in Human Research, and ethical approval was obtained from the Human Ethics Low Risk Committee at La Trobe University, Australia (approval number HEC24265). Data for Rounds 1 and 2 were collected between 7 October 2024 and 13 January 2025.

A link to each Round of the survey was emailed to participants and responses were collected using QuestionPro version 2 (Austin, TX, USA) [32]. Prior to receiving the first survey link, participants were required to sign a participation consent form which included advice to contact their local healthcare provider if they experienced any lasting negative emotions after taking part in the study. Links to international helplines were also provided. Each survey was initially open for two weeks, with a short time for data analysis scheduled between rounds to maintain participant engagement and reduce attrition. Closure of both survey rounds was extended by 10 days (Round 1) and one month (Round 2) in order to allow for increased participation, and account for the busy December holiday period (Round 2). Email reminders were sent to participants that had not yet completed the survey two days before the initial survey closure date, and then again after the initial closure date to inform remaining participants of the extended deadline.

A summary of responses was circulated to participants following data analysis of each round to allow participants to compare their responses with those of the collective panel. The Round 1 summary document outlined the key barriers and enablers that had been identified from participant responses, as well as the mean ease-of-management rating for each risk and protective factor. After Round 2, the summary document provided an overview of the ease and effectiveness ratings for solutions proposed in Round 1, as well as highlighting notable findings from the data.

2.5. Data Analysis

Data from open ended questions in Round 1 were analysed using NVivo version 15 (Denver, CO, USA) [33] and coded using conventional content analysis [34] to identify and describe the emerging categories. This approach is recommended when existing research on the area is limited, as it identifies patterns and recurrent viewpoints among participant responses to open-ended questions, without exposing participants to preconceived theories or ideas [34]. An iterative approach was taken where one author (AC) read the responses in full and then reviewed them multiple times to identify and refine categories and sub-categories until no novel phenomena emerged. In contrast to thematic analysis which relies on interpretive analytical approach by the researcher to contextualise the data, content analysis takes a descriptive analytical approach, coding and categorising data to identify trends and patterns of words [35]. Risk of bias resulting from the epistemological perspectives of the researcher is, therefore, much lower. Debriefs were conducted between the primary author and the last author (VR) to ensure that context and clarity of the data were accurately represented in the coding, and to further reduce the risk of bias.

Data from open ended questions in Round 2 were analysed using directed content analysis [34] to validate and extend the existing findings from Round 1. Directed content analysis utilises existing themes, which were developed in Round 1, to provide a framework with which to design and analyse questions based on the existing categories [34]. The same iterative process was followed to categorise data into the existing codes developed in Round 1, with debriefs to increase validity of the process [34].

Quantitative data from Rounds 1 and 2 were analysed using descriptive statistics, with means and standard deviations reported for each item. Missing data were managed by calculating the central tendency based on the number of participant responses to each item and excluding missing responses. Percentages and frequency counts for each Likert scale rating were also calculated and used to determine whether consensus had been reached.

3. Results

3.1. Participants

Forty experts were recruited from the United States of America (USA) ($n = 18$), Australia ($n = 9$), United Kingdom (UK) ($n = 7$), Canada ($n = 4$), and New Zealand ($n = 2$). The majority of participants were VN/Ts ($n = 33$), with the remainder either veterinarians ($n = 3$), or veterinary wellbeing experts without a veterinary clinical qualification ($n = 3$). A total of 32 and 30 participants completed the survey in Rounds 1 and 2 respectively (Figure 2).

3.2. Round 1

Round 1 explored barriers, enablers, and strategies to address risk and protective factors for burnout in VN/Ts. Results for Round 1, summarising the themes identified among barriers and enablers to address risk and protective factors, as well as the mean rating for how easy or difficult participants thought that the risk or protective factor is to manage, can be seen in Table 1.

Perceived ease of management ratings for all risk and protective factors ranged from 2.38 (±1.01) to 3.74 (±1.03) on a scale of 1 (very difficult) to 5 (very easy). Consensus around ease of management was achieved in only three out of 13 items, with scores for the remaining items spread across at least four out of five ratings. The factor that was rated the most difficult to address in Round 1 was Problem 5 'Poor management and leadership of the team'. One participant suggested that *"It is very difficult to address poor management or leadership because that would involve leadership admitting that those things are a problem"*. In contrast, Protective factor 2 'Knowledge of having a positive impact on a patient or client' was rated the easiest protective factor to leverage, with numerous client and feedback systems being proposed that one participant described as *"Pretty easy and low cost!"*.

Analysis of the qualitative data exploring barriers and enablers identified two key overarching themes. First, there is a lack of training and support for leaders as well as few positive role models in this area. One participant noted that this is an ongoing cycle, where *"Leaders in the vet profession don't routinely get exposed to good leadership so learn poor behaviours, then are promoted into the role with no support"*. In addition, there is a lack of, or variability in, VN/T regulation across all countries represented in the study, which may impact the capacity to effect positive change in several risk areas. One participant highlighted the extent of the impact, noting that *"Out of date/touch regulations and rules with regard to VN/T capabilities that would value add to the business, animal welfare, workload for vets, and job satisfaction for VN/Ts"*. Other frequently cited barriers included workforce shortages, existing levels of burnout in the team or management, hierarchical organisational structures and a lack of workplace resources such as time or money. Enablers included access to technology to support efficiency, professional networks, open and transparent communication, and breadth of skills within the team.

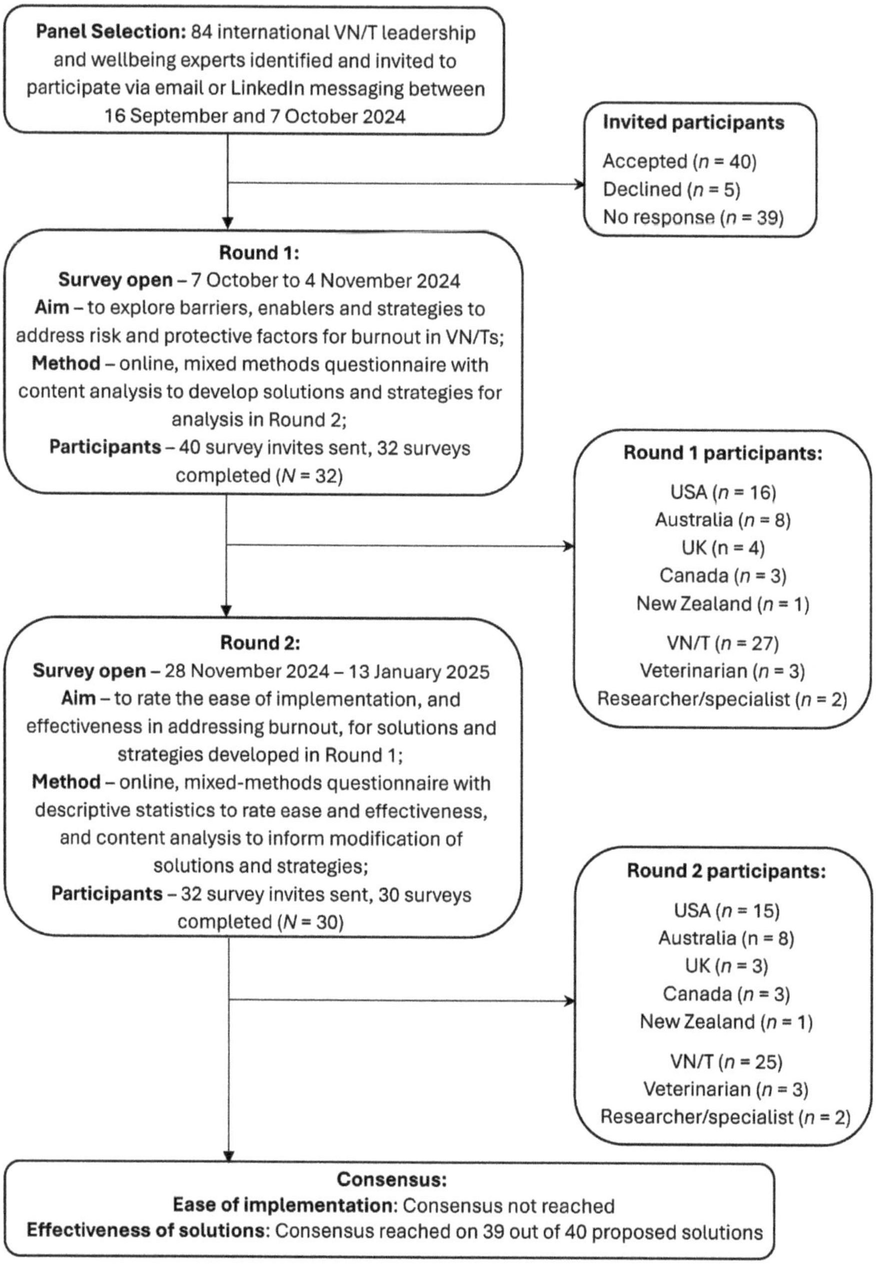

Figure 2. Flow diagram of Delphi study process and participants including country of residence and professional background.

Table 1. Barriers and enablers to addressing risk and protective factors associated with burnout in VN/Ts derived from Round 1.

Risk Factor	Barriers to Addressing the Risk Factor Derived from Content Analysis Themes	Enablers to Addressing the Risk Factor Derived from Content Analysis Themes	Perceived Ease of Management Rating (Mean/5.00 (*SD*))	Consensus Rating (Participant Agreement %)
1. The workload is too high	• Financial constraints of the business • Unpredictable workload • Workforce shortages and existing levels of burnout • Lack of clear systems and procedures to guide workflow • Lack of teamwork and communication	• Necessity forcing clinics to address workflow systems • Collaborative leadership culture • Technologies that support workload streamlining and efficiencies • Flexible scheduling	2.66/5.00 (±0.79)	Consensus: Difficult/neither difficult nor easy (82.93%)
2. There is a lack of opportunities to utilise skills and knowledge for which veterinary nurses/technicians are trained and qualified	• Understaffing leading to a lack of time and support • Lack of trust from veterinarians • Resistance to change • Small clinic size or staff hierarchies	• Professional networks and community support • Broad team skillset for mentorship • Veterinarian awareness of VN/T education and capabilities • Leadership advocacy	3.00/5.00 (±1.14)	Consensus not reached
3. A negative team culture exists (for example: bullying, gossiping, criticism, or general incivility)	• Lack of leadership awareness or accountability • Lack of psychological safety • Fear of losing staff • Industry workforce characteristics (female/mental health/generational differences)	• Industry awareness and education initiatives (e.g., Veterinary Incivility Toolkit) • Budget for resources and training • Regular communication and opportunities for feedback	2.52/5.00 (±0.96)	Consensus not reached
4. There is a lack of, or unclear communication from both management and within the team	• Large clinic or multiple sites • Variance in communication styles and preferences • Time limitations • Organisational hierarchies and multi-level communication	• Culture of psychological safety • Regularly scheduled meetings or discussion forums • Access to communication platforms such as Teams or Slack • Structured and consistent communication channels	3.23/5.00 (±1.07)	Consensus not reached

Table 1. *Cont.*

Risk Factor	Barriers to Addressing the Risk Factor Derived from Content Analysis Themes	Enablers to Addressing the Risk Factor Derived from Content Analysis Themes	Perceived Ease of Management Rating (Mean/5.00 (*SD*))	Consensus Rating (Participant Agreement %)
5. There is poor management/leadership of the team (for example: micromanagement, favouritism, lack of support, or lack of action on team conflict)	• Poor leadership training or support • Poor leadership role models • Negative workplace culture • Lack of reporting or feedback mechanisms for staff	• Access to leadership training and resources • Access to leadership mentoring and professional networks • Shallow organisational hierarchies • Open communication and feedback channels between team and leaders	2.38/5.00 (±1.01)	Consensus not reached
6. There is an expectation of working overtime, not having a break, and a general lack of flexibility in rostering	• Industry cultural norms around prioritising patients over staff wellbeing • Workforce shortages • Unpredictable workload • Resistance to change	• Access to rostering software • Legislation around breaks requirements and maximum shift length (where applicable) • Consistent messaging and advocacy • Wellness resources and initiatives	2.86/5.00 (±0.92)	Consensus not reached
7. Remuneration is poor	• Lack of business expertise • Community attitudes to veterinary fees • Financial limitations or of the business • Lack of industry regulation or clear professional structure	• Workforce shortage driving wages up • Appropriate utilisation of VN/Ts and support staff to reduce costs • Professional advocacy and legislative changes (where applicable) • Management business acumen	2.48/5.00 (±0.99)	Consensus not reached
8. There is a lack of opportunity for progression or development	• Lack of clinic resources (monetary and staffing) • Small clinics lacking need for advanced roles • Lack of industry awareness of VN/T value or potential • Fear of change from veterinarians and leadership	• Abundance of available CE and educational resources • Innovation and opportunities for lateral progression • Leadership awareness of VN/T capabilities and value • Broad team skillset facilitating mentorship and coaching	2.79/5.00 (±0.86)	Consensus: Difficult/neither difficult nor easy (80.65%)

Table 1. *Cont.*

Risk Factor	Barriers to Addressing the Risk Factor Derived from Content Analysis Themes	Enablers to Addressing the Risk Factor Derived from Content Analysis Themes	Perceived Ease of Management Rating (Mean/5.00 (*SD*))	Consensus Rating (Participant Agreement %)
9. Having to deal with rude or abusive clients	• Fear of repercussions (client loss/negative reviews/litigation) • Lack of training in communication and de-escalation • "The customer is always right" mentality • Lack of resources (time/staffing/support) to adequately manage situations	• Positive and well-developed client relationships • Dedicated client support roles (e.g., veterinary social workers) • Availability of training and resources on communication • Access to support (peer networks, Employee Assistance Program)	2.86/5.00 (±1.13)	Consensus: Difficult/Neither difficult nor easy (97.74%)
10. There is a lack of appreciation, feeling valued, or being heard, by management	• Diversity in staff acknowledgement needs and preferences • Burned out managers • Negative or hierarchical workplace cultures • Poor management role models and lack of training	• Professional advocacy efforts on VN/T appreciation • Abundance of existing recognition programs to model • Workplace cultures that support open communication and feedback to management	2.86/5.00 (±1.27)	Consensus not reached
Protective Factor	**Barriers to Leveraging the Protective Factor Derived from Content Analysis Themes**	**Enablers to Leveraging the Protective Factor Derived from Content Analysis Themes**	**Perceived Ease of Leverage Rating (Mean/5.00 (*SD*))**	**Consensus Rating (Participant Agreement %)**
1. Having some control over the schedule or expected tasks	• Hierarchical or negative workplace cultures • High and unpredictable workloads • Staffing shortages • Conflicting team member needs or skill levels	• Flexible staffing models • Collaborative team culture • Cross trained staff to increase task capabilities	3.09/5.00 (±0.89)	Consensus not reached
2. Knowledge of having a positive impact on a patient or client	• Shift work rosters—absence at patient discharge • Lack of client awareness of VN/T role in patient care • Absence of feedback systems • Negativity bias—natural focus on negative outcomes	• Ability to provide high quality care • Room to build connections with clients • Clear and established client, and internal, feedback systems	3.74/5.00 (±1.03)	Consensus not reached

Table 1. *Cont.*

Protective Factor	Barriers to Leveraging the Protective Factor Derived from Content Analysis Themes	Enablers to Leveraging the Protective Factor Derived from Content Analysis Themes	Perceived Ease of Leverage Rating (Mean/5.00 (*SD*))	Consensus Rating (Participant Agreement %)
3. Being trusted with, and involved in, decisions around patient care	• Hierarchical or negative workplace culture • Negative veterinarian attitudes towards VN/T capabilities • Lack of veterinarian experience and/or self-confidence • Lack of, or unclear, professional regulation	• Well-developed veterinarian-VN/T relationships • Culture of shared team values and collaboration • Good patient management record systems	3.13/5.00 (±0.98)	Consensus not reached

Consistent themes were also identified across the proposed solutions. These focused primarily on addressing leadership issues by improving recruitment procedures for leadership roles, providing ongoing leadership training and support, and utilising management consultants where necessary to address gaps in business expertise. In addition, a number of strategies were proposed to support suggested solutions but were beyond the scope of individual clinics to implement. These included public education campaigns to increase awareness of industry challenges such as workload; the promotion of better understanding and acknowledgment of VN/Ts in professional liability insurance policies; and advocacy initiatives to lobby government and industry bodies for better pay standards, mandatory registration, and title protection.

Specific solutions and strategies to address each risk and protective factor were developed based on common themes that emerged from participant responses. A range of broad solutions were identified for each risk factor, with more specific actions proposed to help achieve this solution. For example, to increase opportunities for skills and knowledge utilisation, one proposed solution was 'Implement systems to support delegation'. Suggested actions included: implementing VN/T-to-patient and veterinarian ratios, developing mentoring programs, developing clear standard operating procedures (SOPs) for performing clinical tasks, employing support staff to complete non-clinical tasks, and implementing team rounds to support collaboration. Common themes found across all solutions included improving communication, training and support, and workflow systems.

3.3. Round 2

Round 2 asked participants to rate the solutions and strategies, developed in Round 1, for ease of implementation (solutions and strategies) and effectiveness in addressing burnout (solutions). Results for Round 2, summarising the proposed solutions developed from the Round 1 responses, as well as the mean and consensus ratings for how easy each solution and strategy would be to implement, and how effective each solution would be in addressing burnout, can be seen in Tables 2 and 3.

A broad lack of consensus was found regarding the perceived ease of implementation with scores for 50 out of 51 (98%) of the proposed solutions and strategies spread across at least four different ratings on a Likert scale of one (very easy) to five (very difficult). This lack of consensus could be explained by general qualitative data across all risk and protective factors, which suggested that ease of implementation was expected to vary depending on a range of contextual factors in the affected clinic. Existing workplace climate, including team culture, leadership quality, staff willingness for change, attitudes and behaviours of existing staff, and the ability to effectively design and implement change processes, were identified by participants as aspects that impact the complexity of effecting workplace change. Based on these findings, achieving consensus on ease of implementation was determined to be unlikely due to there being too many variables to determine one, or any, best practice recommendations. Advancement of these questions to further rounds was discontinued.

Table 2. Mean perceived ease of implementation ratings and participant consensus ratings for solutions and strategies to workplace burnout risk and protective factors derived from Round 2.

Risk Factor	Solution	Perceived Ease of Implementation Rating (Mean/5.00 (*SD*))	Consensus Rating (Participant Agreement %)
1. The workload is too high	Hire more staff	2.23/5.00 (±0.57)	Consensus: Difficult/neither easy nor difficult (96.33%)
	Improve staff retention	3.20/5.00 (±1.03)	Consensus not reached
	Implement workload management systems to enhance efficiency and communications around workload issues	3.60/5.00 (±1.07)	Consensus not reached
	Preventative healthcare focus to reduce the number of cases seen	2.62/5.00 (±1.06)	Consensus not reached
2. There is a lack of opportunities to utilise skills and knowledge for which veterinary nurses/technicians are trained and qualified	Provide role clarity on skill level and task expectations of VN/Ts and veterinarians	3.80/5.00 (±1.19)	Consensus not reached
	Support veterinarians to delegate tasks to VN/Ts	3.30/5.00 (±1.06)	Consensus not reached
	Create opportunities for skill utilisation by reducing non-clinical workload and increasing clinical work opportunities	3.30/5.00 (±1.02)	Consensus not reached
	Implement systems to support delegation	3.33/5.00 (±1.12)	Consensus not reached
3. A negative team culture exists (for example: bullying, gossiping, criticism, or general incivility)	Zero-tolerance to incivility at all levels of the workplace	2.67/5.00 (±1.24)	Consensus not reached
	Promote culture change	3.17/5.00 (±1.12)	Consensus not reached
	Set clear expectations on expected behaviour	3.63/5.00 (±1.22)	Consensus not reached
	Provide staff and leadership training and support	3.97/5.00 (±1.00)	Consensus: Easy/Very easy (76.66%)

Table 2. *Cont.*

Risk Factor	Solution	Perceived Ease of Implementation Rating (Mean/5.00 (*SD*))	Consensus Rating (Participant Agreement %)
4. There is a lack of, or unclear, communication from both management and within the team	Increase communication opportunities	3.86/5.00 (±1.01)	Consensus not reached
	Promote and reward good communication	3.57/5.00 (±1.03)	Consensus not reached
	Develop clear communication protocols and reporting lines	3.89/5.00 (±0.96)	Consensus not reached
	Utilise different communication methods	3.64/5.00 (±1.10)	Consensus not reached
5. There is poor management/leadership of the team (for example: micromanagement, favouritism, lack of support, or lack of action on team conflict)	Improve leadership recruitment and training processes	2.67/5.00 (±1.06)	Consensus not reached
	Implement systems to support leaders	3.00/5.00 (±1.02)	Consensus not reached
	Improve workplace communication	3.50/5.00 (±1.01)	Consensus not reached
	Initiate leadership reviews and accountability	3.53/5.00 (±1.04)	Consensus not reached
6. There is an expectation of working overtime, not having a break, and a general lack of flexibility in rostering	Review and adjust staffing to meet clinic needs	2.47/5.00 (±1.04)	Consensus not reached
	Implement clear break and overtime policies	3.23/5.00 (±1.10)	Consensus not reached
	Provide leadership and team training	3.33/5.00 (±1.15)	Consensus not reached
	Review and implement workflow systems to streamline tasks and develop contingency plans	3.00/5.00 (±0.95)	Consensus not reached
7. Remuneration is poor	Offer non-monetary remuneration	2.63/5.00 (±1.19)	Consensus not reached
	Explore opportunities to increase revenue	3.23/5.00 (±1.14)	Consensus not reached
	Implement salary banding and progression pathways	3.60/5.00 (±1.28)	Consensus not reached
	Implement work processes to reduce costs	3.17/5.00 (±1.18)	Consensus not reached

Table 2. *Cont.*

Risk Factor	Solution	Perceived Ease of Implementation Rating (Mean/5.00 (*SD*))	Consensus Rating (Participant Agreement %)
8. There is a lack of opportunity for progression or development	Develop clear progression pathways for VN/Ts	3.33/5.00 (±1.12)	Consensus not reached
	Explore professional growth opportunities	3.43/5.00 (±1.17)	Consensus not reached
	Provide internal VN/T training and support	3.30/5.00 (±1.12)	Consensus not reached
	Promote external VN/T training and support	3.47/5.00 (±1.17)	Consensus not reached
9. Having to deal with rude or abusive clients	Provide clear expectations on client conflict management and empower the team	3.73/5.00 (±1.05)	Consensus not reached
	Create workplace support systems for VN/Ts faced with client abuse	3.40/5.00 (±1.00)	Consensus not reached
	Prepare and train the team for conflict situations	3.53/5.00 (±0.97)	Consensus not reached
	Communicate clear behavioural expectations to clients	3.93/5.00 (±0.83)	Consensus: Easy/very easy (76.66%)
10. There is a lack of appreciation, feeling valued, or being heard, by management	Implement VN/T recognition systems	3.70/5.00 (±0.99)	Consensus not reached
	Increase communication channels between management and VN/Ts	3.67/5.00 (±0.96)	Consensus not reached
	Provide support and training for leaders	3.79/5.00 (±1.05)	Consensus not reached
	Identify what appreciation looks like for individuals	3.90/5.00 (±0.92)	Consensus not reached

Table 2. *Cont.*

Protective Factor	Promotion Strategy	Perceived Ease of Implementation Rating (Mean/5.00 (*SD*))	Consensus Rating (Participant Agreement %)
1. Having some control over the schedule or expected tasks	Adopt a collaborative team scheduling approach	3.37/5.00 (±1.10)	Consensus not reached
	Upskill and cross-train VN/Ts	3.07/5.00 (±1.08)	Consensus not reached
	Develop clear expectations for VN/T tasks and roles	3.93/5.00 (±0.83)	Consensus: Easy/very easy (76.66%)
	Implement work systems to enhance clarity and communications around scheduling	3.53/5.00 (±1.04)	Consensus not reached
2. Knowledge of having a positive impact on a patient or client	Implement peer feedback systems	4.16/5.00 (±0.80)	Consensus: Easy/Very easy (84%)
	Encourage clear and open communication within the team	3.37/5.00 (±1.25)	Consensus not reached
	Provide recognition based on individual VN/T needs	3.69/5.00 (±0.97)	Consensus not reached
3. Being trusted with, and involved in, decisions around patient care	Increase veterinarian and leadership awareness of VN/T training and capabilities	3.27/5.00 (±1.11)	Consensus not reached
	Develop clear VN/T capability and advancement levels	3.47/5.00 (±1.11)	Consensus not reached
	Build veterinarian trust in VN/Ts through fostering a collaborative culture	3.07/5.00 (±1.14)	Consensus not reached
	Support VN/T professional development and learning	3.67/5.00 (±1.06)	Consensus not reached

Table 3. Mean perceived effectiveness ratings and participant consensus ratings for solutions to workplace burnout risk factors derived from Round 2.

Risk Factor	Solution	Perceived Effectiveness Rating (Mean/5.00 (*SD*))	Consensus Rating (Participant Agreement %)
1. The workload is too high	Hire more staff	3.86/5.00 (±0.85)	Effective/very effective (79%)
	Improve staff retention	4.57/5.00 (±0.74)	Effective/very effective (93%)
	Implement workload management systems to enhance efficiency and communications around workload issues	4.18/5.00 (±0.55)	Effective/very effective (93%)
	Preventative healthcare focus to reduce the number of cases seen	2.75/5.00 (±0.84)	Ineffective/neutral (75%)
2. There is a lack of opportunities to utilise skills and knowledge for which veterinary nurses/technicians are trained and qualified	Provide role clarity on skill level and task expectations of VN/Ts and veterinarians	4.21/5.00 (±0.57)	Effective/very effective (93%)
	Support veterinarians to delegate tasks to VN/Ts	4.25/5.00 (±0.70)	Effective/very effective (93%)
	Create opportunities for skill utilisation by reducing non-clinical workload and increasing clinical work opportunities	4.39/5.00 (±0.74)	Effective/very effective (93%)
	Implement systems to support delegation	4.29/5.00 (±0.71)	Effective/very effective (93%)
3. A negative team culture exists (for example: bullying, gossiping, criticism, or general incivility)	Zero-tolerance to incivility at all levels of the workplace	4.14/5.00 (±0.79)	Effective/very effective (83%)
	Promote culture change	4.38/5.00 (±0.68)	Effective/very effective (90%)
	Set clear expectations on expected behaviour	4.14/5.00 (±0.74)	Effective/very effective (86%)
	Provide staff and leadership training and support	4.28/5.00 (±0.65)	Effective/very effective (90%)

Table 3. *Cont.*

Risk Factor	Solution	Perceived Effectiveness Rating (Mean/5.00 (*SD*))	Consensus Rating (Participant Agreement %)
4. There is a lack of, or unclear, communication from both management and within the team	Increase communication opportunities	4.23/5.00 (±0.71)	Effective/very effective (85%)
	Promote and reward good communication	4.08/5.00 (±0.63)	Effective/very effective (85%)
	Develop clear communication protocols and reporting lines	4.12/5.00 (±0.65)	Effective/very effective (85%)
	Utilise different communication methods	3.96/5.00 (±0.6)	Effective/very effective (88%)
5. There is poor management/leadership of the team (for example: micromanagement, favouritism, lack of support, or lack of action on team conflict)	Improve leadership recruitment and training processes	4.38/5.00 (±0.62)	Effective/very effective (93%)
	Implement systems to support leaders	4.31/5.00 (±0.54)	Effective/very effective (97%)
	Improve workplace communication	4.45/5.00 (±0.51)	Effective/very effective (100%)
	Initiate leadership reviews and accountability	4.24/5.00 (±0.74)	Effective/very effective (90%)
6. There is an expectation of working overtime, not having a break, and a general lack of flexibility in rostering	Review and adjust staffing to meet clinic needs	4.17/5.00 (±0.85)	Effective/very effective (79%)
	Implement clear break and overtime policies	4.00/5.00 (±0.89)	Effective/very effective (76%)
	Provide leadership and team training	4.21/5.00 (±0.41)	Effective/very effective (100%)
	Review and implement workflow systems to streamline tasks and develop contingency plans	4.00/5.00 (±0.60)	Effective/very effective (83%)
7. Remuneration is poor	Offer non-monetary remuneration	3.48/5.00 (±0.95)	Effective/ neutral (76%)
	Explore opportunities to increase revenue	3.79/5.00 (±0.62)	Effective/neutral (90%)
	Implement salary banding and progression pathways	4.17/5.00 (±0.6)	Effective/very effective (90%)
	Implement work processes to reduce costs	4.17/5.00 (±0.66)	Effective/very effective (89%)

Table 3. *Cont.*

Risk Factor	Solution	Perceived Effectiveness Rating (Mean/5.00 (*SD*))	Consensus Rating (Participant Agreement %)
8. There is a lack of opportunity for progression or development	Develop clear progression pathways for VN/Ts	4.21/5.00 (±0.73)	Effective/very effective (83%)
	Explore professional growth opportunities	4.10/5.00 (±0.56)	Effective/very effective (90%)
	Provide internal VN/T training and support	4.28/5.00 (±0.53)	Effective/very effective (97%)
	Promote external VN/T training and support	4.03/5.00 (±0.68)	Effective/very effective (79%)
9. Having to deal with rude or abusive clients	Provide clear expectations on client conflict management and empower the team	4.17/5.00 (±1.00)	Effective/very effective (83%)
	Create workplace support systems for VN/Ts faced with client abuse	4.10/5.00 (±0.77)	Effective/very effective (83%)
	Prepare and train the team for conflict situations	4.14/5.00 (±0.74)	Effective/very effective (79%)
	Communicate clear behavioural expectations to clients	3.72/5.00 (±1.19)	Consensus not reached
10. There is a lack of appreciation, feeling valued or being heard, by management	Implement VN/T recognition systems	3.69/5.00 (±0.35)	Effective/neutral (76%)
	Increase communication channels between management and VN/Ts	4.03/5.00 (±0.63)	Effective/very effective (83%)
	Provide support and training for leaders	4.15/5.00 (±0.6)	Effective/very effective (89%)
	Identify what appreciation looks like for individuals	4.45/5.00 (±0.69)	Effective/very effective (90%)

In contrast to ease of implementation, consensus around effectiveness was reached in 39 out of 40 (97.5%) proposed solutions. The majority of solutions (87.5%) were rated as effective/very effective, with three (7.5%) rated as effective/neutral, one (2.5%) rated as ineffective/neutral, and one (2.5%) where consensus was not reached. Qualitative data highlighted three key challenges and considerations that applied broadly across the risk factors and proposed solutions. First, implementation time and strategy must be considered when initiating any change process to set realistic expectations. Solutions that rely on culture change, for example, require long term commitment, with one participant estimating that *"It takes time to engage the team and shift the culture (1–2 years)"*, and another noting that change management processes must be carefully considered *"It needs to be done* with *the people not* to *the people and it needs to be authentic not just words"*. In addition, historical cultural attitudes embedded in the industry also need to shift in order to reduce barriers to change as illustrated by the following response: *"The most difficult part [. . .] is getting past the 'but I have always done it this way' mentality"*. One participant suggested that embedding leadership skills in professional training programs could be of benefit *"The changing of workplace wellbeing, culture and leadership could be quite easy if these issues were addressed within [Doctor of Veterinary Medicine] DVM school trainings as well as technician and assistant schools"*. Finally, in some geographical regions, progress on issues including utilisation, progression opportunities, and remuneration, was reported as being hindered by lack of regulation or title protection, with one participant suggesting that *"Registration and accreditation of [VN/Ts] with delineation of duties based on experience and education will assist professional growth and recognition [. . .] and be covered under registration/insurance just as vets are"*. Another participant noted that the lack of, or unclear, regulation impedes veterinarian's willingness to delegate tasks that VN/Ts are trained to perform *"[Vets] prefer to do things themselves because they know where accountability will land"*.

Out of all risk factors analysed, high workload had the most effective solution: 'Improving staff retention', which was rated as considerably more effective than: 'Hiring more staff'. One participant noted that *"Hiring more staff will always be a problem: 1. As we have a decline in the numbers of both DVMs and VN/Ts interested in serving this field, 2. Until we positively impact culture (which drives retention) and workload management systems"*. Another stated that *"Hiring more staff is most likely not cost effective for many clinics, improving workflow and retention of staff is better"*. High workload also had the least effective solution: 'Preventative healthcare focus to reduce the number of cases seen'. Participants suggested that this was beyond the capacity of an individual clinic to manage, with one noting that *"The public health promotion to clients and consumers would require a HUGE effort from all sectors of the profession and would be extremely challenging for a clinic to do on their own to change client and consumer behaviours"*.

The most highly rated effective solutions overall addressed poor management and leadership of the team, which had been rated the hardest risk factor to address in Round 2. Participants noted that leaders in the veterinary industry are often not selected for leadership qualities, therefore, early support is needed *"In the veterinary industry (VN/T and vet) the leaders are often those that own the practice or 'fall into' the position with length of service or when staff leave. Better or greater focus on leadership and management skills in undergraduate programs would help"*, as well as ongoing peer support *"Leadership peer groups that provide coaching are a much-needed solution"*.

Dealing with clients showing rude and abusive behaviours had the only solution where consensus was not reached: 'Communicate clear behavioural expectations to clients'. Conflicting opinions around this focused on how the solution is implemented, with support for providing clear expectations for both clients and veterinary staff. One participant noted that *"Expectations from clients alone without what they receive in return may be damaging on first impressions"*, and another confirming *"You can post signs for clients about poor behaviour—what do they care? They can just go someplace else"*. A third participant suggested that *"When a client begins at a practice, [they] should be signing some sort of agreement of what the practice will provide for them and the required client behaviours"*.

Analysis of data from open-ended questions in Round 2 was used to revise the proposed solutions and suggested actions derived from Round 1. This included changes to language to promote inclusive practice. For example, for Problem 3, exploring solutions to a negative team culture, the proposed action: 'support calling *out* unacceptable behaviour' was changed to 'support calling *in* of unacceptable behaviour'. It also included changes to promote a growth mindset, acknowledging that individuals have the capacity to change. For example, in Problem 9, exploring solutions to client incivility, 'Having to deal with rude or abusive clients' was changed to 'Dealing with clients expressing rude or abusive behaviours'. In addition, a solution rated as ineffective/neutral was removed, and proposed timelines to guide implementation of solutions were added based on feedback around setting realistic expectations for implementation. The final recommendations can be seen in Table 4.

Proposed strategies and suggested actions to leverage burnout protective factors were also updated based on analysis of Round 2 data and can be seen in Table 5.

Table 4. Proposed solutions and associated actions to address ten workplace burnout risk factors in VN/Ts, ranked in order of effectiveness as rated by Delphi panel members.

Risk factor 1: The workload is too high		
Proposed solutions	**Effectiveness rating** (mean/5.00 (*SD*))	**Examples of actions that may be implemented include**
Improve staff retention	Very high (4.57/5.00 (±0.74))	**Short term:** Implement clear job goal and progression tracking; improve leader-staff communication; implement exit and stay interviews
		Medium term: Improve workplace wellbeing; improve leader responsiveness; empower staff to have a voice; provide leadership and team training on psychosocial hazards and occupational health and safety (OHS) responsibilities
		Long term: Improve workplace culture; provide training and support to improve leadership skills; provide staff training and increase VN/T utilisation
Implement workload management systems to enhance efficiency and communications around workload issues	Very high (4.18/5.00 (±0.55))	**Short term:** Develop clear policies and standard operating procedures (SOPs) to provide guidance on caseload and booking protocols; hold regular team meetings; review current systems to improve workflow
Hire more staff	High (3.86/5.00 (±0.85))	**Short term:** Determine skill gaps and capacity to support training of unskilled VN/Ts; hire more VN/Ts and/or non-VN/T support staff to reduce non-clinical workload—level of experience should be determined by needs assessment
		Medium term: Implement robust induction and training processes
Risk factor 2: There is a lack of opportunities to utilise skills and knowledge for which veterinary nurses/technicians are trained and qualified		
Proposed solutions	**Effectiveness rating** (mean/5.00 (*SD*))	**Examples of actions that may be implemented include:**
Create opportunities for skill utilisation by reducing non-clinical workload and increasing clinical work opportunities	Very high (4.39/5.00 (±0.74))	**Short term:** Introduce VN/T clinics
		Medium term: Utilise technology to manage non-clinical workload—ensuring support is provided; implement progression pathways for VN/Ts
Implement systems to support delegation	Very high (4.29/5.00 (±0.71))	**Short term:** Implement VN/T-to-patient and veterinarian ratios; develop clear SOPs for clinical tasks; introduce team rounds to promote collaboration and increase veterinarian awareness and trust of VN/T capabilities
		Medium term: Implement mentoring programs; hire/utilise non-VN/T support staff for non-clinical tasks
Support veterinarians to delegate tasks to VN/Ts	Very high (4.25/5.00 (±0.70))	**Short term:** Provide support from leadership
		Medium term: Provide veterinarian training on VN/T education and relevant legislation/regulations; provide delegation training
Provide role clarity on skill level and task expectations of VN/Ts and veterinarians	Very high (4.21/5.00 (±0.57))	**Short term:** Develop clear SOPs outlining veterinary and VN/T tasks and responsibilities—specific to experience/specialisation
		Medium term: Introduce VN/T levelling system based on education and experience

Table 4. *Cont.*

Risk factor 3: A negative team culture exists (for example: bullying, gossiping, criticism, or general incivility)		
Proposed solutions	**Effectiveness rating** (mean/5.00 (*SD*))	**Examples of actions that may be implemented include:**
Promote culture change	Very high (4.38/5.00 (±0.68))	**Short term:** Develop team vision and values collaboratively; provide support from leadership; conduct anonymous surveys to measure staff perceptions of culture and identify issues
		Medium term: Introduce culture officer role; promote regular and transparent communication; support low level resolution between individuals; leadership team to model positive culture
		Long term: Promote psychological safety
Provide staff and leadership training and support	Very high (4.28/5.00 (±0.65))	**Medium term:** Provide dedicated time and training for leadership and staff on areas such as communication skills, conflict management, mental health first aid, civility training, human resources management, diversity, equity and inclusion (DEI) awareness, local employment laws
Set clear expectations on expected behaviour	Very high (4.14/5.00 (±0.74))	**Short term:** Develop clear policies and definitions of bullying; introduce a code of conduct
		Medium term: Implement performance improvement plans; implement disciplinary procedures
Zero-tolerance to incivility at all levels of the workplace	Very high (4.14/5.00 (±0.79))	**Short term:** Identify causes of incivility and address issues early; apply zero tolerance policies equitably across all roles
		Medium term: Support calling in unacceptable behaviour; implement disciplinary procedures and termination if necessary
Risk factor 4: There is a lack of, or unclear, communication from both management and within the team		
Proposed solutions	**Effectiveness rating** (mean/5.00 (*SD*))	**Examples of actions that may be implemented include:**
Increase communication opportunities	Very high (4.23/5.00 (±0.71))	**Short term:** Introduce interdisciplinary and individual team meetings; implement team huddles and debriefs at the start and end of the day; implement a leadership open door policy; create feedback opportunities
Develop clear communication protocols and reporting lines	Very high (4.12/5.00 (±0.65))	**Short term:** Implement clear reporting lines; establish a single source of information; develop communication templates; ensure availability of recordings or minutes for those unable to attend; provide training in new protocols and systems
Promote and reward good communication	Very high 4.08/5.00 (±0.63))	**Medium term:** Promote leadership modelling of good communication; provide communication training; celebrate effective communication
		Long term: Promote psychological safety
Utilise different communication methods	High (3.96/5.00 (±0.60))	**Short term:** Seek input on individual preferences for communication; consider personality types, e.g., introverts and adapt bidirectional communication accordingly; implement anonymous and identified feedback systems
		Medium term Utilise technology to increase accessibility—ensuring support is provided; implement a centralised communication hub

Table 4. *Cont.*

Risk factor 5: There is poor management/leadership of the team (for example: micromanagement, favouritism, lack of support, or lack of action on team conflict)		
Proposed solutions	**Effectiveness rating** (mean/5.00 (*SD*))	**Examples of actions that may be implemented include:**
Improve workplace communication	Very high (4.45/5.00 (±0.51))	**Short term:** Implement feedback systems; hold regular team meetings; promote transparency
		Long term: Promote psychological safety
Improve leadership recruitment and training processes	Very high (4.38/5.00 (±0.62))	**Short term:** Adopt recruitment strategies focused on leadership and clinical skills/experience not just clinical seniority
		Medium term: Implement succession planning
		Long term: Provide ongoing training in leadership and human resource management
Implement systems to support leaders	Very high (4.31/5.00 (±0.54))	**Short term:** Promote empowerment and support from upper management; Promote role modelling and introduce mentorship programs
		Medium term: Implement allocated and protected admin time for those in mixed leadership/clinical roles; implement management levelling system to support development
Initiate leadership reviews and accountability	Very high (4.24/5.00 (±0.74))	**Short term:** Develop and communicate clear expectations; implement structured leadership review systems such as 360 reviews
		Medium term: Implement performance management processes
Risk factor 6: There is an expectation of working overtime, not having a break, and a general lack of flexibility in rostering		
Proposed solutions	**Effectiveness rating** (mean/5.00 (*SD*))	**Examples of actions that may be implemented include:**
Provide leadership and team training	Very high (4.21/5.00 (±0.41))	**Medium term:** Provide dedicated time for team training on areas such as communication and teamwork, wellness, workplace legislation; provide dedicated time for leadership training on turnover costs and effective workload management; implement cross-training of team skills to enable greater support
Regularly review and adjust staffing to meet clinic needs	Very high (4.17/5.00 (±0.85))	**Short term:** Implement an on-call per diem roster in the event overtime is required
		Medium term: Perform a needs analysis to determine gaps; hire more VN/Ts and/or non-VN/T support staff to meet workload, including flexible or part time roles to increase coverage at busy periods and float VN/Ts to cover breaks
Review and implement workflow systems to streamline tasks and develop contingency plans	Very high (4.00/5.00 (±0.60))	**Short term:** Implement limited service/bypass protocols (seeing only critical patients and redirecting non-critical cases elsewhere); develop clear policies to prevent overbooking; hold morning team huddles to plan workflow; utilise rostering software to assist; utilise telemedicine and triaging support services
		Medium term: Develop team pipelines to improve workflow; partner with local clinics to share relief or floating VN/Ts

Table 4. *Cont.*

Implement clear break and overtime policies	Very high (4.00/5.00 (±0.89))	**Short term:** Introduce scheduled break times, or break guidelines to be coordinated by shift lead; implement overtime bonus pay structures
		Medium term: Cultivate a casual VN/T bank for last minute support
Risk factor 7: Remuneration is poor		
Proposed solutions	**Effectiveness rating** (mean/5.00 (*SD*))	**Examples of actions that may be implemented include:**
Implement salary banding and progression pathways	Very high (4.17/5.00 (±0.60))	**Short term:** Develop clear job descriptions and skill levels—ensuring growth is not limited to title; promote transparency around salary banding as well as clinic running costs
		Medium term: Implement pay commensurate with skill level; develop progression pathways and support to increase responsibility and skill level
Implement work processes to reduce costs	Very high (4.17/5.00 (±0.66))	**Medium term:** Utilise technology to automate routine tasks—ensuring support is provided; implement appropriate utilisation of VN/Ts to increase veterinarian capacity
Explore opportunities to increase revenue	High (3.79/5.00 (±0.62))	**Short term:** Ensure correct charging; increase prices; promote client education on pet insurance
		Medium term: Introduce new services (e.g., VN/T clinics, telehealth); conduct budget forecasting
Offer non-monetary remuneration	High (3.48/5.00 (±0.95))	**Short term:** Develop a structured and equitable system
		Medium term: Determine individualised options in consultation with staff members as suited to their needs (e.g., childcare support, travel vouchers, time off for study)
Risk factor 8: There is a lack of opportunity for progression or development		
Proposed solutions	**Effectiveness rating** (mean/5.00 (*SD*))	**Examples of actions that may be implemented include:**
Provide internal VN/T training and support	Very high (4.28/5.00 (±0.53))	**Short term:** Implement individual development plans; support time off for study
		Medium term: Implement a development and training officer role; provide leadership training; develop mentoring/coaching programs
Develop clear progression pathways for VN/Ts	Very high (4.21/5.00 (±0.73))	**Short term:** Develop clear progression bands; develop clear VN/T job descriptions with training to support growth within the clinic
		Medium term: Support both leadership and non-leadership progression pathways; implement growth lattices—supporting both vertical and horizontal development
Explore professional growth opportunities	Very high (4.10/5.00 (±0.56))	**Short term:** Identify areas for increased responsibility
		Medium term: Support undertaking specialised qualifications that can be utilised by the clinic; develop specific roles that match individuals' interests or skills

Table 4. *Cont.*

Promote external VN/T training and support	Very high (4.03/5.00 (±0.68))	**Short term:** Identify networking opportunities; signpost funding opportunities and access to CE; identify and approach other industry members for mentoring (e.g., VTS)
		Medium term: Establish a continuing education funding program with requirement for funding recipients to share new knowledge with the team
Risk factor 9: Dealing with clients expressingrude or abusive behaviours		
Proposed solutions	**Effectiveness rating** (mean/5.00 (*SD*))	**Examples of actions that may be implemented include:**
Provide clear expectations on client conflict management and empower the team	Very high (4.17/5.00 (±1.00))	**Short term:** Promote zero tolerance for abuse of staff; develop clear guidelines on what constitutes acceptable and non-acceptable behaviour; develop guidelines and provide training on when to escalate issues; develop and provide training on communication protocols for conflict situations
Prepare and train the team for conflict situations	Very high (4.14/5.00 (±0.74))	**Short term:** Identify and address issues that contribute to poor client experience; ensure staff are never rostered alone; install security systems (e.g., CCTV, duress alarms); develop client information on external financial and emotional support services
		Medium term: Provide regular staff training in de-escalation and emotional intelligence
Create workplace support systems for VN/Ts faced with client abuse	Very high (4.10/5.00 (±0.77))	**Short term:** Provide —and ensure access to—leadership support; implement debriefs after difficult interactions; Implement reporting systems for incidents
		Medium term: Employ social workers in the team with training to manage and support distressed clients
		Long term: Promote teamwork and support through improving workplace culture—refer to risk factor 3
Communicate clear behavioural expectations to clients	High (3.72/5.00 (±1.19))	**Short term:** Develop code of conduct contracts for new and/or existing clients outlining two-way expectations of the client-clinic relationship; introduce waiting room signage; provide clear and transparent information on costs and wait times; outline the consequences of abusing staff
Risk factor 10: There is a lack of appreciation, feeling valued, or being heard, by management		
Proposed solutions	**Effectiveness rating** (mean/5.00 (*SD*))	**Examples of actions that may be implemented include:**
Identify what appreciation looks like for individuals	Very high (4.45/5.00 (±0.69))	**Short term:** Survey the team; implement individual development plans; Include individual motivator discussion as part of new staff inductions
		Medium term: Provide dedicated time for leaders to spend with staff
Provide support and training for leaders	Very high (4.15/5.00 (±0.60))	**Medium term:** Provide training on areas such as effective communication, emotional intelligence, diversity, equity and inclusion (DEI), culture, intrinsic motivators; develop mentoring and peer group programs
Increase communication channels between management and VN/Ts	Very high (4.03/5.00 (±0.63))	**Short term:** Implement feedback systems; hold regular meetings; establish preferred communication channels in consultation with the team; Implement open door policies

Table 4. *Cont.*

Implement VN/T recognition systems	High (3.69/5.00 (±0.85))	**Short term:** Introduce initiatives in collaboration with the team such as newsletters, VN/T of the month, long service awards, staff appreciation days; include recognition as a standing agenda item in meetings
		Medium term: Establish a staff appreciation committee; establish a staff appreciation fund

Effectiveness rating scored out of 5: Very low = 0–1; Low = 1.1–2; Neutral = 2.1–3; High = 3.1–4; Very high = 4.1–5
Duration of implementation: Short term = 0–6 months; Medium term = 6–12 months; Long term = 1–2 years+
Note: Success of many of these strategies relies on effective planning and implementation. If existing expertise is not available within the clinic, the use of—or communication with—external consultants is suggested to increase chance of success.

Table 5. Proposed strategies and associated actions to promote three burnout protective factors in VN/Ts.

Protective Factor 1: Having some control over the schedule or expected tasks	
Proposed strategies	**Examples of actions that may be implemented include:**
Adopt a collaborative team scheduling approach	VN/T representation in management decision making; morning team huddles to plan tasks, breaks, and teamwork; support innovation to improve scheduling or workflow practices
Upskill and cross-train VN/Ts	Increase capacity to perform in all VN/T roles; build confidence to work autonomously; cross-train to increase opportunity to swap shifts
Develop clear expectations for VN/T tasks and roles	Collaborative development of VN/T shift descriptions with tasks and skill levels outlined
Implement work systems to enhance clarity and communications around scheduling	Clear booking policies to prevent overbooking; break and overtime policies; seek VN/T feedback on scheduling issues and collaboratively problem solve
Protective Factor 2: Knowledge of having a positive impact on a patient or client	
Proposed strategies	**Examples of actions that may be implemented include:**
Implement peer feedback systems	Kudos boards; team meeting shout outs; communication systems to pass feedback up to management; make acknowledgement part of team huddles and debriefs
Encourage clear and open communication within the team	Improve culture around good communication; leadership modelling of good communication; create regular and easy feedback systems and habits
Provide recognition based on individual VN/T needs	Survey the team to determine preferences; public vs. private feedback; increase team and leadership awareness of generational and career stage influences on individual needs
Protective Factor 3: Being trusted with, and involved in, decisions around patient care	
Proposed strategies	**Examples of actions that may be implemented include:**
Increase veterinarian and leadership awareness of VN/T training and capabilities	Encourage active involvement of VN/Ts in case discussions providing an opportunity to demonstrate knowledge; education of veterinarians and leaders on VN/T education levels and professional regulation

Table 5. *Cont.*

Develop clear VN/T capability and advancement levels	Clear guidelines around skills and abilities expected at each level; conduct VN/T competency assessments to progress to next level; develop a spectrum of care chart to clearly outline clinical expectations at each level
Build veterinarian trust in VN/Ts through fostering a collaborative culture	Psychological safety; all team patient rounds; veterinarian to VN/T mentoring and reverse mentoring programs; encourage questions and discussion for learning; team debriefing; leadership support; team consulting; collaborative patient care plans
Support VN/T professional development and learning	Individual development plans; in house training; journal clubs; shadowing shifts with experienced VN/Ts; provide clear patient parameter ranges and alert guidelines to inexperienced VN/Ts

4. Discussion

The aim of this study was to develop effective and feasible organisational management strategies to address burnout in VN/Ts. This was achieved by utilising the Delphi method to first identify the barriers and enablers to effecting change and then explore the perceived ease and effectiveness of proposed strategies, to develop recommendations.

4.1. Industry-Wide Barriers

The findings revealed that the same barriers exist across all countries involved in this study. Some barriers, such as inadequate regulation and lack of leadership education in veterinary and VN/T training programs, are beyond the capacity of individual clinics to effect change and require industry-wide or government interventions. The lack of, or uncertainty around, regulation of VN/Ts was a key barrier to addressing multiple burnout risk factors. Whilst current regulatory requirements vary between, and within, countries, participants from all represented countries (USA, UK, Australia, Canada, and New Zealand) reported the impact of inadequate regulation on VN/T utilisation. Local associations not permitting VN/Ts to perform skills they are trained and qualified in, as well as poor veterinarian education on VN/T regulations, have been found to contribute to poor utilisation [36,37]. Guidelines for optimal utilisation of VN/Ts, published by the American Animal Hospital Association (AAHA) [38], outline the positive impact on the whole veterinary team, including improved patient care, staff retention, and financial sustainability of the business, and provide multiple resources to support improved utilisation. Further research, however, is required to measure the impact of these guidelines in the future.

Inadequate support for leaders was also found to be a barrier to addressing numerous burnout risk factors. Previous studies have highlighted the important role that leadership plays in managing veterinary team burnout through actions such as support, advocacy, recognition, and empowerment of staff [1,3]. These findings were replicated in the current study, but it was also revealed that many veterinary team leaders lack the necessary training or time to succeed in the role. Promotion of individuals to leadership roles based on clinical expertise, or length of service, was reported as an embedded cultural problem within the industry, resulting in a lack of positive role models or mentors to drive change. Provision of training or support to leaders was proposed as a solution strategy for over half of the risk factors that were reviewed, which illustrates the extent of the issue. Improved recruitment processes for leadership positions, as well as better support and training for those interested in taking on a leadership role, are vital to reducing burnout in VN/Ts as well as VN/T leaders. Furthermore, non-leadership career progression pathways, other than leaving the industry, must be offered to increase options for advanced VN/Ts in order to prevent people advancing to management roles as the only career progression option.

4.2. Clinic Specific Barriers

Unique barriers within individual clinics focused on the existing workplace climate and therefore, will vary between clinics. Quality of leadership, existing team culture, staff willingness for change, existing level of staff burnout, financial health of the clinic, and the ability to effectively design and implement change processes, are all issues that must be objectively evaluated before determining suitable strategies for implementation.

Addressing poor leadership (Risk factor 5) was found to be a particular challenge as it requires leaders to accept that they are part of the problem. Whilst this poses a critical barrier to effecting positive change for VN/T teams, qualitative data from this study also acknowledged the risk of burnout in leaders. Research suggests that negative leader well-being is associated with negative employee well-being [39]. However much of the literature focuses on the effects of leadership on employee burnout, with limited research exploring burnout in leaders, despite reports of high levels of stress and demands in their role [39,40]. In addition to providing support to improve leadership skills, it is essential that well-being support is also provided to leaders in order to enable them to perform to the best of their ability. Similarly, implementing significant organisational change has been found to contribute to burnout in teams [41]. Whilst pre-existing burnout in the team does not prevent the introduction of new systems, required levels of support, such as time and resources, should be re-evaluated in order to maximise adaptive reserve and resilience within the team and avoid increased burnout and turnover [42].

Reluctance of staff to engage in a change process due to attitudes such as "we've always done it this way", was identified as a barrier in the current study and has also been reported elsewhere [37,43]. Resistance to organisational change has been reported as one of the key reasons why change initiatives fail [44]. Reasons for resistance include perceived loss of control and lack of fairness [44,45], which comprise two of the six key Areas of Worklife found to contribute to burnout [46]. When encountering resistance to change, it is, therefore, essential to understand the underlying reasons for resistance, in order to address these directly [44].

Clinic-specific barriers that are within the capability of individual leaders to address will vary widely between clinics. Consideration must, therefore, be given to the existing workplace climate before selecting which strategies to implement, and indeed, how to implement them, in order to maximise chances of success.

4.3. *Solutions*

4.3.1. Risk Factors

Common themes among the proposed solutions included improving communication, developing a culture of psychological safety, developing progression pathways for VN/Ts with embedded training and support, developing clear policies in collaboration with the team, and reviewing workplace systems to enhance efficiency. Many of the solutions, such as improving workplace culture, will be a long process requiring time, commitment, and resources to ensure that changes are successful and become embedded in the ongoing normality of the clinic [47]. Kotter's [48] change management process suggests that short term wins can help to build morale and momentum to help sustain motivation within larger change efforts. It may be possible, and even beneficial, therefore, to implement a combination of short- and long-term strategies simultaneously to help generate positive change in the short term.

Of the ten workplace risk factors evaluated in the study, high workload and lack of support have been found to be significant contributors to burnout in VN/Ts [16]. In the current study, improving staff retention was considered a more effective strategy for reducing workload (Risk factor 1) than hiring more staff. Reasons for VN/T turnover have been found to include poor financial outlook, lack of career progression opportunities, lack of utilisation, poor workplace culture, and lack of employer support [19,50], all of which have also been found to be risk factors for burnout in VN/Ts [16]. Factors predicting retention in veterinary nurses have been described as multi-factorial and individual [50]. The introduction of 'stay interviews' was one of the proposed actions to achieve this solution in the current study. These short, proactive discussions between leader and individual team member are conducted at regular intervals and establish what works well in their current role and what can be improved and have been shown to have positive results in human nursing teams [51,52].

Improving workplace culture (Risk factor 3) was identified as particularly challenging to address due to the time it takes to establish culture change within an organisation. Research suggests that culture impacts employee engagement, morale, and cooperation, all of which play a key role in the implementation of successful change initiatives [47]. Proposed solutions focused on breaking down barriers within the team through actions such as developing team vision and values collaboratively, establishing support from the leadership team, and promoting regular and transparent communication. Establishing a need for change and developing a shared vision are proposed to be two key stages of successful change management [53]. Research suggests that acknowledging current problems within the team, developing a clear vision, and combined leadership and employee support are all required for culture change to be successful [47]. Whilst these have all been identified as separate actions within the recommendations, it is, therefore, important to ensure that they are implemented collectively in order to maximise the change of success.

4.3.2. Protective Factors

Factors that protect against burnout in VN/Ts include having control over one's work, knowledge of having a positive impact, and being included in patient care decision making [16]. As with risk factors, the ability to leverage each of these will vary between clinics, therefore strategies should be carefully considered before implementation. The perceived effectiveness of these strategies was not measured, as protective factors are aimed at preventing the onset of burnout, rather than reducing existing burnout [54]. However, a notable overlap of themes can be seen between proposed primary prevention strategies (protective factor strategies) and secondary prevention strategies (solutions to risk factors). Teamwork, collaboration, improved communication, support, and development opportunities, can be seen across recommendations for both primary and secondary burnout prevention. As such, it may be beneficial for clinic leaders to consider all recommendations—regardless of which burnout risk factors have been identified in their clinic—in order to take a proactive approach to burnout management within their teams.

4.4. Implementation of Solutions

Change management is challenging, and organisational change initiatives have been reported to fail in 70% of cases, and in up to 90% of cases addressing culture change [55]. Change is, however, essential for improvement and ultimately, the survival of any organisation [55]. The findings from this study showed that a positive and psychologically safe workplace culture is fundamental to the success of a large number of the proposed solutions. Previous research shows that a solid understanding of the operational process of change, as well as establishing upper management support and awareness of the existing issues, are critical to driving successful change [56]. Instruments to measure organisational culture and health may be of use in conducting impartial evaluations and have been designed for use in human healthcare [57,58]. These surveys conduct a full 360-degree evaluation of areas such as leadership and management effectiveness, staff wellbeing, and patient safety, and provide a valuable reference for developing veterinary focused assessment tools. Use of evaluation tools such as these can help to increase leadership awareness of areas where their perceptions of the organisational climate do not align with those of their teams. This understanding will support leaders to select targeted strategies which are more likely to be successful in addressing existing workplace issues.

In addition to assessing workplace climate, the time and effort involved with strategy implementation must be considered and clearly communicated to the team in order to set realistic expectations for both staff and leaders. Employee attitudes towards change have been found to be a key determinant of its long-term success, therefore any change process—regardless of the intended benefits for staff—must be carefully managed [59]. One of the key barriers to addressing burnout in this study was found to be the lack of leadership or management expertise within the industry. In veterinary clinics where knowledge of workplace program design and implementation is lacking, external support such as the use of business management consultants with an in-depth understanding of the veterinary industry should, therefore, be considered to increase the chances of success.

The dissemination of these and future findings is critical to effecting change. Whilst it is beyond the scope of this study, which focused on implementation of change within the workplace, industry wide change is essential to achieving meaningful progress. Including leadership education in veterinary and VN/T training, improving VN/T regulation, and increasing awareness of burnout reduction strategies across the industry can all make a significant contribution to reducing burnout. In addition, tackling misinformation around topics such as VN/T utilisation, and individuals' weaknesses leading to burnout, is imperative and may benefit from platforms such as social media to discredit broad misconceptions [60].

Finally, it should be noted that whilst burnout is the result of workplace stressors and, thus, the workplace has a responsibility to address them where possible, not all burnout contributors can be completely controlled or eliminated [3]. There is, therefore, a shared responsibility for VN/Ts to implement individual coping strategies to strengthen the effects of workplace efforts. Whilst these may be implemented by the individual, however, many, for example work-life balance, counselling, and education, may also require, or benefit from, workplace support [3].

4.5. Limitations and Further Research

This study had some limitations worth noting. First, a high level of consensus around effectiveness of solutions was achieved in Round 2 with only minor proposed modifications which did not justify additional rounds. As a consequence, there was no opportunity to measure stability of the results over successive rounds. There is significant variance among the accepted closing criteria for Delphi studies. Some authors argue that stability must be measured in conjunction with consensus in order to confirm the validity of results [61]. Others argue that either consensus alone, or a pre-determined number of rounds, is a more commonly used criterion for terminating a Delphi study [62]. As such, additional rounds would have enabled the measurement of stability in addition to consensus, but at the risk of extending the study and further imposing on the goodwill of participants. Further Delphi studies would be beneficial to confirm the reliability and proposed effectiveness of these recommendations. Second, whilst all efforts were made to recruit panel members from a range of representative countries, almost 50% of the panel comprised members from one country (USA), whilst the other 50% represented members from the remaining four countries (UK, Australia, Canada, New Zealand). It is, therefore, possible that some proposed solutions may be more applicable to the culture and legislative climate of the USA. In addition, all panel members were recruited from developed countries and therefore data from developing countries was not captured. The findings, therefore, may not translate to the different challenges that may be experienced by VN/T leaders in developing countries and further research would be beneficial to explore the generalisability of these recommendations. Finally, gaining expert opinion fills a gap in existing knowledge on effective organisational strategies to address burnout in VN/Ts. However, further research is required to evaluate and measure the effectiveness of proposed interventions in order to know if the recommendations are actually effective in preventing burnout.

5. Conclusions

Burnout in VN/Ts has negative impacts on the individual, patient, and business, but existing research lacks clear recommendations on workplace strategies to support better management of burnout at the source. This study developed 39 expert-led workplace burnout reduction strategies and recommended actions to guide VN/T managers worldwide in addressing 10 known risk factors for burnout in VN/Ts. To the authors' knowledge, this is the first research to explore expert recommendations to address burnout in veterinary or animal care professionals. Whilst some of the recommendations are uniquely relevant to VN/Ts, many apply across broader animal care professional roles and may therefore help to guide leaders in addressing burnout more widely.

Proposed strategies to address burnout, and associated recommended actions, are specific to each risk factor, but many had similar overarching themes. These included providing support and education to leaders, improving communication, fostering a culture of psychological safety, developing clear guidelines and protocols in collaboration with the team, providing clear progression pathways, and supporting delegation of tasks to VN/Ts, as well as redistributing tasks for which they are overqualified. Successful implementation of strategies relies on first, identifying the presence of workplace risk factors through assessment of burnout among staff, and then, evaluating the existing organisational climate, in order to select the most appropriate strategies. A good understanding of change processes will also help to maximise success. In addition, the study identified the need for broader change initiatives, including development of clearer regulation of VN/Ts, and inclusion of leadership education within veterinary and VN/T training programs, to better support veterinary clinics in achieving positive change within the industry. These findings provide practical guidelines to help veterinary clinics reduce the risk of burnout in VN/Ts, as well as insights for consideration by the broader veterinary industry to support professional growth and a more sustainable future.

Supplementary Materials: The following supporting information can be downloaded at: https://www.mdpi.com/article/10.3390/ani15091257/s1, Supplementary Materials S1: Delphi study Survey—Round 1; Supplementary Materials S2: Delphi study Survey—Round 2.

Author Contributions: Conceptualization, A.J.C., V.I.R. and P.C.B.; methodology, A.J.C., V.I.R. and P.C.B.; formal analysis, A.J.C.; investigation, A.J.C.; data curation, A.J.C.; writing—original draft preparation, A.J.C.; writing—review and editing, A.J.C., V.I.R. and P.C.B.; supervision, V.I.R. and P.C.B.; project administration, A.J.C. All authors have read and agreed to the published version of the manuscript.

Funding: This work was supported by an Australian Government Research Training Program Scholarship.

Institutional Review Board Statement: The study was conducted in accordance with the National Statement on Ethical Conduct in Human Research and approved by the Human Ethics Low Risk Committee of La Trobe University (approval number HEC24265; approved 10 July 2024).

Informed Consent Statement: Informed consent was obtained from all subjects involved in the study.

Data Availability Statement: Data are unavailable to share due to privacy restrictions.

Acknowledgments: The authors would like to acknowledge and thank all of the study participants for their support of this research and contribution of their expert knowledge. Study participants who gave consent for formal acknowledgement are listed below: Amber Foote, CertAVN (Teaching, Coaching and Mentoring) BSc (Hons) RVN C-SQP; Amy Newfield, MS, CVT, VTS (ECC); Erica Honey MBA/MHRM MEmergMgt GradCertPDev BSc (Hons) RVN; Francesca Brown MProfPrac BVSc BSc GradDip Sustainable Practice; Heather Prendergast, RVT, CVPM, SPHR; Jane Bindloss RVN (UK), DipMgt; Kathleen Dunbar, MSW, RSW, RVT, VTS (Clinical Practice-Canine/Feline); Lis Conarton, LMSW, LVT, VTS (Physical Rehabilitation); Liz Hughston, MEd., RVT, CVT, LVT, VTS (SAIM) Lifetime (ECC) Emeritus; Makenzie Peterson, DSW, MSc; Robyn Sutton, RVT, VTS(ECC); Shannon Molloy RVN.

Conflicts of Interest: The authors declare no conflicts of interest.

Abbreviations

The following abbreviations are used in this manuscript:

AAHA	American Animal Hospital Association
DVM	Doctor of Veterinary Medicine
ILO	International Labour Organisation
OHS	Occupational Health and Safety
SOPs	Standard Operating Procedures
UK	United Kingdom
USA	United States of America
VN/T	Veterinary nurse and technician
WHO	World Health Organisation

References

1. Moore, I.C.; Coe, J.B.; Adams, C.L.; Conlon, P.D.; Sargeant, J.M. The role of veterinary team effectiveness in job satisfaction and burnout in companion animal veterinary clinics. *J. Am. Vet. Med. Assoc.* **2014**, *245*, 513–524. [CrossRef] [PubMed]
2. Brscic, M.; Contiero, B.; Schianchi, A.; Marogna, C. Challenging suicide, burnout, and depression among veterinary practitioners and students: Text mining and topics modelling analysis of the scientific literature. *BMC Vet. Res.* **2021**, *17*, 294. [CrossRef] [PubMed]
3. Steffey, M.A.; Griffon, D.J.; Risselada, M.; Scharf, V.F.; Buote, N.J.; Zamprogno, H.; Winter, A.L. Veterinarian burnout demographics and organizational impacts: A narrative review. *Front. Vet. Sci.* **2023**, *10*, 1184526. [CrossRef] [PubMed]
4. Chapman, A.J.; Rohlf, V.I.; Moser, A.Y.; Bennett, P.C. Organizational Factors Affecting Burnout in Veterinary Nurses: A Systematic Review. *Anthrozoös* **2024**, *37*, 651–686. [CrossRef]
5. Volk, J.O.; Schimmack, U.; Strand, E.B.; Reinhard, A.; Hahn, J.; Andrews, J.; Probyn-Smith, K.; Jones, R. Merck Animal Health Veterinary Team study reveals factors associated with well-being, burnout, and mental health among nonveterinarian practice team members. *J. Am. Vet. Med. Assoc.* **2024**, *262*, 1330–1337. [CrossRef]
6. Johnson, J.; Hall, L.H.; Berzins, K.; Baker, J.; Melling, K.; Thompson, C. Mental healthcare staff well-being and burnout: A narrative review of trends, causes, implications, and recommendations for future interventions. *Int. J. Ment. Health Nurs.* **2018**, *27*, 20–32. [CrossRef]
7. Kelly, L.A.; Gee, P.M.; Butler, R.J. Impact of nurse burnout on organizational and position turnover. *Nurs. Outlook* **2021**, *69*, 96–102. [CrossRef]
8. Salvagioni, D.A.J.; Melanda, F.N.; Mesas, A.E.; González, A.D.; Gabani, F.L.; Andrade, S.M.d. Physical, psychological and occupational consequences of job burnout: A systematic review of prospective studies. *PLoS ONE* **2017**, *12*, e0185781. [CrossRef]
9. WHO. *International Classification of Diseases*; 11th Revision; ICD-11; WHO: Geneva, Switzerland, 2023; Volume 11.
10. ILO. Mental Health at Work. Available online: https://www.ilo.org/topics/safety-and-health-work/mental-health-work (accessed on 11 March 2025).
11. WHO. *WHO Guidelines on Mental Health at Work*; World Health Organization: Geneva, Switzerland, 2022; ISBN 978-92-4-005305-2.
12. ILO. Psychosocial Risks and Stress at Work. Available online: https://www.ilo.org/resource/psychosocial-risks-and-stress-work (accessed on 12 March 2025).
13. Chapman, A.J.; Rohlf, V.I.; Moser, A.Y.; Bennett, P.C. Understanding Veterinary Technician and Nurse Burnout. Part 2: Addressing Veterinary Technician Burnout Requires Tailored Organizational Wellbeing Initiatives. *J. Am. Vet. Med. Assoc.* **2025**. *Submitted*.
14. Vasconcelos, A.F. Workplace incivility: A literature review. *Int. J. Workplace Health Manag.* **2020**, *13*, 513–542. [CrossRef]
15. White, B.; Polly, Y.; Louise, C.B.; O'Donoghue, K. Reducing the "cost of caring" in animal-care professionals: Social work contribution in a pilot education program to address burnout and compassion fatigue. *J. Hum. Behav. Soc. Environ.* **2021**, *31*, 828–847. [CrossRef]
16. Chapman, A.J.; Rohlf, V.I.; Bennett, P.C. Understanding Veterinary Technician and Nurse Burnout. Part 1: Burnout Profiles Reveal High Workload and Lack of Support are Among Major Workplace Contributors to Burnout. *J. Am. Vet. Med. Assoc.* **2025**. *Submitted*.
17. Black, A.F.; Winefield, H.R.; Chur-Hansen, A. Occupational stress in veterinary nurses: Roles of the work environment and own companion animal. *Anthrozoös* **2011**, *24*, 191–202. [CrossRef]
18. Foster, S.M.; Maples, E.H. Occupational stress in veterinary support staff. *J. Vet. Med. Educ.* **2014**, *41*, 102–110. [CrossRef]

19. Grant, A.; Kontak, J.; Jeffers, E.; Lawson, B.; MacKenzie, A.; Burge, F.; Boulos, L.; Lackie, K.; Marshall, E.G.; Mireault, A.; et al. Barriers and enablers to implementing interprofessional primary care teams: A narrative review of the literature using the consolidated framework for implementation research. *BMC Prim. Care* **2024**, *25*, 25. [CrossRef]
20. Leclercq, C.; Hansez, I. Temporal Stages of Burnout: How to Design Prevention? *Int. J. Environ. Res. Public. Health* **2024**, *21*, 1617. [CrossRef]
21. Hayes, G.M.; LaLonde-Paul, D.F.; Perret, J.L.; Steele, A.; McConkey, M.; Lane, W.G.; Kopp, R.J.; Stone, H.K.; Miller, M.; Jones-Bitton, A. Investigation of burnout syndrome and job-related risk factors in veterinary technicians in specialty teaching hospitals: A multicenter cross-sectional study. *J. Vet. Emerg. Crit. Care* **2020**, *30*, 18–27. [CrossRef]
22. Kogan, L.R.; Wallace, J.E.; Schoenfeld-Tacher, R.; Hellyer, P.W.; Richards, M. Veterinary technicians and occupational burnout. *Front. Vet. Sci.* **2020**, *7*, 328. [CrossRef]
23. Holowaychuk, M.K.; Lamb, K.E. Burnout symptoms and workplace satisfaction among veterinary emergency care providers. *J. Vet. Emerg. Crit. Care* **2023**, *33*, 180–191. [CrossRef]
24. Varela, M.; Correia, I. Empathy and Burnout in Veterinarians and Veterinary Nurses: Identifying Burnout Protectors. *Anthrozoös* **2023**, *36*, 15–34. [CrossRef]
25. McPherson, S.; Reese, C.; Wendler, M.C. Methodology Update: Delphi Studies. *Nurs. Res.* **2018**, *67*, 404–410. [CrossRef] [PubMed]
26. Reavley, N.J.; Ross, A.; Martin, A.; LaMontagne, A.D.; Jorm, A.F. Development of guidelines for workplace prevention of mental health problems: A Delphi consensus study with Australian professionals and employees. *Ment. Health Prev.* **2014**, *2*, 26–34. [CrossRef]
27. Manzano-García, G.; Ayala, J.C. Insufficiently studied factors related to burnout in nursing: Results from an e-Delphi study. *PLoS ONE* **2017**, *12*, e0175352. [CrossRef] [PubMed]
28. Dalkey, N.; Helmer, O. An experimental application of the Delphi method to the use of experts. *Manag. Sci.* **1963**, *9*, 458–467. [CrossRef]
29. Niederberger, M.; Schifano, J.; Deckert, S.; Hirt, J.; Homberg, A.; Köberich, S.; Kuhn, R.; Rommel, A.; Sonnberger, M.; DEWISS Network. Delphi studies in social and health sciences—Recommendations for an interdisciplinary standardized reporting (DELPHISTAR). Results of a Delphi study. *PLoS ONE* **2024**, *19*, e0304651. [CrossRef]
30. Jorm, A.F. Using the Delphi expert consensus method in mental health research. *Aust. N. Z. J. Psychiatry* **2015**, *49*, 887–897. [CrossRef]
31. Yap, M.B.H.; Pilkington, P.D.; Ryan, S.M.; Kelly, C.M.; Jorm, A.F. Parenting strategies for reducing the risk of adolescent depression and anxiety disorders: A Delphi consensus study. *J. Affect. Disord.* **2014**, *156*, 67–75. [CrossRef]
32. QuestionPro. *QuestionPro API V2*; QuestionPro: Austin, TX, USA, 2023.
33. Lumivero. *NVivo (Version 14)*; Lumivero: Denver, CO, USA, 2023.
34. Hsieh, H.F.; Shannon, S.E. Three approaches to qualitative content analysis. *Qual. Health Res.* **2005**, *15*, 1277–1288. [CrossRef]
35. Vaismoradi, M.; Turunen, H.; Bondas, T. Content analysis and thematic analysis: Implications for conducting a qualitative descriptive study. *Nurs. Health Sci.* **2013**, *15*, 398–405. [CrossRef]
36. Brown, F. Opportunities for New Zealand veterinary practice in the utilisation of allied veterinary professional and paraprofessional staff. *Scope Health Wellbeing* **2022**, *7*, 36–44. [CrossRef]
37. Reinhard, A.R.; Celt, V.P.; Pilewki, L.E.; Hendricks, M.K. The newly credentialed veterinary technician: Perceptions, realities, and career challenges. *Front. Vet. Sci.* **2025**, *12*, 1437525. [CrossRef] [PubMed]
38. Prendergast, H.; Mages, A.; Rauscher, J.; Roth, C.; Thompson, M.; Thompson, S.T.; Yagi, K. *2023 AAHA Technician Utilization Guidelines*; AAHA: Lakewood, CO, USA, 2023.
39. Skakon, J.; Karina, N.; Vilhelm, B.; Guzman, J. Are leaders' well-being, behaviours and style associated with the affective well-being of their employees? A systematic review of three decades of research. *Work. Stress.* **2010**, *24*, 107–139. [CrossRef]
40. Courtright, S.; Colbert, A.; Choi, D. Fired Up or Burned Out? How Developmental Challenge Differentially Impacts Leader Behavior. *J. Appl. Psychol.* **2014**, *99*, 681. [CrossRef]
41. Day, A.; Crown, S.N.; Ivany, M. Organisational change and employee burnout: The moderating effects of support and job control. *Saf. Sci.* **2017**, *100*, 4–12. [CrossRef]
42. Miller, W.L.; Crabtree, B.F.; Nutting, P.A.; Stange, K.C.; Jaén, C.R. Primary Care Practice Development: A Relationship-Centered Approach. *Ann. Fam. Med.* **2010**, *8*, S68–S79. [CrossRef]
43. Moore, I.C.; Coe, J.B.; Adams, C.L.; Conlon, P.D.; Sargeant, J.M. Exploring the Impact of Toxic Attitudes and a Toxic Environment on the Veterinary Healthcare Team. *Front. Vet. Sci.* **2015**, *2*, 78. [CrossRef]
44. Mosadeghrad, A.M.; Ansarian, M. Why do organisational change programmes fail? *Int. J. Strateg. Change Manag.* **2014**, *5*, 189–218. [CrossRef]
45. Georgalis, J.; Samaratunge, R.; Kimberley, N.; Lu, Y. Change process characteristics and resistance to organisational change: The role of employee perceptions of justice. *Aust. J. Manag.* **2015**, *40*, 89–113. [CrossRef]

46. Leiter, M.P.; Maslach, C. Six areas of worklife: A model of the organizational context of burnout. *J. Health Hum. Serv. Adm.* **1999**, *21*, 472–489.
47. Johnson, A.; Nguyen, H.; Groth, M.; Wang, K.; Ng, J.L. Time to change: A review of organisational culture change in health care organisations. *J. Organ. Eff. People Perform.* **2016**, *3*, 265–288. [CrossRef]
48. Kotter, J.P. Generating Short Term Wins. In *Leading Change*; Harvard Business Review Press: La Vergne, TN, USA, 2012; pp. 121–136.
49. Fults, M.K.; Yagi, K.; Kramer, J.; Maras, M. Development of Advanced Veterinary Nursing Degrees: Rising Interest Levels for Careers as Advanced Practice Registered Veterinary Nurses. *J. Vet. Med. Educ.* **2021**, *48*, 242–251. [CrossRef] [PubMed]
50. Jeffery, A.; Taylor, E. Veterinary nursing in the United Kingdom: Identifying the factors that influence retention within the profession. *Front. Vet. Sci.* **2022**, *9*, 927499. [CrossRef] [PubMed]
51. McCoy, M.; Cannedy, S.; Oishi, K.; Canelo, I.; Hamilton, A.B.; Olmos-Ochoa, T.T. Using Stay Interviews as a Quality Improvement Tool for Healthcare Workforce Retention. *Qual. Manag. Health Care* **2024**. [CrossRef]
52. Snyder, A.; Whiteman, K.; DiCuccio, M.; Swanson-Biearman, B.; Stephens, K. Why They Stay and Why They Leave: Stay Interviews with Registered Nurses to Hear What Matters the Most. *J. Nurs. Adm.* **2023**, *53*, 154–160. [CrossRef]
53. Kotter, J.P. Successful Change and the Force That Drives it. In *Leading Change*; Harvard Business Review Press: La Vergne, TN, USA, 2012; pp. 19–36.
54. Edú-Valsania, S.; Laguía, A.; Moriano, J.A. Burnout: A Review of Theory and Measurement. *Int. J. Environ. Res. Public. Health* **2022**, *19*, 1780. [CrossRef]
55. Burnes, B. Introduction: Why Does Change Fail, and What Can We Do About It? *J. Change Manag.* **2011**, *11*, 445–450. [CrossRef]
56. Idogawa, J.; Bizarrias, F.S.; Câmara, R. Critical success factors for change management in business process management. *Bus. Process Manag. J.* **2023**, *29*, 2009–2033. [CrossRef]
57. Nicolay, C.R.; Williams, S.P.; Brkic, M.; Purkayastha, S.; Chaturvedi, S.; Phillips, N.; Darzi, A. Measuring the organisational health of acute sector healthcare organisations: Development and validation of the Healthcare-OH survey. *Int. J. Healthc. Manag.* **2021**, *14*, 64–76. [CrossRef]
58. Simpson, D.; Hamilton, S.; McSherry, R.; McIntosh, R. Measuring and Assessing Healthcare Organisational Culture in the England's National Health Service: A Snapshot of Current Tools and Tool Use. *Healthcare* **2019**, *7*, 127. [CrossRef]
59. Rehman, N.; Mahmood, A.; Ibtasam, M.; Murtaza, S.A.; Iqbal, N.; Molnár, E. The Psychology of Resistance to Change: The Antidotal Effect of Organizational Justice, Support and Leader-Member Exchange. *Front. Psychol.* **2021**, *12*, 678952. [CrossRef]
60. Moran, R.E.; Knesl, O. How can the veterinary profession tackle social media misinformation? *J. Am. Vet. Med. Assoc.* **2025**, *1*, 1–7. [CrossRef] [PubMed]
61. Holey, E.A.; Feeley, J.L.; Dixon, J.; Whittaker, V.J. An exploration of the use of simple statistics to measure consensus and stability in Delphi studies. *BMC Med. Res. Methodol.* **2007**, *7*, 52. [CrossRef] [PubMed]
62. Nasa, P.; Jain, R.; Juneja, D. Delphi methodology in healthcare research: How to decide its appropriateness. *World J. Methodol.* **2021**, *11*, 116–129. [CrossRef] [PubMed]

animals

MDPI

Article

Assessing Gender Equality in Italian Animal Science: A Case Study on Academic Careers and Research Outcomes

Anna Sandrucci [1], Lucia Bailoni [2,*] and Paola Crepaldi [1]

[1] Department of Agricultural and Environmental Sciences- Production, Landscape, Agroenergy, University of Milan, 20133 Milan, Italy; anna.sandrucci@unimi.it (A.S.); paola.crepaldi@unimi.it (P.C.)
[2] Department of Comparative Biomedicine and Food Science, University of Padova, 35020 Legnaro, Italy
* Correspondence: lucia.bailoni@unipd.it

Simple Summary: Gender equality is a goal (Goal 5) of the United Nations Development Programme, yet challenges persist in academia, especially in fields like animal science. This study focuses on gender issues within the Italian Animal Science and Production Association (ASPA), which includes both academic and non-academic researchers involved in animal sciences. Using 2023 data from ASPA and bibliometric information from Scopus and Web of Science, the research highlights a slow but ongoing reduction in the gender gap. However, vertical segregation remains a major issue, with few women holding top positions like full professors. There is also horizontal segregation, as fewer women work in animal science areas closely related to Science, Technology, Engineering, and Mathematics (STEM) disciplines, such as Animal breeding and genetics. At the bibliometric level, men generally perform better in research metrics like publication and citation counts. However, these differences become less significant when considering academic position, scientific sector, and age. Women are still under-represented in prestigious authorship.

Abstract: This paper focuses on gender issues within the Italian Animal Science and Production Association (ASPA), which includes both academic and non-academic researchers involved in animal sciences. Data from the association's archives in 2023 and bibliometric data obtained from Scopus and Web of Science were used. This study highlighted how within the ASPA and in that part of the academic realm falling within the field of animal science, a noticeable gender gap still exists, albeit decreasing over time at a very slow pace. There is clear vertical segregation, with a minority of women occupying full professor positions, and horizontal segregation with a low percentage of women involved in animal science disciplines closer to STEM fields, such as "Animal breeding and genetics". At the bibliometric level, gender differences in bibliometric indicators are observed, favouring men, although these differences are not significant when considering the academic position, scientific sector, and age. In the official journal of the ASPA (*Italian Journal of Animal Science*), women are under-represented in prestigious positions such as first, last, and corresponding authors. Scientific societies, academic institutions, and research organizations are called upon to do their part to accelerate the process of overcoming these inequalities.

Keywords: academic careers; authorship; bibliometrics; gender gap; segregation

1. Introduction

Gender equality constitutes one of the 17 key objectives (Sustainable Development Goals, SDG) outlined in the 2030 Agenda for Sustainable Development, signed by 193 United Nations (UN) member states in 2015. As highlighted in SDG 5, "Gender equality is not only a fundamental human right but a necessary foundation for a peaceful, prosperous and sustainable world". This commitment has to be actively pursued by recognizing and enhancing female skills while ensuring equal leadership opportunities at all levels of the decision-making process. UNESCO also recently published a document proposing global action to address the persistent gender gap in science [1].

In recent years, considerable progress has been achieved and regulatory interventions have emerged. In the United States, the National Strategy on Gender Equity and Equality [2] is the first comprehensive national strategy to advance gender equity and equality. It is built on an intersectional approach that acknowledges the overlapping forms of discrimination related to gender, race, sexual orientation, and socioeconomic status, among other factors, identifying ten interconnected priorities. The EU has implemented comprehensive strategies for gender equality, resulting in the formulation of the Gender Equality Strategy 2020–2025. The Strategy, defined as "a set of commitments and actions that aim to promote gender equality in an organization through a process of structural change", presents policy objectives and actions to make significant progress by 2025 toward a gender-equal Europe [3]. Despite the presence of guidelines in both national and international regulatory frameworks, achieving gender equality in the workplace and professions remains a significant challenge. The Global Gender Gap Report 2024 from the World Economic Forum highlights that significant gender disparities persist [4]. Progress towards closing the gap has been extremely slow, with a slight improvement compared to 2023. At the current pace, it is estimated that it will take 134 years to achieve full gender parity globally. This report highlights significant gender disparities in the labour market. Globally, women represent 42% of the workforce but occupy only 31.7% of senior leadership positions. These disparities are even more pronounced in technical roles and STEM fields, where women hold only 29% of entry-level positions and just 12.2% of executive roles. The lack of full technical contributions from women in scientific fields of animal science, where technological solutions like AI and Agriculture 4.0 are advancing rapidly, limits the ability to find the innovative and sustainable solutions our planet needs.

The gender gap persists prominently in the context of academic and research environments [5,6], ranging from universities to scientific associations. The adoption of gender policies specifically focused on universities and research is relatively recent. Starting in 2022, participation in the new European Framework Programme for Research and Innovation, Horizon Europe, requires public entities, research organizations, and higher education institutions to have a Gender Equality Plan. This requirement was introduced in the "Gender Equality Strategy 2020–2025" by the European Commission [7]. Despite this, concrete advancements in structural changes or the reduction in gender gaps in academia remain a challenge. According to Gallego-Moron and Matus-Lopez [8], university measures to address gender equality vary widely, often shaped by factors like budget constraints and institutional commitment. As a result, these strategies are frequently inadequate and ineffective in achieving meaningful progress. Moreover, even when policies are in place, they appear to have limited results because they mainly address isolated factors rather than taking a multifaceted, integrative approach [9]. For instance, simulations based on Italian data revealed that policies such as compensating for women's reduced productivity during childrearing years, ensuring greater gender balance in promotion evaluation committees, and implementing gender quotas are not fully effective unless they are implemented together in a comprehensive approach [10]. This highlights the importance of continuing to monitor and critically assess the effectiveness of such policies, particularly in highly specialized fields close to STEM, like animal science, where disparities persist.

This paper seeks to address these challenges by analyzing the current state of gender equality within the field of animal science in Italy, with a particular focus on the academic and research contexts. Specifically, it aims to explore the factors contributing to vertical and horizontal segregation and differences in research performances and identify possible actions to foster greater gender equity.

This preliminary study analyses the current gender scenario within the Italian Association for Science and Animal Production (ASPA), which includes researchers from all Italian universities and research organizations (e.g., National Research Council, etc.) dedicated to various aspects of animal science, including livestock production, aquatic animals, pets, sports animals, and wildlife. The ASPA, with its member base and study commissions, endeavours to advance the field of animal sciences and technologies. Its cultural and scientific role extends further, promoting the exchange of knowledge among Italian scientific communities. Indeed, the ASPA is committed to improving scientific communication within Italian society, emphasizing the importance of addressing gender disparities in academic and research environments.

The authors of this paper are the proponents of the ASPA Working Group on gender equity with the aim of fostering awareness among members, promoting and disseminating gender balance through monitoring the situation within the ASPA, and encouraging the development of a constructive debate aimed at identifying useful actions to overcome persistent vertical and horizontal segregation. To the best of our knowledge, this is the first study to analyze the gender equality scenario within the ASPA.

2. Materials and Methods

2.1. Collection of ASPA Member Data

The data on the ASPA members were obtained from the association archive between March and April 2023 and include the following information: name, surname, age, gender, type of membership, position, and affiliation organization. The data for 2024 are not yet available.

The academic positions and scientific sectors of each ASPA member were collected by consulting the archive of the Italian Ministry of University at https://cercauniversita.cineca.it/php5/docenti/cerca.php (accessed on 11 April 2023). In Italy, Scientific Disciplinary Sectors (SDSs) denote specific fields or disciplines of focus for scientists and researchers. These sectors serve to organize and classify academic and research activities. Each SDS corresponds to a distinct area of knowledge, allowing for a systematic categorization of research and expertise. Scientists specialize in one SDS based on their research interests and expertise. Within these SDSs, scientific productivity is evaluated by qualifying competitions based on the possession of different threshold values for different SDSs.

In the field of animal sciences, the Scientific Disciplinary Sectors (SDSs) dedicated to animal husbandry encompass the following:

- Animal breeding and genetics, abbreviated as AGR/17;
- Nutrition and feeding, abbreviated as AGR/18;
- Husbandry techniques, abbreviated as AGR/19;
- Short-cycle animals (fish, poultry, rabbit, laboratory animals), abbreviated as AGR/20.

For the academic regular and aggregate members, the Glass Ceiling Index (GCI) was calculated. The GCI is a relative index comparing the proportion of women in academic environments (grades A, B, and C) to the proportion of women in top academic positions (grade A positions, equivalent to full professorships in most countries) in a given year [11]. The GCI can range from 0 to infinity. A GCI of 1 indicates that there is no difference between women's and men's promotion prospects. A score of less than 1 means that women are over-represented at grade A level and a GCI score of more than 1 points towards a glass ceiling effect where women are under-represented in grade A positions. In other words, the higher the value of GCI score, the stronger the glass ceiling effect and the more difficult it is for women to move into a higher position.

Key bibliographic parameters (n. of publications, h-index, and citation index with and without self-citations) for each ASPA member were collected from Scopus, one of the largest databases containing abstracts and citations of peer-reviewed research literature (consulted at the end of March 2023). The h-index, also known as the Hirsch index, is a metric used to measure both the productivity and impact of researchers' scientific output. The h-index provides a single number that reflects both the quantity (number of publications) and impact (citation counts) of a researcher's work, commonly used as a measure of productivity and influence within academic and research environments.

2.2. Data Collection of Authors with Publications on IJAS

The *Italian Journal of Animal Science* (IJAS), the official open access journal of ASPA, invites all members of the association to support the journal by submitting their manuscripts. Starting from February 2023, IJAS articles authored by Italian researchers, both ASPA members and non-members, were extracted from the Web of Science database [12] for four different years (2002, 2008, 2014, and 2021), refining the search by country/region (Italy). This study identified the prestigious positions of first, last, and corresponding authors, and the number of women and men in these roles was counted for each publication. The corresponding author was only counted if different from the first and last author. Gender determination required access to the full name of each author, including their given name in full (not merely initials) and surname. In Italy, gender can be easily inferred from the full name. In the few ambiguous cases involving foreign co-authors, a specific online search was conducted to identify the researcher's gender.

3. Statistical Analysis

The analyses of bibliographic parameters were conducted on a subset of 293 members, excluding honorary members (aged over 70 years), non-academic members, and members who lacked an indication of a Scientific Disciplinary Sector.

Subsequently, these data were analyzed using JMP® Pro 17.0.0 software, utilizing descriptive statistics, ANOVA and ANCOVA models, and non-parametric tests (Welch's test ANOVA). These analyses aimed at assessing the effect of gender, age, position, and scientific field on bibliographic performances. The Logworth statistics (log transformation of p-value) are reported to explain the contribution of each variable to the ANCOVA models used.

The sample size in the different analyses could be smaller in the different analyses reported due to the lack of some information (age, SSDs) for some members or categories analyzed. For example, the PhD students and fellows do not have an indication of SDs.

4. Results and Discussion

4.1. Gender Distribution of Members in the ASPA

In 2023, the Association for Science and Animal Production counted a total of 491 members, considering only individuals and excluding organizations. Members were classified into three categories: honorary members (retired members), regular members, and aggregate members. According to ASPA's statute, aggregate members are young individuals undergoing training in animal science research, including doctoral students, research fellows, and grant holders. Upon completing their training and transitioning to stable positions as researchers, they become regular members. Figure 1 illustrates the percentage of women within the entire association and across the three membership groups. When considering only aggregate and regular members (excluding honorary members), women account for 46.5%. Among aggregate members, the proportion of women is 52.5%, markedly exceeding the overall average.

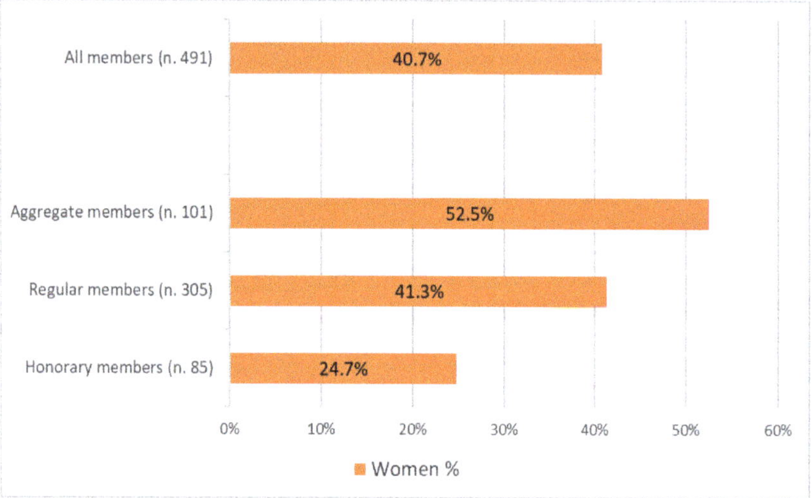

Figure 1. Percentage of women members of the Association for Science and Animal Production in the year 2024.

According to statistics from the European Union (EU), the proportion of women among doctoral graduates has shown a slight increase in the last decade, reaching 48.1% in 2018 (EU-27) [11]. This outcome suggests that, without differentiation by the field of study, gender parity between female and male doctoral graduates has almost been achieved at the European level, indicating gradual progress towards gender equality over time. At the Italian level, the proportion of female doctoral graduates is slightly higher than at the European level, although the evolution between 2010 and 2018 recorded a slight reduction in the percentage of young women obtaining a doctoral degree, from 53.2% to 50.5% [11]. In particular, when examining the specific fields of "Agriculture, forestry, fisheries and veterinary", which are closely related to but not completely overlapping the field of animal sciences, the percentage of women gaining a doctorate in 2018 was 56.8% at the European level (EU-27) and 56.3% at the Italian level. These figures are slightly higher than the 52.5% percentage of aggregate members of the ASPA, which also includes research fellows.

The ASPA was established just over 50 years ago (1973), with only 3 out of its 28 founding members (10.7%) being women. Over time, the percentage of women in the association has steadily increased, rising from 20.6% in 1994 to 40.9% in 2023, reflecting a nearly threefold growth over 30 years.

The association primarily includes scientists from all Italian universities and other research organizations, along with a small number of technicians and professionals. Its members are distributed across eighteen regions in Italy. Membership is exclusively male in two regions, while thirteen regions exhibit a male majority, one achieves gender parity, and two have a female majority.

Academic members constitute the vast majority, representing 88.2% of the association when excluding honorary members. In contrast, among non-academic, non-honorary members, gender parity (50:50) is observed, demonstrating a more balanced distribution compared to their academic counterparts.

The academic members of the association represent almost the entire cohort of Italian academics within the field of animal sciences and technologies, which totals 409 scientists, 46.7% of whom are women.

When classifying academic members (aggregate and regular members) by position and gender, a notable gender disparity emerges in the full professor position (Figure 2). The figure does not include the category of tenured university researchers as this category is being phased out and is no longer renewed. Notably, women represent 57% of the tenured researcher category.

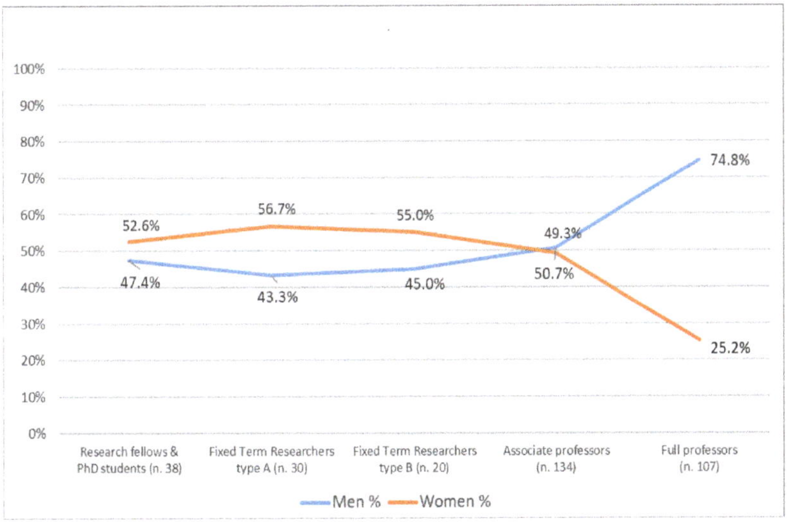

Figure 2. Members of the Association for Science and Animal Production in the year 2023 by position and gender. Only academic regular and aggregate members, excluding tenured researchers, were reported.

The diagram highlights the typical "scissor-like" trend that characterizes the male-to-female ratio at different career levels: the female component consistently dominates in lower-level positions but becomes a minority in higher-level positions, as confirmed also by the glass ceiling index, which is equal to 1.7. The balance point corresponds to the position of associate professor. This trend, with some differences, is also confirmed at the national level concerning academic staff in 2020 [13]. A similar trend among academic staff is also reported at the European level [14]. According to this report, while the overall percentage of women in academic roles is generally close to parity, the representation of women significantly decreases in higher positions. In 2018 (EU-27), the proportion of women declined from nearly half (46.6%) in grade C positions (PhD holders) to 40.3% in grade B (more senior) positions. There was a further decline to approximately one-quarter of women (26.2%) in the grade A positions, which represents the highest grade at which research is typically conducted within the institutional or corporate system. Moreover, it should be emphasized that from 2015 to 2018, the improvement at the European level appears minimal, indicating a prolonged path toward gender parity. In Italy in 2018, only 23.7% of grade A positions in academic environments were held by women.

The gap is particularly noticeable in Scientific Disciplinary Sectors compared to social and humanities disciplines: the proportion of women in category A was 17.9% and 28.5% in Engineering and Technology and Agricultural Sciences, respectively, while, in social and humanities sciences, it exceeded 30% in 2018. In Italy, the situation appears even more imbalanced, with only 13.8% and 19.5% of grade A positions being held by women in the fields of Engineering and Technology and Agricultural Sciences, respectively [11].

The "scissor effect" refers to a prevalent trend of vertical segregation observed across various work domains. However, as highlighted by Farina et al. (2023) and other authors, gender disparities are particularly pronounced in the academic and research spheres, with progress toward overcoming these inequalities advancing at an exceptionally slow pace [14]. The representation of women declines as if there were a "leaky pipeline" during advancement from junior to senior academic positions, with high attrition rates observed [15]. The under-representation of women in higher career positions can be attributed to both the "leaky pipeline" and "glass ceiling" phenomena. The former refers to the effect of women leaving the career pipeline at various stages while the latter pertains to structural barriers such as discrimination and gender bias that hinder women's access to top decision-making and managerial roles [11].

The causes of vertical segregation in academic careers are multifaceted, complex, and interconnected. On one hand, there is a well-documented, lower scientific productivity among women compared to men based on commonly used indicators for assessing scientific output: the number of publications, citations, and citation indexes [16]. The lower scientific productivity of women could be partially attributed to the greater family responsibilities of women, not only childcare but also caring for elderly and disabled family members. These family commitments compete with research activities but also limit opportunities for travelling and the establishment of national and international networks, both crucial factors for accessing funding and publishing scientific work. It is not coincidental that the international mobility of European female doctoral candidates is higher than that of their male counterparts, while among senior researchers, the ratio is reversed, with men exhibiting greater international mobility [11]. The lower mobility of female senior researchers translates into fewer international contacts and opportunities to secure international grants with international teams, leading to diminished chances of publishing and lower visibility in the academic world.

Moreover, within the academic context, women tend to exhibit a stronger inclination than men towards educational activities (teaching and mentoring) and administrative tasks, thus diverting time away from research [17,18]. In addition, several authors have highlighted that female researchers may be more hesitant to participate in competitions due to a lack of self-confidence [19].

According to Filandri and Pasqua (2021), who analyzed career advancement using data from the entire population of researchers and professors in the Italian university system, a significant gender gap in career progression emerges [18]. The analysis revealed that, in this case, the gap cannot be attributed to lower scientific productivity or women's reluctance to seek promotions. Instead, it exposed structural gender biases. These biases, partly conscious and partly unconscious, are likely to contribute to undervaluing the performances and scientific competencies of women. For instance, the study by Jappelli et al. (2017) suggests that research papers authored by women receive less favourable evaluations [16]. Bendels et al. (2018), analyzing 295,557 research articles from 54 journals listed in the Nature index, highlighted that women are authors of fewer articles than men (two articles fewer per year), and articles with female key authors are cited less frequently [20]. The gender difference in citation rates increases as the number of authors contributing to an article increases. The authors concluded that the prognosis for the coming decades predicts a really poor harmonization of disparity between the two genders. Furthermore, additional barriers to career progression include working cultures that lack gender sensitivity and fail to accommodate family commitments, incidents of sexual harassment, bullying, gender-based violence, and differences in individual choices and behaviour based on gender [13].

As a result, lower proportions of women, relative to men, attain full professorship positions, which are considered as a pre-requisite for top-level decision-making roles such as faculty heads or university rectors. These positions are generally associated with "desirable" attributes, including higher salaries, prestige, social security, and adequate pension benefits. In the academic context, the over-representation of men among heads of universities is an example of such vertical segregation. A South Korean study found that gender quotas improved female faculty representation at all tenure levels but not in senior leadership roles like the dean or president. This suggests that entry-level quotas may not suffice to address gender inequality at higher academic levels. Evidence of their effectiveness across disciplines indicates limited and slow progress in fields where women are severely under-represented [21].

In addition to vertical segregation, horizontal segregation was investigated by examining the gender distribution across Scientific Disciplinary Sectors among the association's members. The analysis revealed a clear predominance of men in disciplines related to Animal breeding and genetics (AGR/17; see Figure 3), which are more closely associated with STEM fields. Values indicating closer gender balance were observed in disciplines related to Short-cycle animals, such as fish, poultry, laboratory and fur animals, birds, and rabbits (AGR/20).

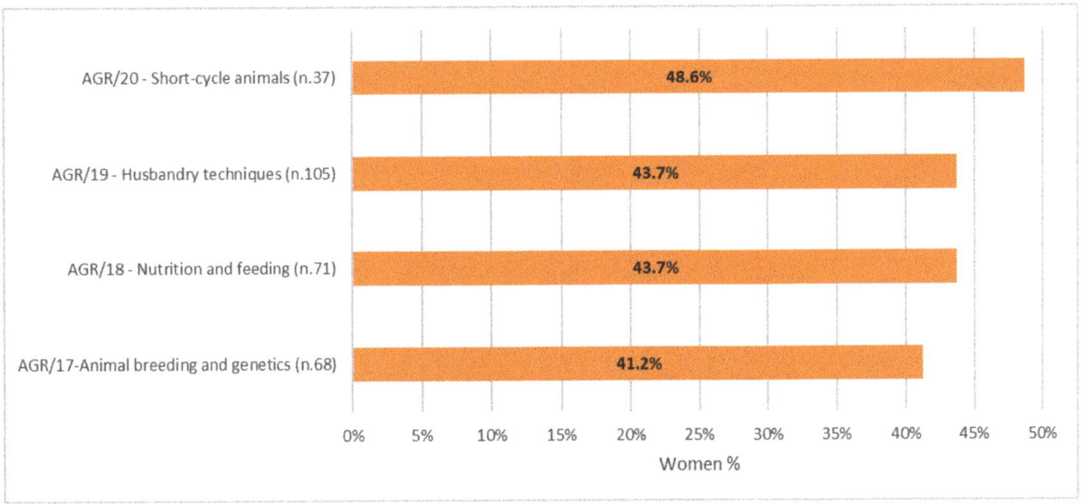

Figure 3. Percentage of women among the academic members of the Association for Science and Animal Production in the year 2023 by the main scientific disciplinary sectors. Only associate and regular members with SDSs were reported (n = 281).

Horizontal segregation refers to the concentration of women and men in different sectors (sectoral segregation) and occupations (occupational segregation) [22]. It can occur within education with over- or under-representation of one gender in specific subjects and employment with over- or under-representation of one gender in specific professions, industries, etc. The issue of horizontal segregation may in turn lead to increased vertical segregation. For instance, undervaluing competencies associated with "women's work" may limit women's prospects for career advancement [11].

Out of the 281 academic regular members, 44% are women. Within the SDSs, women represent 41.2% in Animal breeding and genetics and 48.6% in Short-cycle animals.

Although in the field of Animal breeding and genetics (AGR 17) a smaller percentage of women is observed, this value is not significantly different from the overall average of 44% of women across all SDSs. However, it can be noticed that in three out of the four SDSs considered (AGR17, AGR18, AGR19), there is a strong vertical segregation, with the number of female full professors significantly lower compared to men. Only in the AGR20 sector, gender differences across academic positions are minimal and not statistically significant. In the field of Animal breeding and genetics (AGR/17), the strongest vertical segregation is observed, with a very low percentage of women in full professor positions (10%) compared to other SDSs (Figure 4), probably linked to a stronger gender prejudice that considers statistics and calculation as a prerogative of men, as in other STEM disciplines. This is particularly concerning given the growing reliance of animal science and the wider agricultural sector on precision livestock farming and artificial intelligence tools, making these fields increasingly interconnected with STEM disciplines. A lack of female representation may limit diverse perspectives in a sector that is advancing rapidly through technological and scientific innovations. This perspective is invaluable as we aim to develop innovative solutions that not only increase productivity but also support broader goals of ecological and social sustainability [23]. In-depth analyses of the role of women in promoting environmental and social sustainability have been published recently in various fields [24,25].

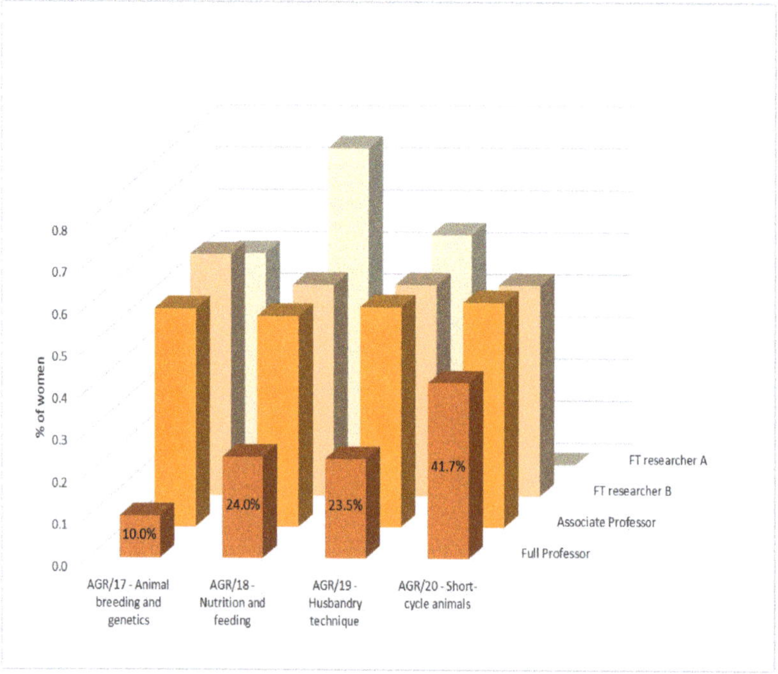

Figure 4. Percentage of women among the academic members of the Association for Science and Animal Production in the year 2023 by the scientific disciplinary sectors and position. Only regular and aggregate members, excluding tenured researchers (n. 281). FT = fixed-term.

The percentages of women reported in Figure 4 reflect the proportion of women present in the four SDSs at the national level in the Italian university system. Overall, women constitute 45.9% of the total, and the percentage of women among full professors is 12.5% in AGR/17, 30.8% in AGR/18, 26.3% in AGR/19, and 58.3% in AGR/20, based on data from the official website of the Italian university system [26,27]. It is worth noting that the EU defines gender parity as a 50:50 ratio and gender equality as a proportion between 40 and 60%. In the case of full professors, there is an evident inequality as confirmed by the glass ceiling index which exceeds 1 in three out of the four SDSs.

Vertical segregation in the SDSs of animal science in Italy could be calculated as the proportion of women and men who are full professors over the total number of women and men in academic environments (from full professors to tenure track researchers and fixed-term type B and A researchers). This results in a significant difference (p-value = 0.0014) with percentages of 15.7% and 34.3% for women and men, respectively. The opportunity for women to become full professors, calculated as relative risk, was 0.44 in 2023, whereas, in 2013, it was 0.27 (when the percentages of women and men full professors were 9.6% and 35.2%).

Vertical segregation could also be seen from the glass ceiling indexes, equal to 2.2 for AGR/17, 1.8 for AGR/18, 1.6 for AGR/19, and 0.9 for AGR/20. These indexes show that in three out of the four SDSs with a value higher than 1, a strong vertical segregation is currently present. The GCIs for the above sectors in 2013 were 1.7, 2.2, 5.3, and 1, respectively. Although in some SDSs, the GCI has improved over the last 10 years; by calculating the GCI for the four SSDs together in the same 10 years, it moves from 1.7 to 1.6.

When comparing the values of 2023 with those of 2013, there has been an increment of approximately 0.6% per year in the number of women full professors and a decrease of 0.1 in the GCI. It can be estimated that it will take approximately 60 years, given the same trends, to have equal opportunities for women and men to access top positions in the four SDSs in animal science.

The probability for a woman to become a full professor is significantly lower (p-value < 0.05) in three out of the four SDSs evaluated. Women (and men) in AGR17, 18, and 19 show values of 7.7% (40.4%), 17.4% (38.3%), and 15.9% (34.1%), respectively. Only in the AGR/20 sector is there a higher but not statistically different value for women (vs. men), equal to 23.3% (17.2%). Overall, women have a probability of becoming full professors equal to 0.44 while men have 2.3 times that probability. These values underline a persistent inequality of opportunity for women to reach the position of full professor, contributing to a gender gap in salaries and retirement pensions that accumulate disadvantages throughout the entire career of a woman scientist. It would also be interesting to evaluate these data with respect to academic age, defined as the age at which individuals achieve different career milestones; however, the necessary data are not available.

While animal sciences, as a whole, may not fall entirely within the STEM category (Science, Technology, Engineering, and Mathematics), certain disciplinary areas within it encompass STEM skills. Research in the field of Animal breeding and genetics now demands proficiency in mathematics, statistics, and computer science. Despite improvements in recent years, women working in STEM fields are still in the minority. According to the 2023 report on gender equality in the EU [26], the proportion of women graduating in STEM disciplines is persistently lower than that of men and is relatively stable: there are two men graduating in tertiary education in STEM disciplines for every woman. The ratio is slightly better at the master's or equivalent level and at the doctoral level (respectively, 1.5 and 1.8 men for every woman in 2020) [27].

As previously highlighted, when discussing doctoral graduates, at both European and Italian levels, women graduates were over-represented in the field of Education and under-represented in the broad fields of ICT and Engineering, Manufacturing, and Construction [11]. For instance, in Italy, out of 100 female students who enrol in university, only 21 choose STEM degree courses. Moreover, among all those enrolled in STEM faculties, female students represented only 37% [28]. This gender gap is present not only in Italy but also in Europe and around the world. As teaching and learning cultures can be influenced by gender stereotypes and unconscious biases, this may constitute a barrier to women's progression in STEM fields [29]. Some of the contributing factors to this situation include gender stereotypes, lack of female role models in STEM disciplines, and differences in education and perception of these disciplines [30].

In the EU, men dominate 85% of all top-level positions in STEM fields [28]. These data suggest that the extent of vertical segregation in career paths for women in academic environments is more pronounced in the field of STEM. Particularly in STEM, women face barriers including biases from hiring committees, lack of mentoring, social marginalization, inhospitable group cultures, lower salaries, fewer resources, less respect, lower likelihood of promotion, and even overt opposition to hiring female faculty members [31].

4.2. *ASPA Governance and Committees*

Regarding aspects related to the governance of the association, since 1973, the year of its foundation, ASPA presidents have always been men, and the board of directors has had an almost exclusively male composition. Only since 2013 has the board, consisting of five members, including the president, seen the presence of one or two female members. This phenomenon is largely associated with the different proportion of women reaching the position of full professor because, as previously highlighted, certain apex positions and roles are almost exclusively held by full professors.

The ASPA also has permanent or temporary internal study committees that look into specific topics within the field of animal production and promote activities such as seminars, conferences, and scientific and informative publications. These committees arise from a proposal by a member, which is first examined by the Board of Directors and then circulated among the other members. Membership in these committees is voluntary but regulated to avoid overly large groups. It is possible to be part of more than one committee. In 2023, ASPA hosted 11 study committees with a total of 168 members, averaging 15.3 members per committee, from a minimum of 8 to a maximum of 26. Women constitute 40.5% of the committee members and 41.7% of the committee coordinators. Since membership is voluntary, it was expected that the percentage of women in the committees would be similar to the overall percentage of women in the association. However, it is noteworthy that even within the committees, evidence of vertical segregation is apparent, with a higher female presence in the study committee on "Companion animal breeding" (75%) and a lower presence in committees dedicated to more technical topics such as "Precision Livestock Farming" and "Statistical Methodology and Experimental Design" (18.8 and 23.1% resp.).

4.3. *Bibliometrics of the ASPA Members*

The scientific performances of the ASPA academic members belonging to the three main categories (fixed-term researchers type A and B, associate professor, and full professor) were analyzed by examining key bibliometric parameters (no. of publications, h-index, no. of citations, and no. of self-citations). These data were collected by Scopus in March 2023.

When considering only gender as a source of variation, statistically significant differences between women and men are observed for the four variables considered and age (Table 1). Men outperform women in all the variables considered, with a statistically significant average (and median) difference in favour of men equal to 17.3 (9.5) documents, 2.5 (2.0) points of h-index, 391.5 (189.5) citations, and 66.3 (13) self-citations. Moreover, the average age of male authors is 3.5 years higher than that of females. This model explains only 2.3 to 3.3 percent of the observed variability. The differences remain significant even when using Welch's test for the variables that show unequal variances (publication numbers, citations, and self-citations).

Table 1. Main descriptive statistics for biometric parameters and age by gender.

	Gender	Women	Men	(W-M)	Statistical Parameters	
Publication	Sample size (n)	121	172		r2	0.033
	Mean	63.9	81.2	−17.3	*p*-value	0.0006
	Median	57	66.5	−9.5	Welch's *p*-value	0.0003
	S.D.	34.6	50.1			
h-index	Sample size (n)	121	172		r2	0.026
	Mean	18.1	20.6	−2.5	*p*-value	0.0039
	Median	17	19	−2.0	Welch's *p*-value	
	S.D.	7.1	8.2			
Citation n.	Sample size (n)	121	172		r2	0.025
	Mean	1224.3	1615.9	−391.5	*p*-value	0.005
	Median	1003	1192.5	−189.5	Welch's *p*-value	0.0033
	S.D.	1024.6	1376.4			
Self-citations n.	Sample size (n)	121	172		r2	0.023
	Mean	126.6	192.8	−66.3	*p*-value	0.0068
	Median	98	111	−13.0	Welch's *p*-value	0.0033
	S.D.	140.2	252.7			
Age (years)	Sample size (n)	121	172		r2	0.025
	Mean	51.6	55.2	−3.5	*p*-value	0.0038
	Median	53	58	−5.0	Welch's *p*-value	
	S.D.	11.3	10.6			

r2: coefficient of determination of the ANOVA model. Welch's *p*-value is reported when the assumption of ANOVA is not satisfied.

This effect is clearly shown in Figure 5, where a higher number of male outliers in terms of the number of documents can be observed. For this metric, out of the 24 top researchers in the first 10% of the distribution, 33% are women. All of the top male researchers hold full professor positions, whereas among women, only 75% are full professors. This observation aligns with findings from previous studies [32], indicating that gender disparities in academic environments can largely be attributed to the extremes of the distribution, notably the disproportionate representation of men among the highest-achieving scientists.

Owing to the low variability explained by the previous model, which considers gender as the sole source of variation, a three-way ANCOVA model was applied, including gender, academic position, and scientific sector as fixed factors with age as a covariate.

It is worth noting that a logarithmic transformation for the variables citations and self-citations was also explored to address the funnel pattern observed in the residuals. However, this transformation did not alter the significance of the factors. Firstly, a saturated model incorporating two- and three-way interactions was applied, but none of these interactions proved statistically significant and were thus removed from the model.

With this model, gender consistently showed no significance for the four bibliometric variables considered (Table 2). On the contrary, academic positions, including fixed-term researchers type A and B, associate and full professors, consistently yielded high significance, emerging as the most important source of variation, as demonstrated by the highest Logworth value. In addition, the SDSs were significant, although the Logworth was lower, except for the h-index. The covariate age also proved significant for all the metrics considered, with Logworths lower than those for the SDSs. The r2 of the model increased for all four variables, with the highest value (0.36) for the h-index and the lowest (0.21) for the self-citations.

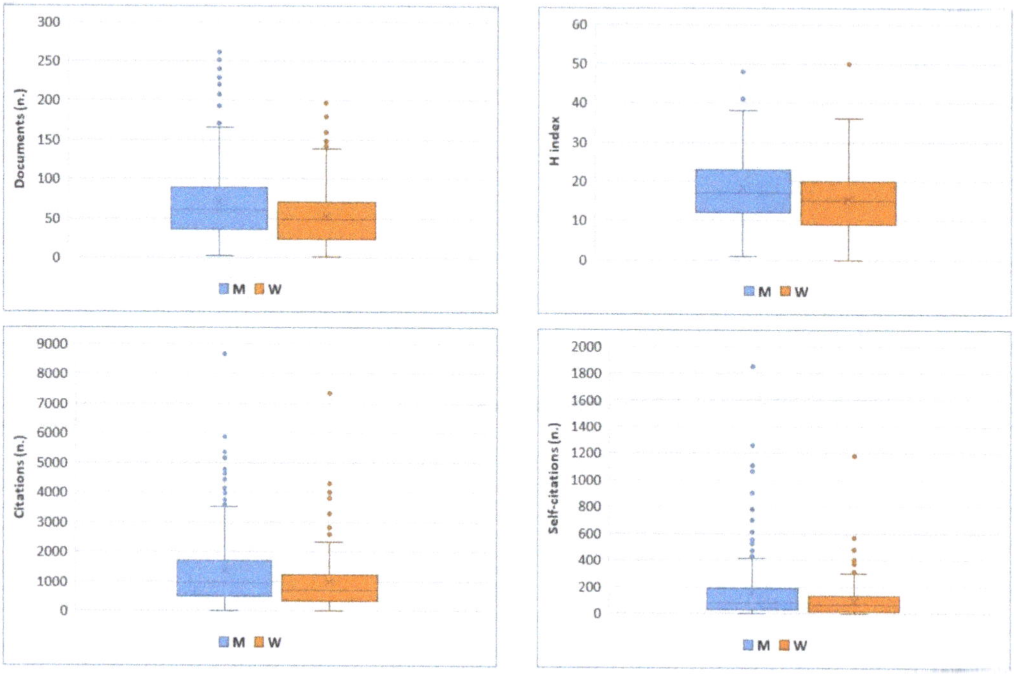

Figure 5. Distribution of bibliometrics by gender for ASPA academic members. The whiskers of the box plot extend from the box to the minimum and maximum data points that are not considered soft outliers (outside 1.5 times the Interquartile indicated by dot).

Table 2. Effects and r2 of the three-way ANCOVA model used.

Y Variables		**Effects**				
Obs. n. 280		**Positions**	**Age (Year)**	**S.S.D.**	**Gender**	r^2
Document n.						0.32
	Logworth	15.13	2.72	2.64	1.01	
	p-value					
h-index						0.36
	Logworth	16.06	4.20	1.28	0.48	
	p-value	<0.0001	0.0001	0.0530	0.3324	
Citations n.						0.29
	Logworth	11.401	3.991	1.022	0.665	
	p-value	<0.0001	0.0001	0.09511	0.21642	
Self-citations n.						0.21
	Logworth	9.32	3.12	1.80	0.80	
	p-value	<0.0001	0.00076	0.01603	0.15866	

The results concerning positions and age align with expectations: as careers progress, the parameters under consideration tend to increase, as illustrated in Figure 6. Notably, among male full professors, there are more outliers in the younger age bracket, hinting that men often advance more swiftly in their careers and attain higher positions earlier compared to women. Several longitudinal studies have linked the gender gap in bibliometric performance to women's shorter career durations [33], a higher representation of women in teaching-intensive and part-time positions [34], and fewer women in the top positions where both genders achieve the highest performance [35].

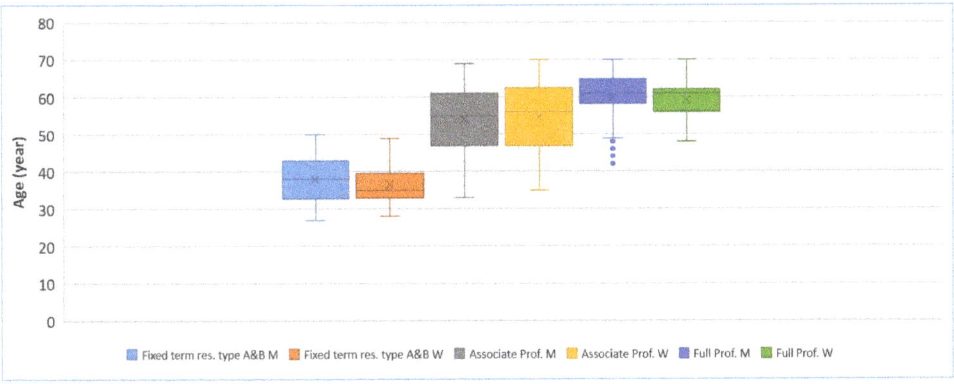

Figure 6. Age by position and gender. The whiskers of the box plot extend from the box to the minimum and maximum data points that are not considered soft outliers (outside 1.5 times the Interquartile indicated by dot).

Analyzing a model that incorporates academic age at various career stages by gender would be beneficial, but regrettably, such data are unavailable.

The position emerged as the most crucial factor. Indeed, the exclusion of the full professor category, dominated by older men at 75%, eliminates statistical gender differences. On the other hand, when considering age alone, gender becomes statistically significant, although with a low explained variability when using gender alone in the simplest model.

In Figure 7, where the Least Square Mean (LSM ± SE) by positions and gender are reported, it is evident that gender is not statistically significant.

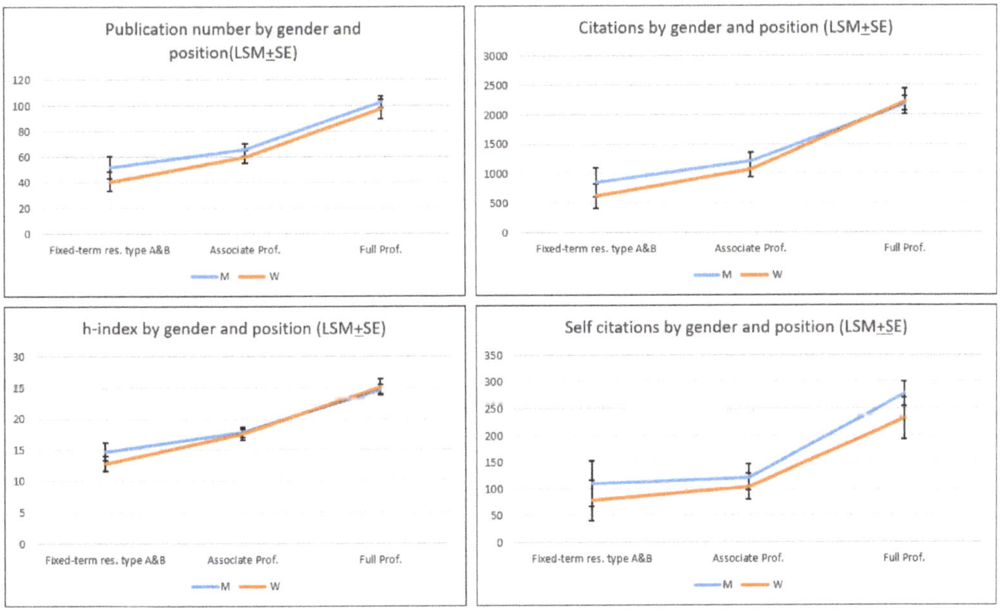

Figure 7. Least Square Means (LSM ± SE) of the bibliometric parameters by gender and position.

Although differences by gender are not statistically significant (Figure 7), the main descriptive statistics of the distribution by gender and position (Table 1 and Supplementary

Table S1) show differences starting from early career stages. These disparities persist across the higher positions, although diminished for some metrics. This pattern highlights both the "sticky floor" and "glass ceiling" theories, especially evident in outliers among young male full professors but absent among young female full professors.

To summarize, considering both academic positions and age, statistical parity emerges between men and women in terms of performance. However, academic positions appear as the primary determinant of bibliometric performance. Specifically, the early attainment of full professor positions enhances opportunities for securing research funding, fostering collaborations, and building professional networks.

As Abramo et al. (2021) note, an intriguing question arises: could the employment of bibliometric indicators contribute to a more equitable assessment of female researchers? [32] Various strategies have been suggested, with the most radical proposal put forward by Abramo et al. (2016) [35], involving the establishment of performance rankings that differentiate between genders. This proposal stems from the observation, corroborated by our own data, that "when comparing the research performance of individuals within the same gender category, distinct rank positions emerge compared to those rankings that disregard gender distinctions".

This concept parallels the practice in sports, where gender-specific rankings are common to ensure fair competition and recognition of individual achievements within distinct categories.

4.4. Gender Distribution of Authors on IJAS

The number of papers published on the IJAS by Italian scientists increased over the years (from 27 to 75 papers in the last two decades). In 2002, only 30% of authors were women and the percentage of prestigious positions covered by female scientists was 22%, the lowest value obtained in the four years included in the survey.

The gap between the percentage of female authors and the prestigious positions held by women widened even more in 2008 (−13%) when about one-third of women covered prestigious positions even though the percentage of female authors was nearly 50%. In 2014, the total number of papers published on IJAS increased significantly in comparison to 2008 but the gender distribution remains unchanged. A trend towards achieving a gender balance was observed only in 2021, with a sharp increase in prestigious positions covered by women (41%) despite the lower percentage of female authors (36%) compared to the two previous surveys.

Abramo et al. (2009) studied the research productivity of the Italian academic system between 2001 and 2003 using the Italian Observatory of Public Research (ORP) [36]. The percentage of Italian female scientists in the disciplinary area of Agriculture and Veterinary Sciences was 27%, and this value is close to the gender distribution of authors in IJAS in 2002 (30%). The authors discovered that in the same period, women were more active (more than one paper per year) than men (52.7% compared to 47.5%). In the report by the European Commission (2018), the women-to-men ratio of authorship in the field of Agricultural Sciences (including animal science) increased from 0.9 to 1.0 in Italy between the five-year periods 2008–2012 and 2013–2017 [30]. These ratios are similar to the value found in this study in 2008 (0.92) but lower than that of 2014 (0.72), which is closer to the EU-28 ratios (from 0.7 to 0.8 in two periods). According to Ross et al. (2022), women in research teams are significantly less likely than men to be credited with authorship [37]. An investigation into the gender balance in STEM subject areas in Portugal showed that, among all researchers in any author position, women wrote fewer publications than men and this gap was largest in 2003 or earlier, although it decreased over the years, reaching parity in the five-year period 2014–2018 [38]. In addition, Bendels et al. (2017), analyzing almost 300.000 articles from 54 journals listed in the Nature index from 2008 to 2016, found that women comprise, on average, 47.6% of all authorship in Italy [20]. This value is very similar to that obtained in this study considering the two central years (2008 and 2014).

The percentage of female first authors increased sharply from 2002 to 2008 (15 to 41%) and this increase continued linearly in 2014 and 2021 when the 50% threshold was reached. Therefore, the growing role of women in the authorship of scientific articles has been confirmed over the years. Conversely, the percentage of women as last authors remained stable or decreased over time (from 30 to 25%). Typically, the last position is held by the author responsible for acquiring funds and other resources necessary to carry out the experiments. Therefore, these data may reflect some difficulties of women in accessing public and private funding and performing the role of principal investigator.

Johnson et al. (2021) observed that the percentage of reviewed research abstracts with a female last author, during the period 2006–2018 at the Pediatric Orthopedic Society of North America annual meeting, was very low (17.8% of the total) but, in addition, abstracts with women as last authors were significantly less likely to reach publication compared to those with men (59.6 vs. 67.9%; $p < 0.05$) [39]. In the paper by Bendels et al. (2017), women are, on average, 33.1% of the first authors and 18.1% of the last authors at the global level [20]. The highest average annual growth rate from 2008 to 2016 was found for the last authorship (1.4%) followed by the first authorship (0.7%). This positive trend is confirmed in this study only for the female first authors while, for the female last authors, the percentage is stable (on average 25% in the last three years considered).

Nevertheless, the percentage of women in the role of corresponding author (considered only if this position is different from the first or last author) increased threefold (from 15 to 45%) over the years. This trend is not linked to a corresponding increase over the years in the total number of women involved in the publication of articles (+6%) and could be justified by the fact that women are traditionally believed to have a greater aptitude for managing, rearranging, and proofreading manuscripts, following the stereotype that women are more organized and more persevering than men. This gender stereotype is derived from the unequal distribution of men and women in social roles both in the household and the workplace [40].

In a recent publication on gender disparities in high-quality research revealed by the Nature index, the writers, who did not have access to the researchers' academic positions, reported lower productivity for female authors [20]. In the same publication, the writers also reported that articles with female key authors (first and last) are cited less frequently than articles with male key authors.

This difference in citation rates increases as the number of authors contributing to an article increases, probably due to the strong competition for key positions among female authors. Furthermore, they observed distinct differences at the level of journal, journal category, continent, and country.

5. Conclusions

This study highlighted that within the association for animal sciences and the broader field of animal sciences, there is still a noticeable gender gap that has reduced over the years but at a very slow pace. In particular, there is a vertical segregation with a minority of women occupying full professor positions and a horizontal segregation with a low percentage of women involved in technical disciplines closer to STEM. At the bibliometric level, differences in bibliometric indicators between women and men are observed, favouring the latter, although these differences are not significant when taking into account academic position and scientific sector as fixed factors, with age as a covariate. Considering the authorship of scientific papers, women are under-represented in prestigious positions such as the first, last, and corresponding author.

This study provides evidence of barriers hindering women's advancement in science despite recent policy efforts for equality. However, some limitations must be acknowledged. It focuses on a single disciplinary field, examines only the Italian context, and does not include variables such as academic age due to data unavailability. Despite these constraints, the findings offer valuable insights for understanding gender disparities in academia.

The question of why so few women reach top positions and why progress is slow remains. The roots of this imbalance are deeply entrenched in local and historical contexts, perpetuating systemic inequalities. Effective policy efforts to increase women's participation in science must address complex social, cultural, economic, and political factors. Each country must identify and tackle the mechanisms perpetuating past inequalities, as neglecting the intellectual contributions of half the population cannot be justified.

Overcoming the gender gap in academic and research environments requires action not only within universities, research centres, and associations but also in broader societal realms. Cultural evolution, education of new generations against stereotypes, family support, and welfare policies are essential. However, the academic and scientific community is also called upon to play its part in the process toward gender equality, a process that is currently advancing too slowly. Efforts should prioritize equity in power roles within institutions, visibility in scientific events, and authorship in scientific publications. Research groups should strive to achieve gender balance across all disciplines, and balanced teams should be incentivized. Departments and universities should be encouraged to adopt resource distribution criteria that consider gender balance in leadership and decision-making roles. Furthermore, selection panels for research projects and editorial boards should ensure balanced gender representation and receive training to mitigate biases that contribute to the under-representation of women. As highlighted by several authors, the simultaneous implementation of all policies is essential; otherwise, progress may be significantly delayed. Scientific associations, such as universities, should adopt regular gender balance monitoring, using indicators to measure and drive progress. Establishing an annual evaluation system tailored to gender in academic environments could aid in addressing the issue.

Supplementary Materials: The following supporting information can be downloaded at https://www.mdpi.com/article/10.3390/ani15030390/s1, Table S1: Description of bibliometrics distributions by gender and positions.

Author Contributions: Conceptualization, A.S., P.C. and L.B.; methodology, P.C. and A.S.; software, P.C.; formal analysis, P.C.; investigation, L.B., A.S. and P.C; data curation, A.S. and P.C.; writing—original draft preparation, A.S., P.C. and L.B.; writing—review and editing, A.S., P.C. and L.B.; visualization, L.B.; supervision, L.B., A.S. and P.C. All authors have read and agreed to the published version of the manuscript.

Funding: This research received no external funding.

Institutional Review Board Statement: Not applicable.

Informed Consent Statement: Not applicable.

Data Availability Statement: Data is contained within the article.

Acknowledgments: The authors thank Nicolò Pietro Paolo Macciotta for his support, and Giorgina Kuzminsky and Mariangela Zarbo for their operational assistance in data retrieval.

Conflicts of Interest: The authors declare no conflicts of interest.

References

1. UNESCO Call to Action: Closing the Gender Gap in Science. Available online: https://www.sciencecentres.org.uk/documents/752/UNESCO_Call_to_action_closing_the_gender_gap_in_science.pdf (accessed on 15 January 2025).
2. The White House. National Strategy on Gender Equity and Equality. The White House. 2021. Available online: https://faolex.fao.org/docs/pdf/usa223274.pdf (accessed on 13 September 2024).
3. Communication from the Commission to the European Parliament, the Council, the European Economic and Social Committee and the Committee of the Regions. A Union of Equality: Gender Equality Strategy 2020–2025. Available online: https://eur-lex.europa.eu/legal-content/EN/TXT/PDF/?uri=CELEX:52020DC0152 (accessed on 13 September 2024).
4. World Economic Forum. Global Gender Gap Report 2024. Available online: https://www.weforum.org/publications/global-gender-gap-report-2024/ (accessed on 13 September 2024).
5. European Research Area Policy Agenda: Overview of Actions for the Period 2022–2024. Available online: https://commission.europa.eu/system/files/2021-11/ec_rtd_era-policy-agenda-2021.pdf (accessed on 13 September 2024).
6. Deiana, G.; Dettori, M.; Muresu, N.; Puci, M.V.; Saderi, L.; Piga, M.L.; Sias, V.; Pisu, D.; Foddai, M.A.; Gazzolo, T.; et al. Gender equality in the Italian academic context. Results from the IGEA project. *Front. Public Health* **2023**, *11*, 1125496. [CrossRef] [PubMed]
7. Striving for a Union of Equality: The Gender Equality Strategy 2020–2025. Available online: https://ec.europa.eu/newsroom/just/items/682425/en (accessed on 10 January 2025).
8. Gallego-Moron, N.; Matus-Lopez, M. Exploring self-exclusion as a gendered barrier in Spanish universities. A mixed methodological study. *Women's Stud. Int. Forum* **2023**, *99*, 102797. [CrossRef]
9. Kapareliotis, I.; Miliopoulou, G.Z. Gender bias in academia: An attempt to render the intangible tangible. *Divers. Within Divers. Manag.* **2019**, *22*, 247–271. [CrossRef]
10. Filandri, M.; Pasqua, S.; Priori, E. Breaking through the glass ceiling. Simulating policies to close the gender gap in the Italian academia. *Socio-Econ. Plan.Sci.* **2023**, *88*, 101655. [CrossRef]
11. European Commission. *She Figures 2021: Gender in Research and Innovation—Statistics and Indicators*; Publications Office of the European Union: Brussels, Belgium, 2021. [CrossRef]
12. Web of Science Database. Available online: https://www.webofscience.com (accessed on 11 October 2024).
13. Gaiaschi, C. *Doppio Standard: Donne e Carriere Scientifiche Nell'italia Contemporanea*; Carocci Editore: Roma, Italy, 2022; ISBN 978-88-290-1541-2.
14. Farina, S.; Iafrate, R.; Boccia, S. Unveiling the gender gap: Exploring gender disparities in European academic landscape. *Lancet. Reg. Health Eur.* **2023**, *34*, 100752. [CrossRef]
15. Avargil, S.; Shwartz-Asher, D.; Reiss, S.R.; Dori, Y.J. Professors' retrospective views on chemistry career choices with a focus on gender and academic stage aspects. *Sustain. Chem. Pharm.* **2023**, *36*, 101249. [CrossRef]
16. Jappelli, T.; Nappi, C.A.; Torrini, R. Gender effects in research evaluation. *Res. Policy.* **2017**, *46*, 911–924. [CrossRef]
17. Angervall, P. The academic career: A study of subjectivity, gender and movement among women university lecturers. *Gender Educ.* **2018**, *30*, 105–118. [CrossRef]
18. Filandri, M.; Pasqua, S. 'Being good isn't good enough':gender discrimination in Italian academia. *Stud. High. Educ.* **2021**, *46*, 1533–1551. [CrossRef]
19. De Paola, M.; Ponzo, M.; Scoppa, V. Gender differences in the propensity to apply for promotion: Evidence from the Italian scientific qualification. *Oxf. Econ. Pap.* **2017**, *69*, 986–1009. [CrossRef]
20. Bendels, M.H.K.; Müller, R.; Brueggmann, D.; Groneberg, D.A. Gender disparities in high-quality research revealed by Nature Index journals. *PLoS ONE* **2018**, *13*, e0189136. [CrossRef] [PubMed]
21. Park, S. Seeking changes in ivory towers: The impact of gender quotas on female academics in higher education. *Women's Stud. Int. Forum.* **2020**, *79*, 102346. [CrossRef]
22. European Institute for Gender Equality. *Gender Equality Index 2023: Towards a Green Transition in Transport and Energy*; Publications Office of the European Union: Luxembourg, 2023; ISBN 978-92-9486-099-6.
23. Hamrita, T.K. *Women in Precision Agriculture: Technological Breakthroughs, Challenges and Aspirations for a Prosperous and Sustainable Future*; Springer: Cham, Switzerland, 2021; ISBN 978-3-030-49243-4. Available online: http://cercauniversita.cineca.it (accessed on 12 September 2024).
24. Mahmood, Z.; Kouser, R.; Masud, M.A.K. Women in the boardroom and corporate environmental sustainability: Evidence from emerging economies. *Bus. Strategy Environ.* **2023**, *32*, 1014–1029.
25. Ullah, I.; Majeed, M.A.; Fang, H.X.; Khan, M.A. Female CEOs and corporate environmental investments: Evidence from the US. *Bus. Strategy Environ.* **2022**, *31*, 362–377.
26. European Commission. *2023 Report on Gender Equality in the EU*; Publications Office of the European Union: Luxembourg, 2023; ISBN 978-92-76-99066-6; ISSN 2443-5228.

27. European Commission. *Education and Training Monitor*; Publications Office of the European Union: Luxembourg, 2022; ISBN 978-92-76-54156-1.
28. Osservatorio Talents Venture e STEAMiamoci sul Gender Gap nelle Facoltà STEM. Available online: https://www.assolombarda.it/media/comunicati-stampa/osservatorio-talents-venture-e-steamiamoci (accessed on 12 October 2024).
29. Thege, B.; Schmeck, M.; van Elsacker, M. *Gender-Sensitive Teaching: An Introduction for Teaching Staff in STEM*; Baltic Gender Coordination Office: Kiel, Germany, 2020.
30. European Commission. *She Figures 2018: Research and Innovation*; Publications Office of the European Union: Brussels, Belgium, 2019; ISBN 978-92-79-86715-6.
31. Howe, M.E.; Kim, M.M.; Pazicni, S. Graduate Student Women's Perceptions of Faculty Careers: The critical role of departmental values and support in career choice. *JACS Au.* **2022**, *2*, 1443–1456. [CrossRef]
32. Abramo, G.; Aksnes, D.W.; D'Angelo, C.A. Gender differences in research performance within and between countries: Italy vs Norway. *J. Informetr.* **2021**, *15*, 101144. [CrossRef]
33. Huang, J.; Gates, J.; Sinatra, R.; Barabási, A.L. Historical comparison of gender inequality in scientific careers across countries and disciplines. *Proc. Natl. Acad. Sci. USA* **2020**, *117*, 4609–4616. [CrossRef]
34. Eagly, A.H. Do the social roles that women and men occupy in science allow equal access to publication? *Proc. Natl. Acad. Sci. USA* **2020**, *117*, 5553–5555. [CrossRef]
35. Abramo, G.; D'Angelo, C.A.; Rosati, F. Gender bias in academic recruitment. *Scientometrics* **2016**, *106*, 119–141. [CrossRef]
36. Abramo, G.; D'Angelo, C.A.; Caprasecca, A. Gender differences in research productivity: A bibliometric analysis of the Italian academic system. *Scientometrics* **2009**, *79*, 517–539. [CrossRef]
37. Ross, M.B.; Glennon, B.M.; Murciano-Goroff, R.; Berkes, E.G.; Weinberg, B.A.; Lane, J.I. Women are credited less in science than men. *Nature* **2022**, *608*, 135–145. [CrossRef] [PubMed]
38. Gender in the Portugal Research Arena: A Case Study in European Leadership. Available online: https://assets.ctfassets.net/zlnfaxb2lcqx/7u4YKppKMUePpuEAdzgWCO/2e455e490cd53367929123d241783709/portugal-gender-report.pdf (accessed on 9 October 2024).
39. Johnson, M.A.; Mulvey, H.; Parambath, A.; Anari, J.B.; Wall, L.B.; Shah, A.S. A Gender Gap in Publishing? Understanding the Glass Ceiling in Pediatric Orthopaedic Surgery. *J. Pediatr. Orthop.* **2021**, *41*, e484–e488. [CrossRef] [PubMed]
40. Hentschel, T.; Heilman, M.E.; Peus, C.V. The Multiple Dimensions of Gender Stereotypes: A Current Look at Men's and Women's Characterizations of Others and Themselves. *Front. Psychol.* **2019**, *10*, 11. [CrossRef] [PubMed]

animals

MDPI

Article

The Role of Comparative Psychology in the Training of Veterinarians

Brooke A. Boughton and Charles I. Abramson *

Laboratory of Comparative Psychology and Behavioral Biology, Oklahoma State University, Stillwater, OK 74078, USA; bbought@okstate.edu
* Correspondence: charles.abramson@okstate.edu

Simple Summary: Comparative psychology is the oldest of the social sciences, and is one of the natural science branches of psychology. This article is the first to suggest that comparative psychology be incorporated into the vet school curriculum. Many aspects of comparative psychology form natural links with the training of veterinary students. These links include the study of ethics, animal behavior, research methodology, and animal welfare.

Abstract: This article highlights some of the advantages that comparative psychology offers the veterinary student and veterinary education generally. Comparative psychology is the oldest of the social sciences and, as such, has accumulated over three centuries of experience in such areas as research design, animal–human interactions, and animal behavior. To establish whether comparative psychology is taught in veterinary schools, we survey all course catalogs of U.S. veterinary schools. None of the schools surveyed offered a course in comparative psychology, and inconsistencies were noted among the schools in regard to courses in animal–human interaction, animal behavior, and ethics. Suggestions are provided on how to incorporate principles of comparative psychology in veterinary education at both the undergraduate and graduate levels.

Keywords: comparative psychology; veterinary education; teaching

1. Introduction

One of the most important challenges facing veterinary science is the training of veterinary students. In the United States (U.S.), the veterinary curriculum is usually four years, at the end of which the student receive the degree of Doctor of Veterinary Medicine. Throughout the four years, students receive training in a variety of areas, including anatomy, animal–human interaction, biochemistry, comparative anatomy and physiology, endocrinology, ethics, neurobiology, nutrition, parasitology, pharmacology, and a host of other specialized courses.

The purpose of this article is to recommend that veterinary students take a course at either the undergraduate or graduate level in comparative psychology. Comparative psychology (CP) is the oldest of the organized social sciences, with the term first used in 1778 [1]. As the oldest of the social sciences, CP has the most experience of any behavioral science working on the fundamental issue of animal behavior including ethics, animal–human interaction, and experimental design [2,3].

CP has been defined as the "application of the comparative method to problems in psychology" [4,5]. As such, it is a general psychology with methods and results applicable to both human and non-human animals. Indeed, one of the goals of CP is to conduct a variety of comparisons of humans with non-human animals. CP is one of the few natural science branches of psychology and is arguably the only behavioral science that specifically compares human and non-human animals. As such, we believe that many of the principles, methods, and data of CP are a natural fit with veterinary education. As far as we can determine, the present article is the first to suggest that a link between veterinary education and a course in comparative psychology would be beneficial to veterinary students.

CP differs from fields such as animal behavior and comparative cognition. While some aspects of CP may overlap with other animal behavior courses/disciplines, they are not identical [5]. Students of CP receive combined training in the principles of behavior and methods of comparative analysis. Of relevance to veterinary education is that CP courses contain components related to animal–human interactions, the use of conditioning methods, and the role of animals in the therapeutic process. Seldom, if at all, are these topics covered in any other course that focuses on animal behavior. Moreover, in the best CP courses, students receive laboratory experiences where they directly compare the behavior of various animals, including humans.

We believe that CP has much to recommend for veterinary training. First, as a general psychology, CP offers students a variety of perspectives, many of which are directly related to veterinary training. These include a focus on ethics, animal–human interaction, the use of animals as a therapeutic adjunct, and the use of clinical psychological methods to treat animals for depression and other behavioral ailments. Moreover, as CP is psychology-based, students also receive instruction in the more social aspects of dealing with animals and interacting with fellow humans. Recently, it has been suggested that an interaction between CP and clinical psychology would be beneficial to both fields [6]. This emphasis on the social interactions of human animals is perhaps unique to psychology-based courses.

Second, a course on CP contains information on how to use classical and operant conditioning methods to train a variety of animals in a variety of situations. For instance, conditioning methods are routinely used not only to increase the production of farm animals, but also to improve their welfare [7,8]. Moreover, the training of companion animals is also based upon some form of conditioning. The fact that veterinary students have little to no theoretical and practical experience in classical and operant conditioning puts them at a distinct disadvantage when confronted with the behavioral problems of their clients.

Third, the research designs used in CP will help the veterinary student better understand good research, and recognize poor and misleading veterinary research. For those veterinary students interested in conducting research, a thorough understanding of comparative research methods will dramatically increase the reliability of their findings [2]. Even a cursory understanding of the research methods used in CP will help the student better understand research, and make them better researchers and consumers of veterinary science.

Consider, for example, that one of the most fundamental research methods in CP is the ethogram (also known as a behavioral profile). A veterinarian may be confronted with a situation where the human caregiver may state that their pet "always engages in the problem behavior". A veterinarian with a background in CP will immediately know that this is not true, as there are "behavioral patterns". The veterinarian will then request that the human caregiver keep a detailed record of, for example, the time of occurrence, the intensity of occurrence, and what was happening the moment the problem behavior was expressed. In effect, the human client becomes a citizen scientist [9]. With such a detailed record, both the veterinarian and the human caregiver are in a better position to treat the behavioral problem. A Google search will reveal that there are literally hundreds of ethograms on all aspects of animal behavior that the veterinarian can refer to. Moreover, there are videos on how to prepare an ethogram. The senior author (CIA), for example, co-developed an ethogram to evaluate enrichment devices for elephants [10].

Fourth, because CP contains a significant social science aspect, the veterinary student will be in a better position to understand the social bond between the animal and the human caregiver. As mentioned earlier, animal–human interaction is a significant research area in CP. No other psychology or animal behavior course maintains such a focus.

2. Search Methodology

To determine if CP is currently covered in veterinary schools, we looked at the course catalogs of all 32 veterinary schools in the United States (U.S.). We restricted our search to U.S. veterinary schools, as we could not access data from non-U.S. schools. We looked at three areas covered in a typical CP course to determine whether some aspects of CP are covered. These areas are animal welfare, animal behavior, and ethics. The results are below, and clearly show that these fundamental aspects of CP are seldom, if at all, included in the veterinary school curriculum.

All university course catalogs were accessed and evaluated (omitting the University of Florida, because student login credentials were required). Courses in welfare, ethics, and behavior were all recorded on an Excel spreadsheet. Course numbers and course descriptions, as well as whether the course was offered as an elective or core class, were also recorded in the spreadsheet.

3. Results

The data we obtained from our search of veterinary school catalogs is presented below. The catalogs were examined from November 2022 to January 2023. We believe they are the most current catalogs at the time this article was submitted. The first graph represents the number of schools offering courses related to animal welfare. The second graph represents the number of schools offering courses in animal behavior. The last graph represents the number of ethics-related courses offered by veterinary schools.

Animal Welfare Course Data: Figure 1 shows that, of the 32 AVMA-accredited veterinary colleges that allowed access to course catalogs, six (19%) required an animal welfare course to be taken by the veterinary students. Only four (12%) colleges offered a welfare class as an optional elective course, and the remaining 22 (69%) colleges do not offer a welfare course.

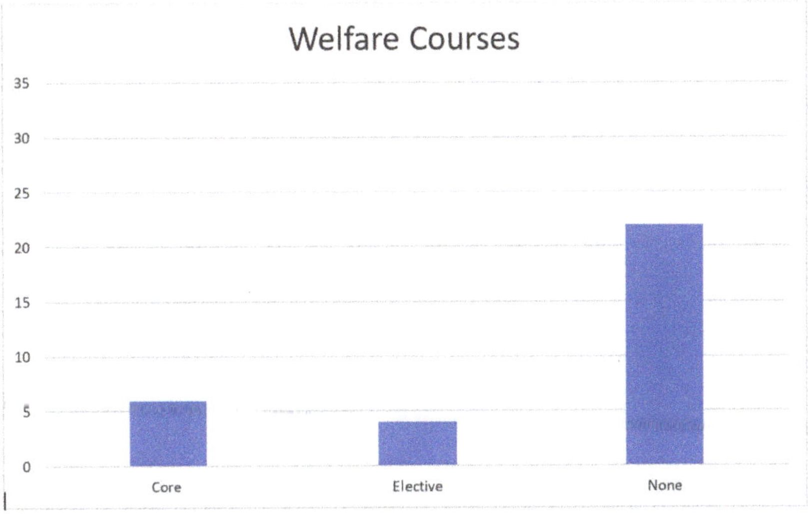

Figure 1. Distribution of animal welfare courses for schools of veterinary medicine.

Behavior Course Data: Figure 2 shows that, of the 32 AVMA-accredited veterinary colleges that allowed access to course catalogs, 12 (37%) required a behavior course to be taken by the veterinary students. Seven (22%) colleges offered a behavior course as an optional elective, and the remaining 13 (41%) universities do not offer a behavior course.

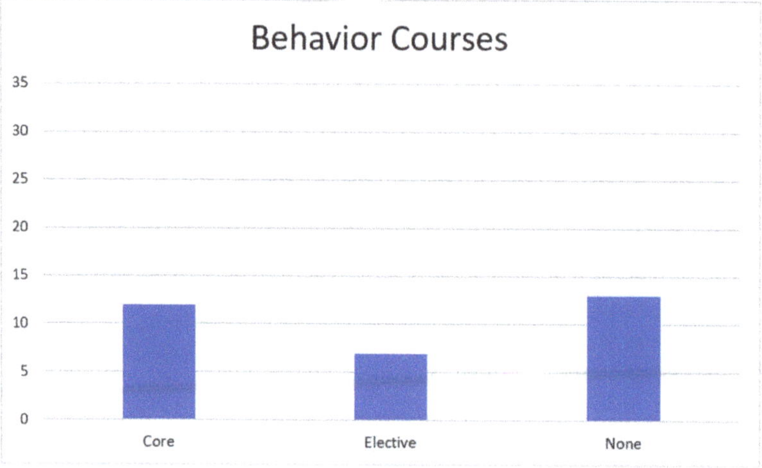

Figure 2. Distribution of animal behavior courses for schools of veterinary medicine.

Ethics Course Data: Figure 3 shows that, of the 32 AVMA-accredited veterinary colleges that allowed access to course catalogs, only 11 (35%) require a core class in ethics to be taken. Two (6%) of the colleges offer ethics as an optional elective course, and the remaining 19 (59%) do not offer any sort of ethics course.

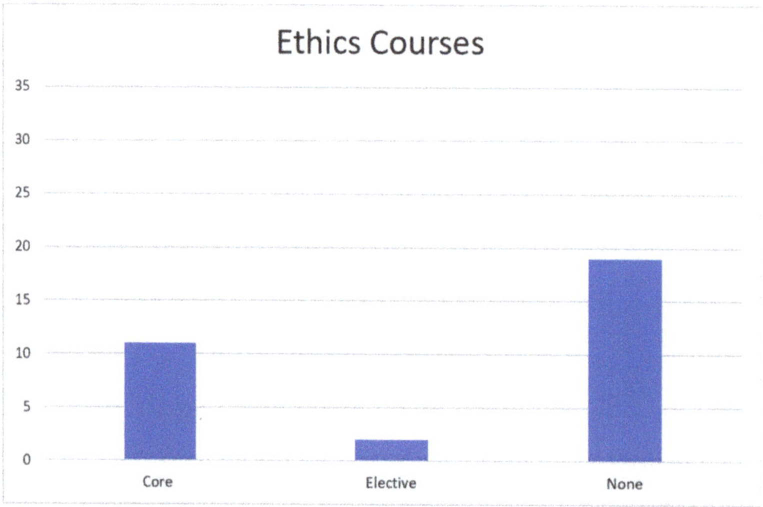

Figure 3. Distribution of animal ethics courses for schools of veterinary medicine.

4. Resources

It is beyond the scope of this paper to provide specific exercises that can be incorporated into a veterinary school curriculum. Many resources can be found in the open-access journal *The International Journal of Comparative Psychology* (*IJCP*) (https://escholarship.org/uc/uclapsych_ijcp accessed on 3 July 2023). In addition to free access to articles related to CP, *IJCP* recently published two special issues related to teaching (Volume 33) and the state of CP (Volume 31), respectively. These two special issues will be particularly important for those educators wanting to either develop a CP course specifically designed for veterinary students and/or incorporate elements of CP into an existing course. These resources can also serve as independent readings, and as a base for discussion at the administrative level for those programs considering integrating CP into their curriculum on a formal basis.

The special issue related to teaching (https://escholarship.org/uc/item/78468853 accessed on 3 July 2023) includes 12 papers summarizing over 50 classroom-tested inquiry-based exercises. A wide variety of invertebrates and vertebrates are used, ranging from tardigrades to humans. The activities range from experiments on basic conditioning to the construction of ethograms. Of particular interest are papers describing how to construct apparatus using 3D printers, and how to construct low-cost robotic animals [11].

The current state of comparative psychology is the focus of the second special issue [12]. This issue contains 13 articles that cover a wide range of topics. These topics include comparative methodology, data analysis, equine therapy, and the philosophy behind CP (https://escholarship.org/uc/item/0mn8n8bc accessed on 3 July 2023). One paper provides general resources including books, review articles, history, websites, and teaching exercises [5].

5. Benefits of CP to Both Undergraduate and Graduate Veterinary Students

Incorporating CP at the graduate level offers veterinary students several advantages. Many of these we have already mentioned, including the study of ethics, the implementation of research design, and the use of conditioning methods. Moreover, the "social" nature associated with a psychology course will better prepare students for interacting with the public and, perhaps, better understanding themselves.

As just one example, consider how conditioning methods are used to improve the lives of farm animals and to increase their production. Abramson [13] shows how classical and operant conditioning is used to modify the behavior of farm animals, and Baldwin [7] reports on how operant techniques are used by animals to regulate their environment. Functional knowledge of conditioning methods is not only useful for veterinarians working with hoofed animals, but also for those working with companion animals exhibiting behavior problems.

Moreover, conditioning methods can be used to improve the lives of animals by reducing environmental stress. In an unpublished experiment, the senior author (CIA) trained a llama to poke its head through a "hula hoop" for a food reward. Head poking was automatically recorded, and a food bin was programmed to operate when the llama met specific contingencies. This method, which was later adapted for horses [14], was subsequently used by the llama to tell the researcher which food it preferred, to turn on and off a water, spray, and to turn on and off a fan. The latter two rewards were particularly useful in the hot Oklahoma summers, where temperatures can reach in excess of 100° Fahrenheit (37.8° Celsius).

For veterinarian students focusing on research, there is no behavioral science that has more experience designing and interpreting animal behavior experiments than CP [2]. Consider the following example. The senior author, who is a comparative psychologist (CIA), was asked to join a team to evaluate the digestive properties of dog chews such as Greenies™. Rather than test the product on a dog, he modified the original method of Pavlov [15] by placing the digestive juices in a test tube along with the product. The degradation of the product could now easily be determined by weighing the remaining sample as a function of time. This procedure has the added advantage that it permits the parametric manipulation of several independent variables, such as the amount of gastric juices. This procedure eliminated any possible stress in test animals, as none were used [16].

Other examples where the methods of CP were used to gather data of interest to veterinarians include a study on the use of silver vine (*Actinidia polygama* Maxim) as an enrichment aid for cats [17], the development of a survey instrument to match a human's personality characteristics to those of their pets [18], issues related to equine therapy [19], an analysis of reproductive endocrinology and musth in a captive Asian elephant [20], a comparison of food vs. human contact as a reward for horses [21], and a study investigating the ability of horses to measure time [14].

The above examples focus on traditional research areas familiar to veterinarians. However, an understanding of CP can be used in areas not normally considered by veterinarians. These include the relationship of CP to pet industry litigation [22], and how consumer products affect animal behavior [23].

At the undergraduate level, we would encourage pre-vet majors to take a course in comparative psychology. Such a course, in combination with those typically required for a pre-vet major, will significantly enhance their preparation for graduate training. The results of our survey of veterinary schools show the graduate training of veterinary students in the area of ethics, behavior, and animal welfare is not consistent. These topics are part of any competent undergraduate course in CP.

6. Limitations and Challenges

This article advocates incorporating CP in the training of veterinarians at the graduate and at undergraduate levels. We also suggest that CP be incorporated into the training of veterinary professional associates (VPA). The development of VPA fills a much-needed gap in veterinary practice [24]. We would advocate that those veterinarian policymakers charged with developing VPA programs consider adding a course in comparative psychology.

Despite the many advantages of CP [3–5], there are challenges associated with finding CP programs. A major challenge is that few psychology departments associated with universities that maintain veterinary schools offer CP courses to their undergraduates. In our previous data set, we omitted the University of Florida because a login was required. No such restriction was present to access the course listing in the psychology department. Of the 33 total AVMA-accredited veterinary colleges in the United States, seven (21%) offered comparative psychology courses to their undergraduate students, and seven (21%) additional universities offered an animal behavior course, but did not include comparative psychology in the course title. The remaining 19 (58%) universities did not offer any comparative psychology or animal behavior courses to their undergraduate students.

The situation is perhaps more dire when graduate programs in CP are considered. Of the 33 total AVMA-accredited veterinary colleges in the United States, not a single university offers a strictly CP program. Eight (24%) universities offer an animal-behavior-focused graduate program, and the remaining 25 (76%) universities do not offer any CP or animal-behavior-focused graduate programs.

The lack of CP programs is not restricted to universities that maintain veterinary schools. The problem is nationwide. Of the 650 universities and colleges surveyed, including those that maintain veterinary schools, only 82 (12%) offered an undergraduate course in CP [5]. This absence of CP programs is reflected by the fact that there is only one currently available textbook [25].

7. Recommendations and Discussion

As mentioned in the Introduction, we believe this is the first article to suggest that comparative psychology be incorporated into the veterinary school curriculum. To provide some supporting evidence for our assertation, we looked at volumes 25 (2001) through 50 (2023, numbers 1 and 2) of the *Journal of Veterinary Medical Education*. Discounting, letters to the editor, editorials, and book reviews, of 1,360 articles, only three fall into the general area of CP [26–28].

Despite the limitations and challenges, we believe that incorporating CP into the veterinary school curriculum will benefit both CP and the teaching of veterinary students. Given the lack of comparative psychology courses and graduate programs, we suggest that those interested in incorporating CP:

1. Work closely with a comparative psychologist to develop curricula. The International Society for Comparative Psychology operates a Listserv (http://www.comparativ

epsychology.org/accessed on 3 July 2023) and Division 6 (Society for Behavioral Neuroscience and Comparative Psychology) of the American Psychological Association (APA) maintains a list of comparative psychologists. Moreover, the APA has an educational consulting service consisting of individuals specializing in evaluating and developing educational resources;
2. Commission a CP textbook specifically designed for veterinary students;
3. Develop an online CP course for veterinary students;
4. Integrate CP courses into the undergraduate pre-vet curriculum;
5. Assign CP readings for veterinary students without access to CP programs;
6. Hire comparative psychologists as faculty members/consultants;
7. Design an intensive one-week "mini-course" in comparative psychology.

Although the data and ideas discussed in this paper are based on U.S. institutions, we believe that the situation is similar in other parts of the world. Several papers have been written advocating for CP in Africa [29,30] and Asia [31]. These papers, and the present contribution, can help colleagues in these parts of the world better understand CP, and stimulate them to incorporate CP into their countries' veterinary training.

In conclusion, we believe that, with some effort, CP can significantly add to the training of veterinarian students.

8. Conclusions

The partnership between comparative psychology and aspects of veterinary training seems a natural one. Both have a stated interest in the ethical treatment of animals, a focus on behavior, and a concern for animal welfare. Moreover, both share an interest in animal–human interactions and the use of behavioral techniques. Behavioral techniques are used to treat problem behaviors and to increase the output of farm animals, by establishing appropriate conditions of reward and designing suitable environments conducive to production. Moreover, the research designs associated with CP are some of the oldest available, and help the veterinarian student plan better experiments and recognize good behavioral science.

Integrating CP into veterinary school curricula will not be easy. Few veterinary schools have associated psychology departments offering CP courses. There are also few graduate programs. We have provided several suggestions, such as independent readings, developing a CP textbook designed for veterinarian students, and creating an online course.

Author Contributions: Conception C.I.A.; data gathering B.A.B. and C.I.A.; writing, C.I.A. and B.A.B.; review and editing C.I.A. and B.A.B. All authors have read and agreed to the published version of the manuscript.

Funding: The participation of Charles Abramson was funded in part by NSF REU grant 1950805 and NSF PIRE grant 1545803.

Institutional Review Board Statement: Not applicable.

Informed Consent Statement: Not applicable.

Data Availability Statement: The data presented in this study are available on request from the corresponding author.

Conflicts of Interest: The authors declare no conflict of interest.

References

1. D'isa, R.; Abramson, C.I. The origin of the phrase comparative psychology: An historical introduction. *Front. Psychol.* **2023**, *14*, 1174115. [CrossRef] [PubMed]
2. Abramson, C.I. Research methods in comparative psychology: A tutorial. *J. Mind Behav.* **2023**, *44*, 111–135.
3. Abramson, C.I. Why the study of comparative psychology is important to neuroscientists. *Front. Behav. Neurosci.* **2023**, *16*, 1095033. [CrossRef]
4. Abramson, C.I. A crisis in comparative psychology: Where have all the undergraduates gone? *Front. Psychol.* **2015**, *6*, 1500. [CrossRef] [PubMed]

5. Abramson, C.I. Let us bring comparative psychology back. *Int. J. Comp. Psychol.* **2018**, *31*. Available online: https://escholarship.org/uc/item/81j662cd (accessed on 3 July 2023). [CrossRef]
6. Marston, D.; Gopaul, M.T. Considerations for an integrated undergraduate comparative and clinical psychology course. *Int. J. Comp. Psychol.* **2020**, *33*. Available online: https://escholarship.org/uc/item/41j4c087 (accessed on 3 July 2023). [CrossRef]
7. Baldwin, B.A. Operant Conditioning in Farm Animals and its Relevance to Welfare. In *Indicators Relevant to Farm Animal Welfare. Current Topics in Veterinary Medicine and Animal Science*; Smidt, D., Ed.; Springer: Dordrecht, The Netherlands, 1983; Volume 23. [CrossRef]
8. Varnon, C.A.; Martin, A.L.; Abramson, C.I. Conditioning methods for farm animals: A mini-review. *Uludağ Univ. J. Fac. Vet. Med.* **2012**, *31*, 1–10.
9. Abramson, C.I.; Bowser, T.J. In-home animal product evaluation using the Citizen Scientist™ program. In *Nutritional Biotechnology in the Feed and Food Industries, Proceedings of Alltech's 22nd Annual Symposium, Lexington, KY, USA, 23–26 April 2006*; Lynons, T.P., Jacques, K.A., Hower, J., Eds.; Nottingham University Press: Nottingham, UK, 2006; pp. 251–254.
10. Abramson, C.I.; Carden, M. The use of the ethogram to assess enrichment experiences for elephants. *J. Elephant Manag. Assoc.* **1998**, *9*, 206–209.
11. Abramson, C.I. The teaching of comparative psychology: Exercises, experiences, and philosophy: A introduction to the special issue. *Int. J. Comp. Psychol.* **2020**, *33*. Available online: https://escholarship.org/uc/item/78468853 (accessed on 3 July 2023). [CrossRef]
12. Abramson, C.I.; Hill, H.M. The State of Comparative Psychology Today: An Introduction to the Special Issue. *Int. J. Comp. Psychol.* **2018**, *31*. Available online: https://escholarship.org/uc/item/0mn8n8bc (accessed on 3 July 2023). [CrossRef]
13. Abramson, C.I.; Kieson, E. Conditioning methods for animals in agriculture: A mini-review. *Ciênc. Anim. Brasileira.* **2016**, *17*, 359–375. [CrossRef]
14. Craig, D.P.A.; Varnon, C.A.; Pollock, K.L.; Abramson, C.I. An assessment of horse (*Equus ferus caballus*) responding on fixed interval schedules of reinforcement: An individual analysis. *Behav. Process.* **2015**, *120*, 1–13. [CrossRef] [PubMed]
15. Pavlov, I.P. *Conditioned Reflexes: An Investigation of the Physiological Activity of the Cerebral Cortex*; Oxford University Press: Oxford, UK, 1927.
16. Bowser, T.J.; Abramson, C.I.; Bennett, D. Low-cost in vitro screening method for digestibility of pet chews. *Am. J. Anim. Vet. Sci.* **2006**, *1*, 23–26. [CrossRef]
17. Abramson, C.I.; Lay, A.; Bowser, T.J.; Varnon, C.A. The use of silver vine (*Actinidia Polygama* Maxim, Family Actinidiaceae) as an enrichment aid for felines: Issues and prospects. *Am. J. Anim. Vet. Sci.* **2012**, *7*, 21–27. [CrossRef]
18. Curb, L.A.; Abramson, C.I.; Grice, J.W.; Kennison, S. The relationship between personality match and pet satisfaction among dog owners. *Anthrozoös* **2013**, *26*, 395–404. [CrossRef]
19. Kieson, E.; Abramson, C.I. Horses are not people: Research, parallels, and problems using equines as relationship models in EAP. In *A Horse is a Horse, of Course 2018: 2nd International Symposium for Equine Welfare and Wellness (Minds-n-Motion Symposium Compendium Book 3)*; Parent, I., Ed.; MiMer: Torna Hallestad, Sweden, 2018; pp. 61–73.
20. Duer, C.; Abramson, C.I.; Tomasi, T. Reproductive endocrinology and musth indicators in a captive Asian elephant (*Elephas maximus*). *Psychol. Rep.* **2016**, *119*, 839–860. [CrossRef]
21. Kieson, E.; Felix, C.; Webb, S.; Abramson, C.I. The effects of a choice test between food rewards and human interaction in a heard of domestic horses of varying breeds and experiences. *Appl. Anim. Behav. Sci.* **2020**, *231*, 105075. [CrossRef]
22. Abramson, C.I.; Black, T.E. Importance of comparative psychology in pet industry litigation. *J. Soc. Sci.* **2017**, *13*, 118–123. [CrossRef]
23. Kieson, E.; Abramson, C.I. Exploring the relationship between animal behavior and consumer products: Developing critical awareness through classroom and home-based experimentation. *Cont. Psychol.* **2015**, *4*, 23. [CrossRef]
24. Kogan, L.R.; Stewart, S.M. Veterinary professional associates: Does the profession's foresight include a mid-tier professional similar to physician assistants? *J. Vet. Med. Educ.* **2009**, *36*, 220–225. [CrossRef] [PubMed]
25. Papini, M. *Comparative Psychology: Evolution and Development of the Brain*, 3rd ed.; Routledge: New York, NY, USA, 2015.
26. Kogan, L.R.; Salman, M.D.; Ruch-Gallie, R. Applied animal behavior obedience training course: A model for veterinary curricula. *J. Vet. Med. Educ.* **2002**, *29*, 241–244. [CrossRef]
27. McGreevy, P.D.; Della Torre, P.K.; Evans, D.L. Animal behaviour learning environment: Software to facilitate learning in canine and feline behaviour therapy. *J. Vet. Med. Educ.* **2003**, *30*, 308–317. [CrossRef]
28. Pearson, G.; Connor, M.; Keen, J.; Reardon, R.; Waran, N. Incorporation of equine learning theory into the undergraduate curriculum. *J. Vet. Med. Educ.* **2021**, *48*, 351–360. [CrossRef]
29. Abramson, C.I.; Kitching, P. The importance of comparative psychology to Africa: Some reflections and sources. *Afr. J. Soc. Sci. Humanit. Res.* **2018**, *1*, 57–73. Available online: https://abjournals.org/african-journal-of-social-sciences-and-humanities-research-ajsshr/wp-content/uploads/sites/9/journal/published_paper/volume-1/issue-1/AJSSHR_gC3nxeh2.pdf (accessed on 3 July 2023).
30. Abramson, C.I.; Radi, M. Comparative psychology in Egypt. Some reflections and sources. *Egypt. J. Psychol.* **2019**, *122*, 93–114.
31. Stauch, K.N.; Somers, A.; Song, Y.; Kieson, E.; Abramson, C.I. Why Asia needs comparative psychology: Applications in canine-human, and equine-human interactions. *Asian J. Interdiscip. Res.* **2019**, *27*, 27–36. [CrossRef]

animals

MDPI

Article

Survey on Psychosocial Conditions of Official Veterinarians in Germany: Comparison with Other Professions and Differences between Age Groups, Gender, and Workplace Characteristics

Katharina Charlotte Jensen * and Roswitha Merle

Institute of Veterinary Epidemiology and Biostatistics, Center for Veterinary Public Health, School of Veterinary Medicine, Freie Universität Berlin, 14163 Berlin, Germany; roswitha.merle@fu-berlin.de
* Correspondence: charlotte.jensen@fu-berlin.de

Simple Summary: Veterinarians often suffer from mental diseases. Related studies have mostly regarded veterinarians working in practice, so little is known about veterinarians working for authorities (official veterinarians). Official veterinarians control animal husbandries or food producers to ensure animal welfare, freedom from infectious diseases, and food safety. We assessed the psychosocial wellbeing of official German veterinarians and compared it to that of employees in other professions using an online questionnaire. The results indicated that official veterinarians experience high demands during their work and are regularly exposed to offensive behavior during their activities. They also felt exhausted more often than employees in other professions. They also considered their work as meaningful and had more freedom than other employees concerning working time and how they performed their jobs. The results indicate that official veterinarians may require protection and support.

Abstract: Background: Even though the mental health of veterinarians has raised concerns, little is known about the wellbeing of official veterinarians ensuring animal welfare, food safety, and control of infectious diseases and performing other tasks for veterinary public health. Therefore, the aim of this study was to assess the psychosocial conditions of official German veterinarians and to compare them with those of other employees. Methods: An online survey was conducted including 82 items of the Copenhagen Psychosocial Questionnaire (COPSOQ III) and additional questions on workplace and demographics. Results: The answers of 838 respondents were analyzed, representing 26% of the target population. The average values for the dimensions *Quantitative Demands, Emotional Demands*, and *Burnout Symptoms* were substantially higher than those for German employees in other professions. Official veterinarians mainly working in animal welfare frequently experienced physical violence (6.7%) or threats of violence (53%). However, the profession also provides advantages: official veterinarians reported higher average values concerning the dimensions *Control over Working Time* and *Influence at Work* than other employees. Most participants stated that they experienced their work as meaningful, and the *Job Insecurity* dimension was low. Conclusions: Official veterinarians frequently experience offensive behavior and high-level demands. Therefore, measures to support and protect official veterinarians are needed. The positive aspects of this job should be emphasized to recruit and retain veterinarians in this field of the profession.

Keywords: mental health; COPSOQ III; veterinary authorities; survey; welfare controls; job satisfaction; psychosocial conditions; One Health; wellbeing

1. Introduction

The mental wellbeing of veterinarians is a cause for concern. Veterinarians more often suffer from stress and depression and are more likely to commit suicide than the general population [1,2]. This phenomenon has been observed for several decades worldwide [3–9].

However, the awareness, discussion, and research of this topic have focused on veterinarians working as practitioners. Concerning veterinarians working for the authorities in cities, districts, federal states, or federal ministries (hereafter referred to as official veterinarians), little is known. Additionally, official veterinarians might suffer from work-related mental health problems; for instance, two official veterinarians committed suicide in Germany in 2015, one after being threatened by farmers [10].

Official veterinarians provide several different functions in the context of One Health such as controlling compliance with laws and other regulations. In Germany, they ensure the health of humans by inspecting food of animal origin in slaughterhouses as well as in shops or restaurants, monitor infectious diseases in livestock and pets, and inspect households and farms to ensure animal welfare. Moreover, official veterinarians inspect or control animal by-products, animal experiments, veterinary pharmacies, and the trade of animals and food of animal origin at the border. In 2021, 10% of all veterinarians (3224 of 32,930) were employed as official veterinarians in Germany [11]. Worldwide, no current information is available on the field of work of 10 million veterinarians [12]. In 2003, approximately 25% of veterinarians worked for the government (also including veterinarians performing animal health services funded by the government [13]).

Several risk factors have been identified regarding the mental health of veterinarians working in practice. For instance, dealing with bereaved clients [14], long working hours [15], and performing euthanasia [7] are associated with distress, anxiety, and/or sadness. However, the working life of official veterinarians is different from that of practicing veterinarians; therefore, these factors may not fully apply to official veterinarians. For instance, official veterinarians do normally not perform euthanasia but may have to order and/or perform the culling of thousands of animals to control infectious diseases. In these as well as in other situations, official veterinarians are highly accountable and must weigh different interests and aspects. Unannounced controls concerning animal welfare or food safety are part of the everyday work for most official veterinarians, which can be stressful [16] as the situations are unforeseen. The persons facing these controls are often stressed and sometimes ready to use violence, such as when pet owners fear that their pet will be taken away or when farmers fear losing their livestock, which are their source of income and a part of their identity. In Germany, several attacks on official veterinarians have recently been reported. The most severe cases were caused by farmers: an official veterinarian was killed in 2015, two official veterinarians were injured with an iron rod in 2016, and an official veterinarian was shot in 2017 [17]. Official veterinarians often have to balance the interests of animals and humans, which can lead to moral distress [18]. Animal welfare incidents are often associated with the social, health, and/or psychological difficulties of the owners. Determining an adequate response is challenging for official veterinarians [19]. However, how strongly these factors influence the wellbeing of official veterinarians is unknown.

A second factor that might be demanding for official veterinarians is that all controls and conversations have to be documented to enable their use as proof in court proceedings. In addition, workload impacts the wellbeing of veterinarians as well as other types of employees [20,21]. The work tasks of official veterinarians have probably increased in the recent years due to different factors: new regulations that have been enacted, such as the Animal Health Law in 2021 [22]; more emphasis being placed on animal welfare; and, finally, the prevalence of new or reoccurring infectious diseases, e.g., the highly pathogenic avian influenza and African swine fever. In Germany, the veterinarian workload also increased in official veterinary service due to skills shortages and job vacancies [23,24]. All these factors, including high levels of responsibility, conflicts, requirements for court-proofed documentation, moral distress, and high workload, have presumably resulted in high job demands. However, scientific research on the demands faced by official veterinarians in their jobs is limited. Worldwide, to the best of our knowledge, only one scientific study has been conducted on the wellbeing of official veterinarians [16]. Ultimately, knowledge must be obtained to keep as many official veterinarians in their jobs as possible and to attract more veterinarians to these positions to ensure food safety, animal health, and animal welfare [24]. Therefore, the structural benefits and demands the professionals experience must be understood. As such, the aim of this study was to assess the status of the demands, social relationships, leadership, influences, and potential at work; conflicts and violence; as well as the job satisfaction and (mental) health of official veterinarians using the Copenhagen Psychosocial Questionnaire (COPSOQ III). Where possible, the results were compared with those of employees in other professions to identify differences. In particular, we hypothesized that official veterinarians experience high levels of cognitive and emotional demands and often experience conflicts and offensive behavior during their work. Finally, we analyzed whether the emotional and cognitive demands as well as the burnout symptoms differ between age groups, genders, persons in leadership positions, and different fields of work (animal welfare or others).

2. Materials and Methods

The questionnaire used in this study was developed from the third version of the Copenhagen Psychosocial Questionnaire (COPSOQ III) described by Burr et al. [25]. This questionnaire is a generic instrument used to assess the different dimensions of psychosocial conditions and is applicable for all kinds of jobs [25]. The COPSOQ III is not a ready-to-use questionnaire but a catalog of questions that are grouped into three different levels: core, middle, and long. For this study, all 31 core, 13 middle-level, and 38 long-level questions were used (Table S1). The questions belonged to the different dimensions of psychosocial conditions, e.g., *Job Satisfaction* and *Emotional Demands* [25]. The 82 questions used in this version were from 40 different dimensions. We used most of the items and the phrasing of the validated German Standard Version (GSV [26]). The GSV questions were supplemented using questions from the COPSOQ III that were considered relevant for the purposes of our study. In particular, questions relating to conflicts and offensive behavior were added. Participants were asked about their experiences in the last 12 months concerning gossip and slander, conflicts and quarrels, cyber bullying, sexual harassment, threats of violence, and physical violence. If a person reported that they experienced such behavior, they were asked by whom (owner of animals, food producer, coworker, supervisor, or someone else). Moreover, demographic information (gender, age, and federal state), information concerning professional experience and current workplace, and the availability and the attitude toward certain measures that might reduce work-related demands were requested. All questions except the open questions were mandatory. In total, the questionnaire comprised 139 questions and is available in Supplementary File S2 in the original language (German). The questionnaire was pretested by a colleague with expertise in psychology as well as by three official vets. Feedback was received either by email or voicemail. After the pretest, only minor changes were made.

This study's design and questionnaire were approved by the Ethics Committee of the Freie Universität Berlin (ZEA-Nr.: 2022-024). Each participant was informed of the aims of the study and that some questions might evoke memories of demanding situations. They were further informed of the personal-related data such as gender that would be collected. The possibility of quitting the survey without further consequences was mentioned. IP addresses or other individual-related data were not collected. All participants actively agreed to participate. The data of the participants were treated confidentially.

The questionnaire was implemented in LimeSurvey Cloud and was accessible via an internet link (https://vetepi.limesurvey.net/935244?lang=de accessed on 11 June 2024). A short introduction informed the participants concerning the aim of the study and data protection measures. Questions were displayed on 12 pages. At the end of the survey, the participants had the opportunity to provide comments. The survey was available from 1 November 2022 to 23 of January 2023. The invitation to participate was shared on a Facebook group of official veterinarians and was published in the Journal of the Veterinary Chamber in Germany. Moreover, the association of official veterinarians of

Germany (Bundesverband der beamteten Tierärzte e.V.) distributed the invitation via e-mail to their members.

The answers were exported to Microsoft Excel© (16.0) and imported to Statistical Analyses Software (SAS© Version 9.4), which was used for data handling as well as statistical analyses. Figures were created using Microsoft Excel© (16.0). The answers were checked for plausibility, where possible. The answers from persons who stated they did not work as an official veterinarian and those who did not complete at least half of the questionnaire were excluded.

All questions from the COPSOQ III were answered with a 5-point Likert scale, except the General Health item (1–10) and items of the *Self-Efficacy* dimension (4-point Likert scale). The categories were replaced with the equivalent numbers provided in the guideline (0-25-50-75-100 or 0-33-67-100) [24]. Then, the values of the dimensions were determined by calculating the mean over the corresponding items. For instance, for the *Role Conflicts* dimension, the mean of the answers to the questions "Are contradictory demands placed on you at work?" (item CO2; Table S1) and "Do you sometimes have to do things which seem to be unnecessary?" (item CO3) was calculated. Corresponding to the items, all dimensions ranged between 0 and 100. If an item was missing, the dimension was set to missing. As the questionnaire used in this study also included questions other than the those in the GSV, six dimensions were calculated in two different ways: first, including all items that were used in our study; second, including only those items that were used in the GSV [26] to ensure comparability to the reference data. For example, in our study, the *Emotional Demands* dimension included items ED1, EDX2, and ED3. ED1 was not part of the GSV. Therefore, we first calculated the dimension with all three items and second with only EDX2 and ED3 as in the GSV. The descriptive analyses included the mean and its 95% confidence interval. The means and confidence intervals were compared with those of a reference population [26], including at least 148,435 German employees. Statistical tests could not be conducted as the data were not freely available. For some data, the median as well as 25% (Q1) and 75% (Q3) percentiles were also calculated. The dimensions had one to four corresponding items (Supplementary File S1). Those dimensions consisting of only one item were not continuous as they could only contain the five different values. However, to ensure comparability, we followed the guideline but also reported the percentage of participants within each category. The Mann–Whitney U-test and Kruskal–Wallis test were used to identify differences between subgroups concerning different dimensions (e.g., gender and *Emotional Demands*). The associations between subgroups and categorical data (e.g., main field of work and experience with violence) were tested with chi square tests. p-values < 0.05 were regarded as statistically significant.

3. Results

3.1. Participants

Overall, 886 persons opened the survey and answered at least the first question. A total of 19 persons reported not working as an official veterinarian (defined as working for the government in the fields of animal welfare, food safety, infectious diseases, in the slaughterhouses, or having other responsibilities of authorities), and 28 persons did not finish at least half of the questionnaire. These persons as well as one other person who provided clearly wrong answers were excluded from further analyses. Therefore, the answers of 838 participants were analyzed. This represented 26% of the target population [11].

An average of 21 min was required to complete the questionnaire (median; Q1: 16 min; Q3: 30 min). The information on demographics and job characteristics is displayed in Table 1. Where possible, the percentage in the study was compared with that of the target population [11] or reference population [26]. Nearly 80% of participants were women, which is a higher proportion than in the target population. Two-thirds of the participants worked full-time. The percentage of civil servants was higher in the study population than in the target population, and 22% of the study participants were 55 years or older. The median work experience was 10 years (Q1: 4 years, Q3: 19 years). Most of the participants worked mainly in the field of animal welfare (Table 1). Approximately 41% (n = 348) of the participants reported performing a supervisory function for other official veterinarians.

Table 1. Demographic information and job description from a survey assessing the psychosocial conditions of official veterinarians (n = 838).

	n	Percentage	Percentage in Target Population [1]	Percentage in Reference Population [2]
Gender				
Female	658	78.5	69.7	48.3
Male	179	21.4		51.7
Diverse	1	0.1		
Age				
<35 years	106	12.7		28.7
35–44 years	288	34.4		29.9
45–54 years	258	30.8		17.7
>54 years	186	22.2		13.0
Employment				
Civil servant	403	48.1	33.3	
Employed (temporary or tenure)	437	51.0	66.7	
Miscellaneous	8	1.0		
Working hours				
Part-time	274	32.9		26.1
Full-time	560	67.2		73.9
Level				
State	12	1.4		
Federal state	28	3.3		
City or province	798	95.2		
Main field of work				
Animal welfare	368	43.9		
Food safety	176	21.0		
Infectious animal diseases	140	16.7		
Ante- and postmortem inspection procedures (slaughterhouse)	64	7.6		
Other	87	10.4		
Work on weekends or public holidays (≥once/month)				
Yes	309	36.9		44.1
No	529	63.1		55.9
Work during evening/night (≥once/week)				
Yes	224	26.7		41.2
No	614	73.3		55.9
Possibility of working from home				
Yes	392	46.8		
No	446	53.2		
Work on the road/inspections				
Yes	748	89.3		
No	90	10.7		

[1] Compared with all German official veterinarians (Bundestierärztekammer e.V. 2022 [11]). [2] Compared with a reference population of German employees in different professions (Lincke et al., 2021: COPSOQ III in Germany: validation of a standard instrument to measure psychosocial factors at work [26]; n: 148,435–254,551).

3.2. *Demands*

The descriptive results of the dimensions are shown in Table 2, and the comparison with the reference population is displayed in Figure 1. Most participants stated that their job was highly demanding: concerning the *Cognitive Demands* dimension, most participants reported to often or always have to track and remember many things and that they often or always have to make difficult decisions. This resulted in a mean value of 82 for *Cognitive Demands* (Table 2). The mean score of 71 for *Emotional Demands* was substantially higher than that the reference population (48; Figure 1). Further analyses were conducted for these two dimensions to gain deeper insights. The score for *Emotional Demands* did not vary among genders or age groups, but veterinarians working in animal welfare reported experiencing significantly higher emotional demands (Table 3). Veterinarians in a leadership position for other veterinarians reported higher levels in the *Cognitive Demands* dimension (Table 3). The main field of work did not influence the degree of strain.

Table 2. Descriptive analyses of psychosocial dimensions from survey of 838 German official veterinarians using COPSOQ III.

Dimension	Item [1]	Positive Value	*n*	Mean	STD
DEMANDS					
Work Pace	WP1, WP2	low	838	67.8	18.3
Quantitative Demands	QD2, QD3	low	838	75.1	22.8
Cognitive Demands	CD1, CD2, CD4	low	838	81.7	11.6
Emotional Demands	ED1, EDX2, ED3	low	838	66.0	16.5
Demands for Hiding Emotions	HE2	low	838	64.4	20.7
Work Privacy Conflicts	WF2, WF3	low	838	51.7	23.8
INFLUENCE AND POSSIBILITIES					
Influence at Work	INX1, IN3, IN4, IN6	high	836	55.9	15.4
Possibilities for Development	PD2, PD3	high	838	73.8	17.2
Control over Working Time	CT1, CT2, CT4, CT5 *	high	837	63.6	13.9
Meaning of Work	MW1	high	838	73.3	20.5
SOCIAL RELATIONSHIPS AND LEADERSHIP					
Predictability	PR1, PR2	high	838	53.4	20.2
Recognition	RE1	high	823	50.9	28.2
Role Clarity	CL1, CL3	high	838	60.3	20.3
Role Conflicts	CO2, CO3	low	838	48.0	21.8
Illegitimate Tasks	IT1	low	838	52.6	22.1
Quality of Leadership	QL2, QL3, QL4	high	798	46.8	25.3
Social Support from Supervisor	SSX2	high	809	65.7	28.7
Social Support from Colleagues	SC1	high	822	79.6	20.4
Sense of Community at Work	SW1	high	823	79.5	17.2
JOB SECURITY AND SATISFACTION					
Job Insecurity	JI1, JI3	low	822	17.1	21.0
Insecurity over Working Conditions	IW1	low	821	21.7	24.8

Table 2. *Cont.*

Dimension	Item [1]	Positive Value	*n*	Mean	STD
Job Satisfaction	JS1, JS4, JS5, JSX	high	820	60.9	17.2
Commitment to Workplace	CW1, CW2, CWX3	high	838	55.5	20.0
Work Engagement	WE2	high	814	45.7	23.3
(MENTAL) HEALTH					
Self-rated Health	GH2	high	813	6.3	1.8
Sleeping Troubles	SL1	low	814	56.1	26.3
Burnout	BO1, BO2, BO3	low	814	57.6	20.7
Stress	ST1, ST3	low	814	60.6	21.8
Somatic Stress	SO1, SO2	low	814	29.4	22.0
Cognitive Stress	CS1, CS3	low	814	42.3	20.1
Depressive Symptoms	DS1, DS2, DS3, DS4	low	814	37.3	21.0
Self-Efficacy	SE2, SE4	high	814	66.7	19.7

* reversed scale. [1] See Table S1 or COPSOQ Guideline (https://www.copsoq-network.org/guidelines; [27] accessed on 17 October 2023); STD: standard deviation.

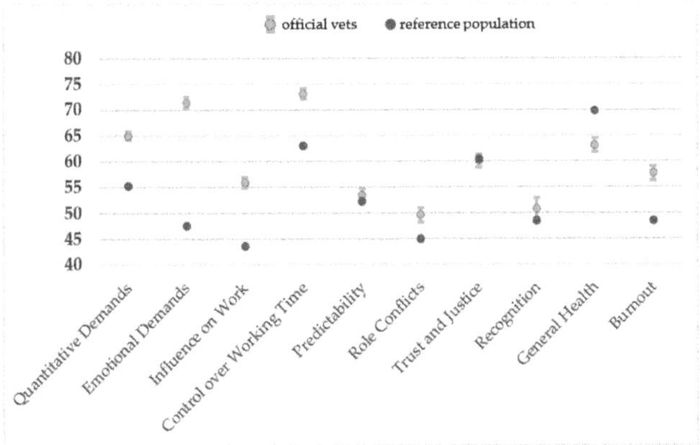

Figure 1. Means with 95% confidence intervals of scores for sociopsychological dimensions from a survey of official veterinarians in Germany (n: 813–838) compared with those of a reference population of German employees in different professions (Lincke et al. 2021: COPSOQ III in Germany: validation of a standard instrument to measure psychosocial factors at work [26]; n: 148,435–254,551); the dimensions included the following items: Quantitative Demands: WP1, WP2, QD2, QD3, CT5; Emotional Demands: EDX2, ED3, Influence at Work: INX1, IN3, IN4; CT: CT1, CT2; Predictability: PR1, PR2; CO: CO2, CO3, IT1; Trust and Justice: TM1, TMX2, JU1, JU4; Recognition: RE1; General Health: GH2*10; Burnout Symptoms: BO1, BO2, BO3; see Supplementary Table S1).

3.3. *Influences and Possibilities for Development*

The assessments concerning the *Influence at Work* and *Possibilities for Development* dimensions were relatively positive, with mean scores of 56 and 74, respectively (Table 2). This result means that, on average, the veterinarians often had a strong influence on decisions, and they often could influence what they performed and how they did it. However, they had less of an influence on the amount of work assigned to them (item IN3): here, 23%, 44%, 26%, and 8% of the participants answered "never/hardly ever", "seldom", "sometimes", and "often" or "always", respectively. The *Control over Working Time* dimension was assessed higher by the study population than by the reference population (Figure 1).

Moreover, the participants stated they worked less often at night and on the weekend than the reference population (Table 1). Additionally, the *Meaning of Work* dimension was positively assessed, as 41% and 28% of participants stated that they felt their work was meaningful "often" and "always", respectively.

Table 3. Differences in *Emotional Demands, Cognitive Demands,* and *Burnout Symptoms* dimensions according to gender, age group, and main field of work of 838 official German veterinarians.

	Emotional Demands					*Cognitive Demands*					*Burnout Symptoms*				
Category	*n*	Mean	LCI	UCI	*p*-Value	*n*	Mean	LCI	UCI	*p*-Value	*n*	Mean	LCI	UCI	*p*-Value
Sex															
Female	658	66.4	65.1	67.6	0.256	658	81.8	81.0	82.7	0.555	640	59.2	57.7	60.8	<0.001
Male	179	64.7	62.3	67.1		179	81.0	79.2	82.8		173	51.3	48.3	54.3	
Age															
<35 years	106	67.8	65.0	70.6	0.806	106	81.6	79.4	83.8	0.897	104	56.1	51.8	60.4	0.016
35–44 years	288	66.6	64.8	68.3		288	82.2	80.9	83.5		279	60.2	57.9	62.4	
45–54 years	258	65.3	63.1	67.5		258	81.4	79.9	82.8		253	58.9	55.9	61.0	
>54 years	186	65.3	62.9	67.7		186	81.2	79.5	83.0		178	53.1	50.0	56.3	
Main field of work															
Animal Welfare	106	70.7	69.3	72.2	<0.001	106	81.7	80.6	82.7	0.922	358	57.4	55.3	59.6	0.774
Else *	288	62.3	60.8	63.9		288	81.6	80.5	82.8		456	57.7	55.8	59.6	
Supervisor of other veterinarians															
Yes	348	68.0	66.3	69.6	0.006	348	84.3	83.2	85.4	<0.001	336	57.7	55.5	59.9	0.984
No	490	64.6	63.1	66.1		490	79.7	78.7	80.8		478	57.5	55.6	59.3	

* Includes infectious animal diseases, food safety, ante- and postmortem meat inspections, and miscellaneous.

3.4. *Social Relationships and Leadership*

Most participants reported always receiving social support from their colleagues if needed and described the working atmosphere with their colleagues (*Sense of Community at Work* dimension) as good (Table 2). The responses for the *Quality of Leadership, Social Support by the Supervisor,* and *Recognition by the Management* dimensions varied more than those for the other scales (Table 2). This finding indicates that some participants were satisfied with their supervisor, while others were not. The scores concerning the *Role Clarity, Role Conflicts, Illegitimate Tasks,* and *Organizational Justice* dimensions varied less, around 50 points. This means that most participants agreed only partly to terms such as "Do you receive all the information you need in order to do your work well?" or "Does your work have clear objectives?" (*Role Clarity* dimension). However, the assessments of the study population concerning the *Recognition, Role Conflicts, Predictability,* and *Trust and Justice* dimensions resembled those of the reference population (Figure 1).

3.5. *Job Security and Job Satisfaction*

The participants reported feeling rather secure concerning their employment (Table 2). This finding can be explained by the high percentage of civil servants participating in the study (Table 1).

Most participants stated that they were "satisfied" or "neither satisfied nor unsatisfied" with the different aspects of their work, resulting in a mean score of 61 on the *Job Satisfaction* dimension (Table 2). The answers varied concerning the different job aspects: 70% chose the answers "satisfied" or "very satisfied" concerning their salary, but only 42% were "satisfied" or "very satisfied" with their management.

Regarding workplace commitment, the agreement with the item "Do you enjoy telling others about your place of work?" was lower than that with the other two items. The reason for this finding might be that, in some cases, the information is confidential or other persons do not like to hear stories about animal abuse, slaughter, or hygiene deficiencies.

3.6. (Mental) Health

All questions concerning the health of the participants related to their general wellbeing during the last four weeks, as health status could be assigned to only personal or only work-related reasons, so this must be kept in mind when interpreting our results.

The assessment of the general health of the study population was slightly lower than that of the reference population (Figure 1), which might have been related to the study population being older (Table 1). However, the study population also scored higher in the *Burnout* dimension (Figure 1). The average *Burnout* score of 58 indicated that most of the participants reported feeling worn out and physically and emotionally exhausted (most) part of the time. Between 7% and 10% of the participants answered these questions with "all the time". The results of further analyses revealed that in contrast with cognitive and emotional demands, the *Burnout* assessment differed among genders and age groups but not concerning the job characteristics (Table 3). Women reported a higher level of *Burnout* symptoms than men, and persons in the age group 35–44 years reported a higher level of *Burnout* than those older than 54 years.

3.7. Conflicts and Offensive Behavior

More than half of the participants reported being involved in gossip and slander and more than 80% in conflicts and quarrels in the last 12 months (Figure 2). This was mostly the case with animal owners (61% and 68%) but also with colleagues (43% and 41%) or supervisors (20% and 24%; multiple choices possible).

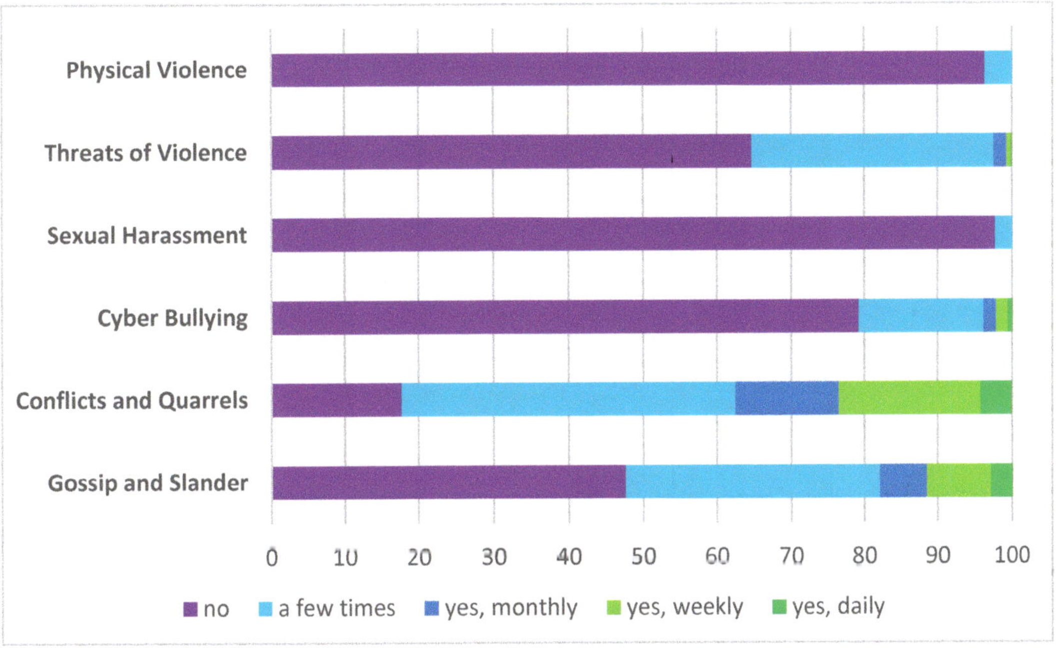

Figure 2. Experiences with concerning conflicts and offensive behavior in the last 12 months reported by official German veterinarians (*n* = 807) on a survey based on COPSOQ III.

A total of 19 persons reported that they had been sexually harassed by animal owners (*n* = 9), colleagues (n = 3), food producers (n = 2), supervisors (n = 2), and others (*n* = 3). Approximately one-third of participants (35%) reported experiencing threats of violence, 93% (*n* = 264 of 285) of them by animal owners and only rarely by food producers (*n* = 28) or others (*n* = 10). Veterinarians working mainly in the field of animal welfare were more likely to be threatened (53% vs. 21%, $p < 0.001$) than those working mainly in other fields. A total of 30 persons reported experiences with physical violence, 24 of whom were working mainly in animal welfare. The veterinarians were harmed by 6 food producers and 25 animal owners.

4. Discussion

Our findings showed that official veterinarians in Germany experienced high work demands but also strongly influenced their work. The relationship with supervisors/management differed, whereas the relationships with colleagues were good in most cases. Finally, more than one-third of the veterinarians reported experiences with threats of violence.

4.1. Study Design and Selection Bias

More than 800 official veterinarians participated in this study. However, as three-quarters of the target population did not respond, selection bias cannot be ruled out. The results of the comparison of the study population with the target population showed that women were more likely to participate. This phenomenon has also been observed in other studies [4,6,28]. The participation in an open online survey depends on the personal interest of the addressed persons. Women were maybe more likely to participate as they felt more addressed, because women are more likely to suffer from mental illnesses (gender gap in mental health [29]) and maybe also talk more openly about difficulties. Nevertheless, concerning cognitive and emotional demands, no differences were apparent between women and men. Different from other surveys among veterinarians [4,30,31], older veterinarians were not under-represented. The association of official veterinarians in Germany, which originally represented the official veterinarians employed as civil servants, distributed the link to our survey. This might be the reason why the participation from civil servants and thereby older persons was higher (Table 1). The results might thus overestimate the level of job security because civil servants were over-represented.

In general, the COPSOQ III is a well-established instrument used to assess different dimensions of psychosocial conditions among employees [25–27]. However, as the COPSOQ III is not a ready-to-use instrument, the surveys vary. Therefore, caution is warranted when comparing the results with those of other surveys, as dimensions with the same names might contain different items. We controlled for this problem by calculating the dimensions by following Lincke et al. [26]. We did not include all items of the GSV in our questionnaire to ensure the survey would not be too long. Therefore, the calculations for only a small proportion of dimensions were the same as those for the reference population. Due to the additional questions, survey completion required approximately 21 min to complete, a time span that should not be exceeded [32], as this might result in more dropouts and lower-quality answers [33].

4.2. Demands

Our results showed that official veterinarians in Germany experienced high job demands. A too-high workload for official veterinarians was also reported by Väärikkälä et al. [16]. Official veterinarians also reported experiencing higher emotional demands than the reference population (Table 3) and slightly higher demands than the employees working in healthcare, the social sector, and teaching and educating (mean = 69) [26]. These high demands might be caused by different circumstances: the official veterinary profession experiences a shortage of staff [24]. Due to the energy crisis and other factors, cities and districts are often in a precarious financial situation. Additionally, the workload presumably increased due to increases in the number of cases of animal neglect following inflation, new regulations such as the Animal Health Law, and the spread of African swine fever and avian influenza. Additionally, the increased workload could be an aftereffect of the COVID-19 pandemic. According to McKee et al. [34], approximately 50% of veterinarians in academic positions reported increased work as well as quantitative and emotional demands due to the COVID-19 pandemic.

A review by Stetina and Krouzecky [35] indicated a gender gap in mental health in veterinary medicine, as elsewhere: women veterinarians experience slightly higher demands [36], are more likely to use negative stress management practices [37], and suffer more often from suicidal ideation, which are more often related to the work situation [31]. In this study, the *Emotional* and *Cognitive Demands* dimensions did not vary among the genders or age groups. Even though different characteristics are assigned to the Baby Boomers, Generation X, and Generation Z [38], all generations of official veterinarians reported experiencing high emotional and cognitive demands. The results of our study contribute to preventing recriminations among genders and generations.

In contrast to these demographic factors, job characteristics significantly influenced the demands (Table 3). Welfare inspections, especially, were reported to be stressful [16]. In this study, veterinarians working mainly in animal welfare reported significantly higher emotional demands (Table 3). This finding is understandable as most of the conflicts, threats, and violence arose from situations involving animal owners. Moreover, veterinarians are confronted with both human and animal misery. Official veterinarians, as empathetic human beings, face challenges in dealing with human and animal suffering [39]. In the work of Devitt et al. [39], official veterinarians also reported an uncertainty: they felt unqualified to provide the necessary support to animal owners, e.g., in cases of farmers experiencing serious mental health problems. In contrast to persons working in, e.g., youth welfare services, knowledge regarding mental health and social support for a person in crisis is not yet always part of the education for official veterinarians in Germany. Here, courses and networks should be offered.

4.3. Influences and Possibilities for Development

Until now, research on the influences and possibilities for development and the control over working time of official veterinarians has been limited. In the work of Väärikkälä et al. [16], 70% of veterinarians reported working from home. In this study, the percentage was substantially lower (Table 1), even though our study was conducted after the COVID-19 pandemic, which increased the possibilities of working from home. The *Possibilities for Development* dimension consisted of two questions concerning the ability to use available expertise and to learn new things. The work of an official veterinarian is highly specialized, and regulations and conditions changing over time explain the relatively high scores (Table 2). The participants also rated their work as meaningful. Meaning and purpose are important drivers of work engagement, especially for Generation Z [40].

4.4. Social Relationships and Leadership

The relationships with colleagues were rated as good in most cases, whereas those with the supervisor and management differed among participants (Table 2). We obtained results similar to those of a survey of veterinarians employed in various fields of work [41]: whereas a good working atmosphere and good relationships with colleagues were mentioned the most often as positive aspects of work, the relationship with the employer/supervisor was reported as being sometimes difficult. In most studies on the stress and mental health of veterinarians, the relationships with colleagues and supervisors were not analyzed or reported [1]. Here, further research is needed because positive social relationships and support from supervisors and colleagues contribute to coping with stress: Väärikkälä et al. [16] found that support availability was associated with a higher work commitment, less feelings of loneliness, and even fewer sleeping disorders.

4.5. Job Security and Job Satisfaction

The veterinarians in this study felt secure in their positions probably due to the shortage of skilled labor and their long-term employment. This security is presumably a driver for this field of the profession, e.g., as long-term work contracts are rarely available in the academic field of veterinary medicine [41].

The overall job satisfaction reported in this study (Table 2, mean = 61) mirrors the job satisfaction of the reference population (mean = 63; [26]). Notably, the job satisfaction scale in the work of Lincke et al. [26] included three additional questions. Therefore, the comparability of these results is limited. In a recent study, the job satisfaction of veterinarians working in the noncurative sector was higher than that of those working in practice in Germany [41]. This finding can be explained by two factors: a higher salary and less time providing on-call services [42]. However, veterinarians might be less attracted by the salary for official services as salaries in the curative sector rise, which could be a reason for the shortage of younger official veterinarians.

4.6. Conflicts and Offensive Behavior

One of the motivations of this study was to assess the level of offensive behavior experienced by official veterinarians. In the work of Väärikkälä et al. [16], 88% of the participants experienced threatening situations during work in the previous 12 months. In our study, "only" 53% of official veterinarians working in animal welfare reported having been threatened. This difference might have multiple reasons: First, the definition of being threatened may vary among individuals and societies. Second, the wording or translation of the question might have biased the results. However, with an incidence of 30 physical attacks in 12 months, official veterinarians regularly experienced violence. Here, further research is needed concerning measures to prevent these events and to protect and support official veterinarians during and after their work. As an insight from this study, participants also assessed the availability and usefulness of certain measures (manuscript under preparation).

5. Conclusions

This is one of the first studies on the wellbeing of official veterinarians ensuring animal welfare, food safety, and control of infectious diseases and performing other tasks for veterinary public health. This study showed high job demand levels for official veterinarians in Germany. Moreover, those working mainly in animal welfare regularly experienced offensive behavior. Further insights are needed into how these demands influence job satisfaction and mental health. Additional approaches to support veterinarians during their work are necessary. Finally, further research is needed to explore similarities to and differences from the psychosocial situations of the official veterinarians in other countries.

Concerning the relationship with management/supervisors, further analyses including free-text answers or subsequent qualitative studies might provide further insight regarding the sources of problems and cooperation.

Positive organizational behavior (POB) focuses not on the weaknesses or mental illnesses of employees but, following the lead of positive psychology, on strengths and resources. Thereby, employees are not just prevented from experiencing mental illness but hopefully gain satisfaction, self-efficacy, and security within their jobs. The positive aspects of the work of official veterinarians in this study were the atmosphere and support from colleagues. Moreover, most participants experienced their work as meaningful and felt secure concerning their employment. These aspects should be highlighted to motivate veterinarians to work in this field. By reducing the demands and strengthening the positive aspects, more official veterinarians can hopefully be recruited and retained, thereby helping to ensure animal health, welfare, and food safety.

Supplementary Materials: The following supporting information can be downloaded at: https://www.mdpi.com/article/10.3390/ani14131975/s1, Table S1: Questions from the COPSOQ III used in this survey assessing the psychosocial situation of official veterinarians in Germany; File S2: Questionnaire in German.

Author Contributions: Conceptualization, K.C.J. and R.M.; methodology, K.C.J. and R.M.; software, K.C.J.; validation, K.C.J.; formal analysis, K.C.J.; investigation, K.C.J., data curation, K.C.J.; writing—original draft preparation, K.C.J.; writing—review and editing, K.C.J. and R.M.; visualization, K.C.J.; supervision, R.M. All authors have read and agreed to the published version of the manuscript.

Funding: The publication of this article was funded by Freie Universität Berlin. We acknowledge support by the Open Access Publication Fund of the Freie Universität Berlin for the publication.

Institutional Review Board Statement: This study was conducted in accordance with the Declaration of Helsinki and approved by the Ethics Committee of the Freie Universität Berlin (ZEA-Nr.: 2022-024).

Informed Consent Statement: Informed consent was obtained from all subjects involved in the study. Participation in this survey was voluntary and could be canceled at any time without any consequences. In addition to demographic information, this survey also collected data regarding personal situation. Names, IP addresses, or other information that can be attributed to an individual were not collected. The stored data were used exclusively for scientific purposes and will not be passed on to third parties. Only the persons directly involved in this study have access to the data. The data collected will be stored in accordance with the requirements of Good Scientific Practice (GWP) for at least 10 years in an access-protected manner and will not be passed on to third parties. In accordance with Art. 17 of the GDPR, every participant has the right to have the respective personal data that were collected in connection with this survey, and data that could be clearly assigned to a person were deleted. There is also the right to have data corrected retrospectively (Art. 13 para. 2 lit. B GDPR). However, as this survey was anonymized, this is not possible.

Data Availability Statement: The data presented in this study are available on request from the corresponding author due to privacy reasons.

Acknowledgments: We thank all persons who participated in this study. We also thank Holger Vogel and Miriam Larsson from the Bundesverband beamteter Tierärzte e.V. for the distribution of the survey and their helpful comments.

Conflicts of Interest: The authors declare no conflicts of interest.

References

1. Pohl, R.; Botscharow, J.; Böckelmann, I.; Thielmann, B. Stress and strain among veterinarians: A scoping review. *Ir. Vet. J.* **2022**, *75*, 15. [CrossRef] [PubMed]
2. Moir, F.M.; van den Brink, A. Current insights in veterinarians' psychological wellbeing. *N. Z. Vet. J.* **2020**, *68*, 3–12. [CrossRef]
3. Chan, C.K.Y.; Wong, P.W.C. Predictors of Suicide Risk and Mental Health Outcomes among Hong Kong Veterinarians: A Cross-Sectional Study. *Behav. Sci.* **2023**, *13*, 770. [CrossRef] [PubMed]
4. Schwerdtfeger, K.A.; Bahramsoltani, M.; Spangenberg, L.; Hallensleben, N.; Glaesmer, H. Depression, suicidal ideation and suicide risk in German veterinarians compared with the general German population. *Vet. Rec.* **2020**, *186*, e2. [CrossRef]
5. Mellanby, R.J. Incidence of suicide in the veterinary profession in England and Wales. *Vet. Rec.* **2005**, *157*, 415–417. [CrossRef]
6. Nett, R.J.; Witte, T.K.; Holzbauer, S.M.; Elchos, B.L.; Campagnolo, E.R.; Musgrave, K.J.; Carter, K.K.; Kurkjian, K.M.; Vanicek, C.F.; O'Leary, D.R.; et al. Risk factors for suicide, attitudes toward mental illness, and practice-related stressors among US veterinarians. *J. Am. Vet. Med. Assoc.* **2015**, *247*, 945–955. [CrossRef]
7. Deponti, P.S.; Jaguezeski, A.M.; Pulgatti, D.H.V.; Soares, J.C.M.; Da Cecim, M.S. Veterinarian's perceptions of animal euthanasia and the relation to their own mental health. *Cienc. Rural* **2023**, *53*, e20210578. [CrossRef]
8. Chigerwe, M.; Holm, D.E.; Mostert, E.-M.; May, K.; Boudreaux, K.A. Exploring issues surrounding mental health and wellbeing across two continents: A preliminary cross-sectional collaborative study between the University of California, Davis, and University of Pretoria. *PLoS ONE* **2020**, *15*, e0241302. [CrossRef]
9. Hatch, P.H.; Winefield, H.R.; Christie, B.A.; Lievaart, J.J. Workplace stress, mental health, and burnout of veterinarians in Australia. *Aust. Vet. J.* **2011**, *89*, 460–468. [CrossRef]
10. Jaeger, M. Tod Einer Amtstierärztin: Kampfzone Stall. Frankfurter Allgemeine Zeitung [Online]. 11 August 2015. Available online: https://www.faz.net/aktuell/politik/inland/warum-sich-amtstieraerztin-anya-rackow-umgebracht-hat-13741670.html (accessed on 21 March 2024).
11. Bundestierärztekammer, e.V. Statistik 2021: Tierärzteschaft in der Bundesrepublik Deutschland. Deutsches Tierärzteblatt [Online]. 2022. Available online: https://www.bundestieraerztekammer.de/btk/statistik/downloads/2021.pdf (accessed on 15 November 2023).

12. WOAH. *Implementation of WOAH Standards: The Observatory Annual Report*; Publication Series; World Organisation for Animal Health: Paris, France, 2022; 149p. [CrossRef]
13. Kouba, V. Public Service Veterinarians Worldwide: A Quantitative Analysis. *Acta Vet. Brno* **2005**, *74*, 455–461. [CrossRef]
14. Dow, M.Q.; Chur-Hansen, A.; Hamood, W.; Edwards, S. Impact of dealing with bereaved clients on the psychological wellbeing of veterinarians. *Aust. Vet. J.* **2019**, *97*, 382–389. [CrossRef] [PubMed]
15. Shirangi, A.; Fritschi, L.; Holman, C.D.J.; Morrison, D. Mental health in female veterinarians: Effects of working hours and having children. *Aust. Vet. J.* **2013**, *91*, 123–130. [CrossRef] [PubMed]
16. Väärikkälä, S.; Hänninen, L.; Nevas, M. Veterinarians Experience Animal Welfare Control Work as Stressful. *Front. Vet. Sci.* **2020**, *7*, 77. [CrossRef]
17. Landesregierung NRW. Antwort auf Die Kleine Anfrage 1861 vom 19.12.2018: Was tut Die Landesregierung um Unsere Amtsveterinäre zu Schützen? Available online: https://www.landtag.nrw.de/portal/WWW/dokumentenarchiv/Dokument/MMD17-5009.pdf (accessed on 20 October 2022).
18. Arbe Montoya, A.I.; Hazel, S.; Matthew, S.M.; McArthur, M.L. Moral distress in veterinarians. *Vet. Rec.* **2019**, *185*, 631. [CrossRef] [PubMed]
19. Devitt, C.; Kelly, P.; Blake, M.; Hanlon, A.; More, S.J. Dilemmas experienced by government veterinarians when responding professionally to farm animal welfare incidents in Ireland. *Vet. Rec. Open* **2014**, *1*, e000003. [CrossRef] [PubMed]
20. Glaser, D.N.; Tatum, B.C.; Nebeker, D.M.; Sorenson, R.C.; Aiello, J.R. Workload and social support: Effects on performance and stress. *Human Perform.* **1999**, *12*, 155–176. [CrossRef]
21. MacDonald, W. The impact of job demands and workload on stress and fatigue. *Aust. Psychol.* **2003**, *38*, 102–117. [CrossRef]
22. European Commission. Regulation (EU) 2016/429 of the European Parliament and of the Council of 9 March 2016 on Transmissible Animal Diseases and Amending and Repealing Certain Acts in the Area of Animal Health: Animal Health Law. Available online: https://eur-lex.europa.eu/EN/legal-content/summary/the-eu-animal-health-law.html (accessed on 13 July 2023).
23. Bundesinformationszentrum Landwirtschaft. Wie Oft Werden Tierhaltende Betriebe Kontrolliert? Available online: https://www.landwirtschaft.de/diskussion-und-dialog/tierhaltung/wie-oft-werden-tierhaltende-betriebe-kontrolliert (accessed on 13 July 2023).
24. Wanke, M. Eklatanter Personalmangel Gefährdet Tierwohl in Schlachtbetrieben und Regionale Lebensmittelproduktion. Available online: https://www.amtstierarzt.de/pressemitteilungen/1754-eklatanter-personalmangel-gefaehrdet-tierwohl-in-schlachtbetrieben-und-regionale-lebensmittelproduktion (accessed on 13 July 2023).
25. Burr, H.; Berthelsen, H.; Moncada, S.; Nübling, M.; Dupret, E.; Demiral, Y.; Oudyk, J.; Kristensen, T.S.; Llorens, C.; Navarro, A.; et al. The Third Version of the Copenhagen Psychosocial Questionnaire. *Saf. Health Work.* **2019**, *10*, 482–503. [CrossRef] [PubMed]
26. Lincke, H.-J.; Vomstein, M.; Lindner, A.; Nolle, I.; Häberle, N.; Haug, A.; Nübling, M. COPSOQ III in Germany: Validation of a standard instrument to measure psychosocial factors at work. *J. Occup. Med. Toxicol.* **2021**, *16*, 50. [CrossRef]
27. Llorens, C.; Pérez-Franco, J.; Oudyk, J.; Berthelsen, H.; Dupret, E.; Nübling, M.; Burr, H.; Moncada, S. COPSOQ III. Guidelines and Questionnaire. Available online: https://www.copsoq-network.org/assets/Uploads/COPSOQ-network-guidelines-an-questionnaire-COPSOQ-III-180821.pdf (accessed on 17 October 2023).
28. Perret, J.L.; Best, C.O.; Coe, J.B.; Greer, A.L.; Khosa, D.K.; Jones-Bitton, A. Prevalence of mental health outcomes among Canadian veterinarians. *J. Am. Vet. Med. Assoc.* **2020**, *256*, 365–375. [CrossRef]
29. Campbell, O.L.K.; Bann, D.; Patalay, P. The gender gap in adolescent mental health: A cross-national investigation of 566,829 adolescents across 73 countries. *SSM-Popul. Health* **2021**, *13*, 100742. [CrossRef]
30. Jensen, K.; Schulte-Bahrenberg, S.; Blaschka, C.; Brandebusemeyer, E.; Ewert, M.; Menzel, A.; Munzel, J.; Steingräber, L.; Niggemann, J.; Damhuis, L.; et al. Befragung angestellter Tierärztinnen in Deutschland—Teil 1: Arbeitsbedingungen. *Berl. Und Münchener Tierärztliche Wochenschr.* **2022**, *135*, 1–15. [CrossRef]
31. Dalum, H.S.; Tyssen, R.; Hem, E. Prevalence and individual and work-related factors associated with suicidal thoughts and behaviours among veterinarians in Norway: A cross-sectional, nationwide survey-based study (the NORVET study). *BMJ Open* **2022**, *12*, e055827. [CrossRef] [PubMed]
32. Revilla, M.; Ochoa, C. Ideal and maximum length for a web survey. *Int. J. Mark. Res.* **2017**, *59*, 5.
33. Galesic, M.; Bosnjak, M. Effects of Questionnaire Length on Participation and Indicators of Response Quality in a Web Survey. *Public. Opin. Q.* **2009**, *73*, 349–360. [CrossRef]
34. McKee, H.; Gohar, B.; Appleby, R.; Nowrouzi-Kia, B.; Hagen, B.N.M.; Jones-Bitton, A. High Psychosocial Work Demands, Decreased Well-Being, and Perceived Well-Being Needs Within Veterinary Academia During the COVID-19 Pandemic. *Front. Vet. Sci.* **2021**, *8*, 746716. [CrossRef] [PubMed]
35. Stetina, B.U.; Krouzecky, C. Reviewing a Decade of Change for Veterinarians: Past, Present and Gaps in Researching Stress, Coping and Mental Health Risks. *Animals* **2022**, *12*, 3199. [CrossRef] [PubMed]
36. Mastenbroek, N.J.J.M.; Demerouti, E.; van Beukelen, P.; Muijtjens, A.M.M.; Scherpbier, A.J.J.A.; Jaarsma, A.D.C. Measuring potential predictors of burnout and engagement among young veterinary professionals; construction of a customised questionnaire (the Vet-DRQ). *Vet. Rec.* **2014**, *174*, 168. [CrossRef]
37. Emmett, L.; Aden, J.; Bunina, A.; Klaps, A.; Stetina, B.U. Feminization and Stress in the Veterinary Profession: A Systematic Diagnostic Approach and Associated Management. *Behav. Sci.* **2019**, *9*, 114. [CrossRef]

38. Kapoor, C.; Solomon, N. Understanding and managing generational differences in the workplace. *WW Hosp. Tour. Themes* **2011**, *3*, 308–318. [CrossRef]
39. Devitt, C.; Kelly, P.; Blake, M.; Hanlon, A.; More, S.J. Veterinarian challenges to providing a multi-agency response to farm animal welfare problems in Ireland: Responding to the human factor. *Rev. Sci. Tech.* **2013**, *32*, 657–668. [CrossRef] [PubMed]
40. Scholz, C.; Grotefend, L.-D. (Eds.) *Generations Z in Europe: Generation Z in Germany: The (Un)Typical German?* Emerald Publishing Limited: Leeds, UK, 2019; ISBN 978-1-78973-492-8.
41. Jensen, K.C.; Blaschka, C.; Brandebusemeyer, E.; Hülsebusch, A.; Munzel, J.; Niggemann, J.; Steingräber, L.; Remien, D.; Wunderlich, C.; Schulte-Bahrenberg, S. Befragung angestellter Tierärztinnen in Deutschland—Teil 2: Arbeitszufriedenheit. *Berl. Und Münchener Tierärztliche Wochenschr.* **2022**, *135*, 1–18. [CrossRef]
42. Ewert, M. Untersuchung der Arbeitsumstände und Zufriedenheit Nicht-Kurativ Tätiger Tiermediziner*Innen in Deutschland (2018). PhD. Thesis, Freie Universität Berlin, Berlin, Germany, 2021.

animals

MDPI

Article

Evaluation of the Role of Veterinarians for Outcomes Related to the Health and Production of Dairy Small Ruminants in Greece

Daphne T. Lianou and George C. Fthenakis *

Veterinary Faculty, University of Thessaly, 43100 Karditsa, Greece
* Correspondence: gcf@vet.uth.gr

Simple Summary: This study, which was carried out as a large-scale investigation in 444 farms throughout Greece, explores the beneficial effects to small ruminant dairy farms of a steady and professional relationship with a veterinarian. The findings of detailed analyses indicated that, in summary, these benefits related to lower parasitic burden in animals of the farms and higher production of better-quality milk, as shown by the assessment of outcomes related to the health and production of animals. Moreover, the welfare of the animals in the farms was also improved, as evidenced by the lower incidence of painful diseases (e.g., clinical mastitis) and the effective use of relevant pharmaceutical products (e.g., non-steroid inflammatory drugs). The results attest that the application of veterinary advice and veterinary clinical services in sheep and goat dairy farms contributes to the improved health, production and welfare of animals.

Abstract: The objective of the present study was to evaluate the potential benefits of veterinarians in improving the health and welfare of dairy sheep and goats by studying the associations of management practices employed in the farms with production- or health-related outcomes in sheep and goat farms in Greece. This work explored associations with 'professional relationship with a veterinarian' at 444 small ruminant dairy farms in an investigation performed around Greece, where 106 variables, related to infrastructure, animals, production outcomes, health management, health problems and human resources, were assessed. In 384 (86.5%) farms, a professional relationship with a veterinarian was maintained. The median value of visits made annually by veterinarians to these farms was five. In farms with a professional relationship with a veterinarian, significant differences were found in 24 variables (35.8%) related to management practices and 6 (30.0%) production- or health-related outcomes. In multivariable analysis, the following emerged with a significant association: epg counts in faecal samples ($p = 0.014$), average annual milk production per ewe/doe ($p = 0.015$), somatic cell counts in bulk-tank milk ($p = 0.037$), and annual incidence of clinical mastitis ($p = 0.044$). Moreover, associations of the characteristics of veterinarians emerged with somatic cell counts in bulk-tank milk: the gender ($p < 0.0001$) and the age ($p = 0.004$) of the veterinarians. The results attest that the application of veterinary advice and clinical services in sheep and goat dairy farms contributes to the improved health, production and welfare of animals.

Keywords: epg counts; farmer; mastitis; veterinarian; veterinary practice; veterinary profession; veterinary specialisation

1. Introduction

Veterinarians can play a role in improving the health and welfare of small ruminants through the control of diseases in the farms by means of investigation of problems occurring therein and the application of various (preventive or reactive) interventions. Within their professional capacity, veterinarians are important stakeholders for the welfare of animals, in all their professional roles. For example, in the role of government officials, they participate in the formulation of welfare standards for the transport and slaughter of animals and thus create and assess the standards for a safe food supply to people; they also participate in the creation of codes of conduct for veterinarians, farmers, etc., to address the care of farm animals. In the role of academics, they are responsible for teaching animal welfare, as well as improving animal health, to undergraduate students. In the role of practitioners, they are responsible for explaining to farmers, animal carers and their clients, the importance of animal welfare and to educate them about the necessity to improve animal health and welfare, which is reflected in the quality of the meat and milk produced and ultimately in the income of the farms.

A recent (September 2021) topical search in the Web of Science, using the terms '[improv* AND veterinary*] AND [sheep OR goat*] AND [welfare]' (* is used as a truncation symbol), revealed 73 relevant articles.

Veterinary interventions in small ruminant farms contribute to improving health and welfare of the animals therein. Examples of such interventions include the management of obstetrical problems [1,2], the control of ectoparasitic infestations (psoroptic mange [3–5] and cutaneous myiosis [3,6]), the establishment of veterinarian-related practices as welfare indicators in farms [7,8], the monitoring of biosecurity practices in farms [9–11], the improvement in neonatal survival [2], the control of foot-related lameness [12,13], the administration of local anaesthesia as a means of pain management [14,15], the development of guidelines for handling sheep and goats [16], and the regularisation of welfare requirements in small ruminant farms [17].

Notably, 35 of these articles (47.9%) have been published during the last five years, i.e., since August 2018, thus indicating the increasing interest in the topic. However, most of these studies have been carried out in countries with meat-production sheep farming systems: 21 (28.8%) in the United Kingdom and another 22 (30.1%) in other countries. In contrast, only 16 (21.1%) papers have originated from Mediterranean countries and referred to dairy production systems, indicating the paucity of relevant studies for dairy small ruminant farms.

Veterinary work with small ruminants occupies around 21% of the overall time of veterinarians in Europe [18], with the lowest proportion in Russia (6%) and the highest in Iceland (55%). In fact, small ruminant work is the third most important area of focus of veterinarians in the continent, after small animal and cattle work [18]. Hence, there is interest in understanding the benefits that veterinarians may bring to farms with which they have a professional association.

The objective of the present study was to evaluate the potential benefits of veterinarians in improving the health and welfare of dairy sheep and goats by studying associations with management practices employed in the farms and with production- or health-related outcomes in sheep and goat farms in Greece.

2. Materials and Methods

2.1. Study Design—Collection of Samples and Information

A large countrywide study was performed in 444 small ruminant farms in Greece (325 sheep flocks and 119 goat herds) (Figure 1). The farms were selected on a convenience basis, which referred to the eagerness and consent of the farmers to receive a visit for an interview and collection of samples. All farms were visited by the investigators in order to obtain information and samples. In total, these farms included 110,228 sheep and 30,192 goats [19].

Initially, an interview of the farmer was carried out, always by the same investigator (author D.T.L.). The senior investigator (author G.C.F.) introduced the interviewer to the farmer; he informed the farmers about her identity and her employment, as well as about the objectives of this study [19]. A detailed interview was carried out with the farmer, using a standardised, structured questionnaire, which included questions regarding infrastructure, animals, production outcomes, health management, health problems and human resources in the farm [19].

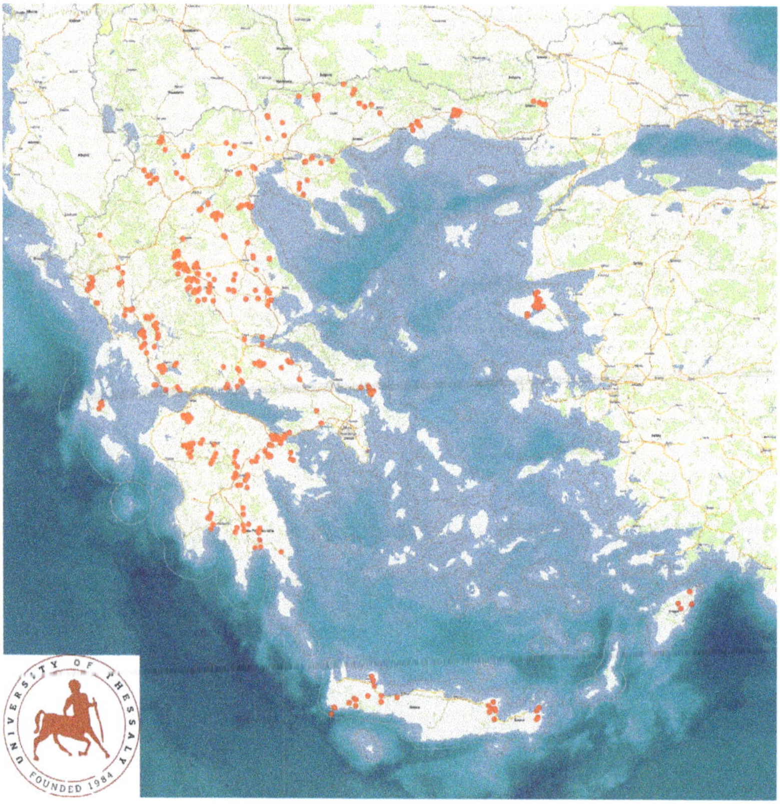

Figure 1. Locations (red dots) of 444 small ruminant dairy farms around Greece, in the 13 administrative regions of the country, which were visited during the countrywide investigation.

Then, on each farm visited, 25 female animals were randomly selected for body condition score evaluation. In order to adhere to the relevant standards [20] and to achieve uniformity of measurements, scoring (0–5, including half scores) was always performed by a certified European Veterinary Specialist in Small Ruminant Health Management.

Subsequently, samples from the bulk-tank milk of the farm were collected for further examinations. Bulk-tank milk samples were obtained for cytological, chemical and bacteriological examination by using aseptic methodology. The samples were collected using sterile plastic single-use pipettes, which were immersed into the tank to withdraw them [21].

Finally, faecal samples were collected directly from the rectum of adult female animals on the farms [21]. In each flock or herd, 20, 30, 40 or 50 ewes of female goats (for farms with ≤165, 166–330, 331–500 or >500 females, respectively) were selected for sampling.

2.2. *Laboratory Examinations*

Initially, bulk-tank milk samples were processed within 4 h of collection for somatic cell counting and measurement of milk composition (fat, protein, added water) by means of an automated counter, as detailed before [21].

Then, they were examined using microbiological techniques for total bacterial counting and for isolation of *Staphylococcus* spp. and *Listeria* spp. [21]. All staphylococcal isolates obtained were subjected to assessment for the detection of antibiotic resistance by employing the automated system BD Phoenix™ M50 [21].

Faecal samples were pooled and the McMaster technique was performed in quadruplicate samples obtained from these samples [21].

2.3. Data Management and Analysis

Data were entered into Microsoft Excel and analysed using SPSS v. 21 (IBM Analytics, Armonk, NY, USA). Initially, the farms were allocated into one of two cohorts: those that maintained a regular and professional relationship with veterinarians, or those that did not. In this context, 'professional relationship' referred to a stable, non-contractual, association with a veterinarian, who, in full accord with and by applying all the relevant professional veterinary conduct codes [22,23], was providing veterinary advice and clinical services in relation to the health and welfare of the animals in the farms.

Univariable analyses were performed initially. A 'professional relationship with a veterinarian' (as defined hereabove) at the farms was considered. A total of 106 variables were assessed (Table A1) and univariable analyses were performed. Comparisons between the results obtained for farms with or without a 'professional relationship with a veterinarian' were made by using the appropriate statistical methods, specifically, Pearson's chi-squared test, Fisher exact test, z-test for proportions, analysis of variance or Mann–Whitney test, as appropriate. Then, parameters related to management practices and to production- or health-related outcomes that were found with a significance of $p < 0.10$ in the above analysis were further evaluated within the cohort of farms with a 'professional relationship with a veterinarian' for potential associations with the gender and the age of the veterinarians, as well as with the annual frequency of veterinary visits to the farm. For the evaluations for potential associations with the gender of the veterinarians, the same techniques as above were used as appropriate. For the evaluations for potential associations with the age of the veterinarians and the frequency of veterinary visits, Spearman's rank correlation was employed.

The above were then followed by multivariable analyses. For the identification of potential associations of a 'professional relationship with a veterinarian' with production- or health-related outcomes, a multivariable model was constructed; variables (production- or health-related outcomes) found with $p < 0.2$ in the preceding univariable analysis were included into this model. Progressively, variables included into the multivariable model were removed from the model by using backwards elimination. The likelihood ratio test was performed to assess the p-value of each parameter; among those found with $p \geq 0.2$, the one with the largest p was removed from the model. The procedure was repeated, until no variable with $p \geq 0.2$ could be removed from the model [24]. The variables included in the final multivariable model constructed are in Table S1. After identifying in the multivariable analysis the production- or health-related outcomes that were significantly associated with the 'professional relationship with a veterinarian', a further multivariable analysis was performed to study associations with the gender and the age of the veterinarians, as well as with the annual frequency of veterinary visits to a farm for each of these outcomes. The variables included in the final multivariable models constructed are in Table S1.

For the results of somatic cell counts and total bacterial counts in milk, appropriate transformations to normalise the data were performed before the analysis [25,26]. For the evaluation of epg counts, only results from farms in which anthelmintic administration had not been performed during the two months prior to sampling (n = 369) were taken into account.

In all analyses, statistical significance was defined at $p < 0.05$.

3. Results

3.1. Descriptive Results

Of the 444 farms visited, in 384 (86.5%, 95% confidence interval (CI): 83.0–89.4%), the farmers indicated that they maintained a professional relationship with a veterinarian. The median value of visits made annually by veterinarians to these farms was 5 (interquartile range: 7).

Veterinary visits were also made to farms where farmers indicated that they did not maintain a professional relationship with a veterinarian. Nevertheless, their frequency was significantly lower; the median value of visits made annually by veterinarians to such farms was 2 (0.25) ($p < 0.0001$).

3.2. *Characteristics of Veterinarians Associated with the Farms Visited*

In total, the farmers maintained a professional relationship with 47 different veterinarians, 17 (36.2%) females and 30 (63.8%) males. The average age of these veterinarians was 42.8 ± 1.5 years.

Male veterinarians were significantly older than females: mean age was 45.4 ± 1.9 years versus 38.1 ± 2.1 years, respectively ($p = 0.019$). Among veterinarians younger than 35 years, there were more females (58.3%), whilst among veterinarians older than 50 years, there were more males (85.7%).

There was no difference between female and male veterinarians in the number of visits made to the farms annually: 5 (7) versus 5 (6.5), respectively ($p = 0.82$).

Most of the veterinarians ($n = 29$, 61.7%) were graduates of the Faculty of Veterinary Medicine of the Aristotle University of Thessaloniki, and fewer ($n = 13$, 28.7%) were graduates of the Veterinary Faculty of the University of Thessaly, whilst a smaller number were graduates of veterinary Faculties of other European countries ($n = 5$, 10.6%). Notably, 17 of the veterinarians (36.2%) had followed some postgraduate training in farm animal health management and diseases.

3.3. *Differences between Farms with or without a Professional Relationship with a Veterinarian*

The detailed results of the univariable analysis for the 106 variables are shown in Table S2. A significant difference between farms with or without a professional association with a veterinarian was found for 38 variables (Table A2).

With regard to variables related to management practices, there was a significant difference in farms with a professional relationship with a veterinarian for 24 (35.8%) practices; further, there was a tendency for significance for 8 (11.9%) practices (Table 1).

Table 1. Summary of the significance in variables related to management practices and production- or health-related outcomes found in 444 small ruminant farms in Greece, in accord with professional relationship with a veterinarian.

Type of Variables	**Difference between Farms with or without Professional Relationship with a Veterinarian in Number of Variables**		
	Significant [1]	**Tending for Significance** [2]	**Not Significant** [3]
Health management	8	2	9
Pharmaceutical treatment	3	0	4
Biosecurity management	2	2	4
Reproductive management	5	3	10
Management in the milking parlour	1	0	5
Nutritional management	5	1	3
Production-related outcomes	2	0	3
Health-related outcomes	3	1	10
Animal condition outcomes	1	0	0
Total	30 variables	9 variables	48 variables

[1]: $p < 0.05$; [2]: $0.05 \leq p < 0.10$; [3]: $p \geq 0.10$.

With regard to production- or health-related outcomes, there was a significant difference in farms with a professional relationship with a veterinarian for six (30.0%) outcomes, and there was a tendency for significance for one (5.0%) outcome (Tables 1 and 2).

Table 2. Production- or health-related outcomes found with a significant association with professional relationship with a veterinarian in this countrywide cross-sectional study in 444 small ruminant farms in Greece.

Farms in Which There Was a Professional Relationship with a Veterinarian (n = 384)	Farms in Which There Was No Professional Relationship with a Veterinarian (n = 60)	p-Value
Average milk production per ewe/doe during the preceding milking period		
199.5 (127.5) L	129.0 (114.0) L	<0.0001
Average number of lambs/kids born per ewe/doe		
1.28 (0.20) newborns	1.20 (0.16) newborns	0.003
Incidence of clinical mastitis during the preceding season		
2.0% (4.5%)	3.0% (4.1%)	0.021
Epg counts in faecal samples		
228 ± 11 epg	320 ± 42 epg	0.011
Body condition score		
2.40 (0.22)	2.26 (0.61)	0.016
Somatic cell counts in bulk-tank milk		
0.543×10^6 (0.504×10^6–0.583×10^6) cells mL^{-1}	0.680×10^6 (0.567×10^6–0.814×10^6) cells mL^{-1}	0.026

In the multivariable analysis, the following production- or health-related outcomes emerged with a significant association with a professional relationship with a veterinarian (Table 3): (a) epg counts in faecal samples (p = 0.012) (Figure 2); (b) average annual milk production per ewe/doe (p = 0.015); (c) somatic cell counts in bulk-tank milk (p = 0.037); and (d) annual incidence of clinical mastitis (p = 0.044) (Figure 3).

Table 3. Results of multivariable analysis of the professional relationship with a veterinarian with production- or health-related outcomes in this countrywide cross-sectional study in 444 small ruminant farms in Greece.

Production- or Health-Related Outcomes	Odds Risk (±se [1])	p
epg counts in faecal samples		0.012
With 'veterinarian' [2]	reference	-
Without 'veterinarian'	1.406 ± 0.147	0.011
Average annual milk production per ewe/doe		0.015
With 'veterinarian'	reference	-
Without 'veterinarian'	1.269 ± 0.109	0.002
Somatic cell counts in bulk-tank milk		0.037
With 'veterinarian'	reference	-
Without 'veterinarian'	1.021 ± 0.012	0.028
Annual incidence of clinical mastitis		0.044
With 'veterinarian'	reference	-
Without 'veterinarian'	1.408 ± 0.429	0.24

[1]: se: standard error; [2]: i.e., a professional relationship with a veterinarian.

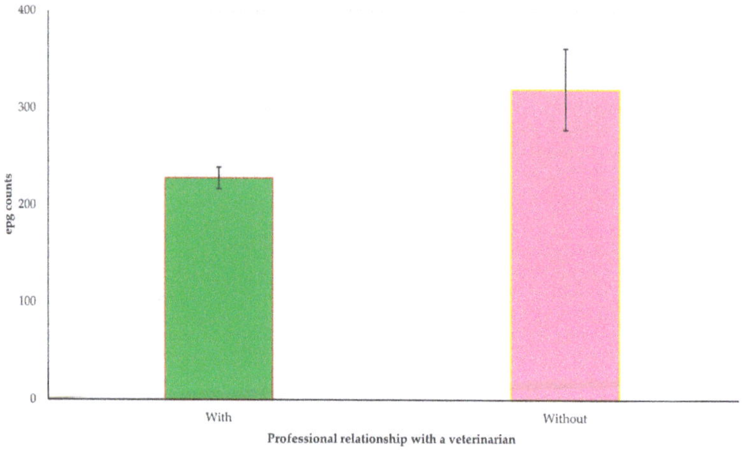

Figure 2. Mean epg counts in faecal samples among farms with (green bar) or without (pink bar) professional relationship with a veterinarian, as found in a countrywide cross-sectional study in 444 small ruminant farms in Greece.

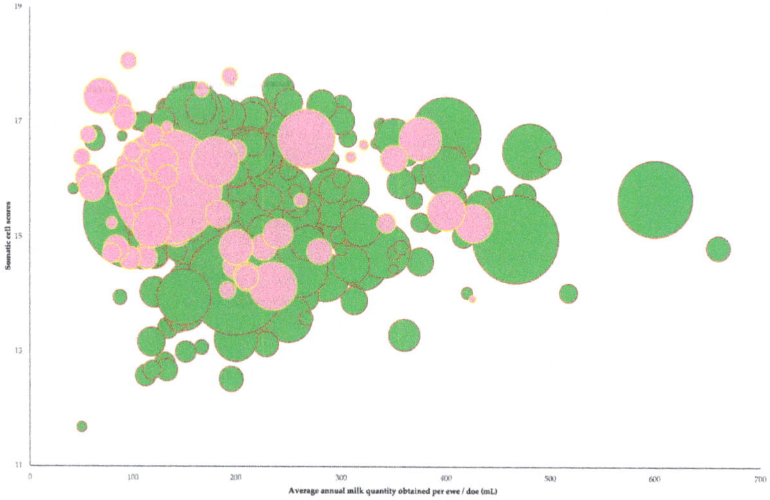

Figure 3. Average annual milk production per ewe/doe (horizontal axis), somatic cell counts in bulk-tank milk (vertical axis) and annual incidence of clinical mastitis (diameter of bubbles) among farms with (green-coloured bubbles) or without (pink-coloured bubbles) a professional relationship with a veterinarian, as found in a countrywide cross-sectional study in 444 small ruminant farms in Greece.

3.4. Differences among Farms with a Professional Relationship with a Veterinarian, in Accord with Characteristics of the Veterinarian

3.4.1. Gender of the Veterinarian

The detailed results of the univariable analysis for association of management practices and production- or health-related outcomes with the gender of the veterinarian are in Table S3. A significant difference between farms related to the gender of the veterinarian with whom there was a professional association was found for ten management practices

($p \leq 0.028$ for all relevant comparisons; details are in Table S3) and for two production- or health-related outcomes ($p \leq 0.026$ for all relevant comparisons; details are in Table 4).

Table 4. Production- or health-related outcomes found with a significant association with the gender of the veterinarian with whom there was a professional relationship in a cross-sectional study in a countrywide cross-sectional study among 384 small ruminant farms in Greece.

Farms in Which There Was a Professional Relationship with a Female Veterinarian (n = 121)	Farms in Which There Was a Professional Relationship with a Male Veterinarian (n = 263)	p-Value
Epg counts in faecal samples		
183 ± 15 epg	250 ± 16 epg	0.024
Somatic cell counts in bulk-tank milk		
0.461×10^6 (0.401×10^6–0.529×10^6) cells mL^{-1}	0.585×10^6 (0.540×10^6–0.638×10^6) cells mL^{-1}	0.026

3.4.2. Age of the Veterinarian

The detailed results of the univariable analysis for the association of management practices and production- or health-related outcomes with the age of the veterinarian are in Table S4. A significant correlation in accord with the gender of the veterinarian, with whom there was a professional association, was found for six variables related to management practices ($p \leq 0.029$ for all relevant comparisons; details are in Table S4) and for two production- or health-related outcomes ($p \leq 0.024$ for all relevant comparisons; details are in Table 5).

Table 5. Production- or health-related outcomes found with a significant association with the age of the veterinarian, with whom there was a professional relationship in a cross-sectional study in a countrywide cross-sectional study among 384 small ruminant farms in Greece.

Variables	r_{sp}	Type of Association	p-Value
Incidence of clinical mastitis	0.116	positive	0.024
Epg counts in faecal samples	0.131	positive	0.020

3.4.3. Annual Frequency of Veterinary Visits to the Farms

The detailed results of the univariable analysis for the association of management practices and production- or health-related outcomes with the annual frequency of veterinary visits to the farms are in Table S5. A significant correlation in accord with the annual frequency of veterinary visits to the farms was found for 16 variables related to management practices ($p \leq 0.045$ for all relevant comparisons; details are in Table S5); however, a significant correlation was not seen for any production- or health-related outcome ($p > 0.07$ for all relevant comparisons; details are in Table S5).

3.5. Associations of Characteristics of Veterinarians with Production- or Health-Related Outcomes

In the multivariable analyses performed, significant associations of the characteristics of veterinarians emerged only for the somatic cell counts in bulk-tank milk, specifically, related to a) the gender ($p = 0.0001$) and b) the age ($p = 0.007$) of the veterinarians (Table 6, Figure 4).

For the other production- or health-related outcomes, no significant associations with the characteristics of veterinarians emerged, i.e., for the epg counts in faecal samples ($p > 0.06$), the annual incidence of clinical mastitis ($p > 0.11$), or the average annual milk production per ewe/doe ($p > 0.13$).

Table 6. Results of multivariable analysis for variables related to the characteristics of veterinarians with a significant association with somatic cell counts in bulk-tank milk among 384 small ruminant farms in Greece.

Variables	Odds Risk (±se [1])	p
Gender of veterinarian		0.0001
Female	reference	-
Male	1.558 ± 1.120	-
Age of veterinarian		0.004
Per year decrease	1.015 ± 1.005	-

[1]: se: standard error of the mean.

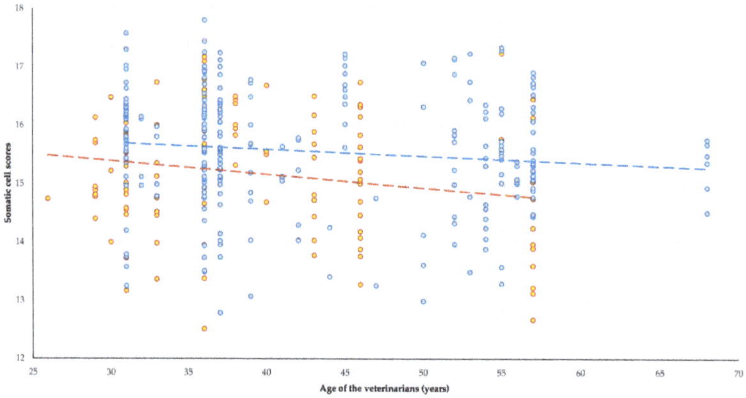

Figure 4. Somatic cell counts in the bulk-tank milk, in accord with the gender (red-yellow dots: female; blue-grey dots: male) and the age of the veterinarians among farms with a professional relationship with a veterinarian, as found in this countrywide cross-sectional study among 384 small ruminant farms in Greece (red and blue dashed lines are respective trendlines).

4. Discussion

4.1. Associations of Professional Relationship with a Veterinarian with Outcomes Related to Milk Production

The findings indicate that the beneficial effects were focused on the production of milk in the farm, as milk production, somatic cell counts in bulk-tank milk and incidence of clinical mastitis were three outcomes significantly improved in farms with a professional relationship with a veterinarian. The improved outcomes regarding milk quantity and quality are the result of the application of a variety of targeted management practices by the veterinarians: preventive use of laboratory diagnostic examinations in samples of milk, vaccination against contagious agalactia, vaccination against staphylococcal mastitis, administration of flunixin in cases of clinical mastitis, and improved general management practices (e.g., better nutritional management). These findings are in line with the production system prevalent in the country, i.e., dairy production [27], as well as with the farmers' consideration of mastitis as the most important problem in their flocks/herds [21]. Therefore, veterinarians comply with the requirements of their clients and contribute to the increase in agricultural production (animal production) relevant to the country.

It is also noteworthy that in a recent scientometrics study of mastitis in sheep [28], the two veterinary faculties of Greece were among the top three establishments internationally with regard to research output on that subject, whilst in another evaluation, it was found that research about sheep and goats in Greece has focused on milk production and diseases of the udder of small ruminants [29]. This indicates the increased interest in the study and control of the infection in the country, as well as the production of relevant knowledge, which is disseminated to field practicing veterinarians. These, in turn, usefully apply that knowledge to the field.

4.2. Associations of Professional Relationship with a Veterinarian with Practices Related to Administration of Pharmaceutical Products

In Greece, veterinarians active in small ruminant health management make most of their income through the sale of veterinary pharmaceuticals, for which they have the exclusive right. Indeed, veterinary services to small ruminant farmers are mostly provided for 'free', considered as a 'professional gift' for the purchase of veterinary products.

The above is reflected in the findings of the evaluation of parameters related to the administration of pharmaceutical products: higher number of occasions of administration of anthelmintic drugs annually, more frequent prescription of (more expensive) injectable solutions for anthelmintic use, more common routine administration of antimicrobials to newborns, more frequent administration of selenium to newborn animals, and more frequent use of flunixin in the treatment of clinical mastitis. Whilst, in some cases, there can be a benefit for these, the financial aspect might always be involved in the decision for prescribing the respective drugs.

The increased prescription and administration of antibiotics to newborns can lead to the development of antibiotic resistance [30–33] and it must thus be discouraged. Moreover, the present results did not show that the more frequent administration of antibiotics to newborns was associated with a lower incidence of pneumonia on diarrhoea in newborns, which are the most significant problems of lambs/kids at that age [34–37]. It is also noted that in sheep and goat farms in Greece, determinants of the administration of antibiotics in the treatment of various infections were found to mostly be the socio-demographic characteristics of farmers rather than management- or animal-related factors in the farms [38]. An improved use of antimicrobials, as underlined by scientific principles and compliance with policies and regulations, is important for an improvement in the welfare of the sheep and goats, as well as for reducing the risk for the development of antibiotic resistance.

The increased number of occasions of anthelmintic administration would have contributed to the lower epg counts found in these farms. Nevertheless, the frequent administration of anthelmintics is a main risk factor for the development of resistance by gastrointestinal nematodes [39–41] and this might have contributed to the presence of extensive and countrywide resistance of *Haemonchus contortus* to benzimidazoles, as found in a recent relevant field investigation [42]. One can also postulate that the frequent prescription of macrocyclic lactones by veterinarians might be practiced as a consequence of the understanding of veterinarians of the possibility of the existence of that widespread resistance.

There are nevertheless some positive facets in this increased administration of pharmaceutics. It is noted that among farms with a professional association with a veterinarian, more frequent use of flunixin was also made. Flunixin contributes to a reduction in the clinical signs of mastitis and alleviates pain [43,44], thus improving the welfare of the animals. That way, veterinarians also contribute to improving animal welfare, given that mastitis has been determined by the European Food Safety Authority to be a disease significantly reducing sheep welfare [45].

All of the above confirm the need to continue the training of professionals and of farmers in the correct usage of veterinary pharmaceuticals. Correct usage should be guided by scientific knowledge and surveying works, with the aim to contribute to a reduction in the resistance of the various pathogens (antibiotics, anthelmintics).

4.3. Characteristics of the Veterinarians

The majority of the veterinarians involved in this study were male. However, the female veterinarians were younger than the male ones, which is a consequence, in Greece and internationally, of most veterinary students over the last 20 years being females. In some faculties, this proportion can even be up to 80% of the total students [18,46,47].

Whilst farm animal veterinary work had been previously considered to be a male-dominated focus of the profession, this has evidently been changing, despite the fact that female veterinary students do not frequently consider such a career [48]. Possibly, this may be due to the changing landscape of veterinary work with farm animals, which nowadays involves an increased advisory and preventive farm health approach rather than clinical work at the individual animal level [48,49]. Additionally, it is also noted that, Europe-wide, of the 54 listed European Veterinary Specialists in Small Ruminant Health Management, 50% are females [50].

In farms with a professional relationship with a female veterinarian, some health-related outcomes were better than in farms with a relationship with a male veterinarian. The final grades of the veterinary degree can be considered a reflection of the knowledge acquired by young graduates during their studies and may thus represent the cognitive level of a new graduate regarding veterinary work [51,52]; this may affect professional actions, including health management in farms. It is thus interesting that an analysis of the final grades of graduates of the Veterinary Faculty of the University of Thessaly revealed that, during the period of 1999 to 2023, female veterinarians graduated with an overall higher final grade than male veterinarians: 6.65 ± 0.02 versus 6.46 ± 0.03 (average $\pm$ standard error of the mean; maximum possible: 10), respectively ($p < 0.0001$).

With regard to age, the application of more frequent management practices by younger veterinarians can be in line with more recent relevant scientific developments. For example, the benefits of the administration of selenium to pregnant ewes/does have only been described in Greece in the last few years [53,54] and have now been disseminated to practicing veterinarians. The present findings are in line with a report that older sheep farmers use fewer of the various management tools available to improve the health of the animals in their farms and less frequently [55].

5. Conclusions

Veterinary practitioners active in farm animal practice have a significant responsibility to the farmers and to the animals within these farms. Their work involves the maintenance of animal health and animal welfare in the farms, and, within this frame, they discuss with farmers the appropriate management practices to improve the health of the animals, to mitigate disease and distress (including pain control) and to maximise productivity.

The results attest that the application of veterinary advice and clinical services in sheep and goat dairy farms contributes to the improved health, production and welfare of the animals. Nevertheless, the training of veterinary practitioners in the correct use of pharmaceuticals should continue, especially given the European initiatives to minimise the administration of drugs in farm animals [56].

Whilst the results provide clear evidence regarding the beneficial role of veterinarians in small ruminant farms, it should be noted that veterinary services to these farmers are underpaid or even not paid at all. Farmers view the veterinary work in their flocks/herds as a 'perk' or 'free benefit' carried out by veterinarians in association with the drugs (pharmaceutical and immunological products) that they sell to the farmers. This may lead to the minimisation of the services provided, especially as veterinary drugs necessary for the farms can be sold to farmers by various veterinarians, even ones that have not provided clinical services to the animals of a farm.

This study presented another facet of the interactions between people and farm animals within the food-producing chain. These people–animal interactions can possibly be considered another approach within the 'One Health' concept.

Supplementary Materials: The following supporting information can be downloaded at: https://www.mdpi.com/article/10.3390/ani13213371/s1, Table S1: Details of multivariable models employed for the evaluation of professional relationship with production- or health-related outcomes in 325 sheep flocks and 119 goat herds in Greece; Table S2: Results of univariable analysis of parameters evaluated for association, in 325 sheep flocks and 119 goat herds in Greece, with the outcome 'professional relationship with a veterinarian'; Table S3: Results of univariable analysis of parameters related to management practices and to production- or health-related outcomes evaluated for association, in 283 sheep flocks and 101 goat herds in Greece, with a 'professional relationship with a veterinarian', in accord with the gender of the veterinarian; Table S4: Results of univariable analysis of parameters related to management practices and to production- or health-related outcomes evaluated for association, in 283 sheep flocks and 101 goat herds in Greece, with a 'professional relationship with a veterinarian', in accord with the age of the veterinarian; Table S5: Results of univariable analysis of parameters evaluated for association, in 283 sheep flocks and 101 goat herds in Greece, with a 'professional relationship with a veterinarian', in accord with the annual frequency of veterinary visits to the farm.

Author Contributions: Conceptualisation, D.T.L. and G.C.F.; methodology, D.T.L. and G.C.F.; formal analysis, D.T.L.; investigation, D.T.L.; resources, G.C.F.; data curation, D.T.L.; writing—original draft preparation, D.T.L.; writing—review and editing, D.T.L. and G.C.F.; visualisation, D.T.L. All authors have read and agreed to the published version of the manuscript.

Funding: This research received no external funding.

Institutional Review Board Statement: The protocols of this study were approved by the academic board of the Veterinary Faculty of the University of Thessaly, meeting 34/03.04.19.

Informed Consent Statement: Informed consent was obtained from all people involved in the study, who willingly and personally accompanied the researchers to the farm visits.

Data Availability Statement: Data associated with this study are presented in the text or in the Supplementary Materials.

Conflicts of Interest: The authors declare no conflict of interest.

Appendix A

Table A1. Variables (n = 106) evaluated for potential association with professional relationship with a veterinarian in a cross-sectional study in 444 small ruminant farms in Greece.

General Management Applied in the Farm
Management system applied in farms (description according to EFSA classification: intensive/semi-intensive/semi-extensive/extensive)
Seasonal transfer of animals to other sites (yes/no)
Infrastructure
Availability of milking parlour (yes/no)
Availability of isolation facilities for animals (yes/no)
Availability of milk replacer facilities and equipment for administration of milk replacer (yes/no)
Animals
No. of female animals in the farm (no.)
Average age of culling females (years: up to 6 years of age/over 6 years of age)
Health Management
Preventive use of laboratory diagnostic examinations in samples of milk (yes/no)
Preventive use of laboratory diagnostic examinations in samples of blood (yes/no)
Preventive use of laboratory diagnostic examinations in samples of faeces (yes/no)
Number of occasions of administration of anthelmintic drugs annually (no.)
Families of anthelmintics administered (description)
Pharmaceutical form of anthelmintics administered (description)
Administration of ectoparasiticides (yes/no)
Vaccination against *Chlamydia* infection (yes/no)
Vaccination against clostridial infections (yes/no)
Vaccination against contagious agalactia (yes/no)
Vaccination against foot rot (yes/no)
Vaccination against contagious ecthyma (yes/no)
Vaccination against paratuberculosis (yes/no)

Table A1. *Cont.*

General Management Applied in the Farm
Vaccination against bacterial pneumonia (yes/no)
Vaccination against staphylococcal mastitis (yes/no)
Total number of optional vaccines administered annually (no.)
Administration of 'dry-ewe' treatment at the end of the lactation period (yes/no)
Duration of the dry period (months)
Record keeping (yes/no)
Pharmaceutical Treatment
Routine administration of antimicrobials to newborns (yes/no)
Maintenance of prescribed withdrawal periods after administration of pharmaceuticals (yes/no)
Means of calculating live bodyweight for the administration of pharmaceutical products (weighing/estimation)
Routine overdosing (compared to dose prescribed) of pharmaceuticals (yes/no)
Number of antibiotics used for treatment of clinical mastitis (number)
Route for administration of antibiotics (systemic/intramammary)
Administration of flunixin in cases of clinical mastitis (yes/no)
Biosecurity Management
Quarantine of new animals arriving at the farm (yes/no)
Isolation of sick animals at the farm (yes/no)
Means for disposal of carcasses of animals that died in the farm (incineration, burial or removal by specialised agent/given to dogs, left unburied, or left in water streams)
Presence of a ditch at the entrance of the farm (yes/no)
Presence of a fence or a wall around the farm (yes/no)
Carrying out disinfections in the farm (yes/no)
Practicing sharing of equipment with other farms (yes/no)
Administration of rodenticides (yes/no)
Presence of spots suitable for reproduction of vectors within 500 m (yes/no)
Reproductive Management
Beginning of the mating period for ewes/does (month)
Application of reproductive control (yes/no)
Changes of rams/bucks into ewes/does during the mating period (yes/no)
Use of artificial insemination (yes/no)
Use of embryo transfer (yes/no)
Use of ultrasound for pregnancy diagnosis (yes/no)
Nutritional modifications before the lambing/kidding period (yes/no)
Grouping of pregnant females during the final stage of pregnancy (yes/no)
Administration of oxytetracycline to the pregnant animals (yes/no)
Administration of selenium to pregnant animals (yes/no)
Induction of lambing/kidding (yes/no)
Recording of births—maintenance of a lambing/kidding book (yes/no)
Newborn care and specific monitoring (yes/no)
Month of the start of the lambing/kidding season (description)
Administration of selenium to newborn animals (yes/no)
Disinfection of navel stump in newborns (yes/no)
Maintenance of a colostrum bank (yes/no)
Tail docking in newborns (yes/no)
Newborn fostering to female animals other than their dams (yes/no)
Age of lamb/kid removal from their dams (days)
Management in the Milking Parlour
Daily number of milking sessions (no.)
System pulsation rate (p. min^{-1})
System pressure (kPa.)
Use of teat disinfection after milking (yes/no)
Temperature of cleaning water after the milking sessions (°C)
Frequency of changing teatcups (description)

Table A1. *Cont.*

General Management Applied in the Farm
Nutritional Management
Provision of hay as fodder to animals (yes/no)
Average quantity of hay provided daily to animals during the preceding season (kg)
Provision of straw to animals (yes/no)
Provision of silage to adult animals (yes/no)
Provision of finished feed (concentrate) to adult animals (yes/no)
Provision of finished feed (concentrate) to adult animals throughout the year (yes/no)
Type of finished feed (concentrate) provided to adult animals (description)
Average quantity of finished feed (concentrate) provided daily to animals during the preceding season (kg)
Person responsible for nutritional management (description)
Production- or Health-related Outcomes
Average milk production per ewe/doe during the preceding milking period (litres)
Average number of lambs/kids born per ewe/doe (no.)
Incidence of clinical mastitis during the preceding season (%)
Incidence of abortion during the preceding season (%)
Incidence of lameness during the preceding season (%)
Incidence of mange during the preceding season (%)
Incidence of obstetrical problems during the preceding season (%)
Incidence of deaths, of any cause, in adult animals during the preceding season (%)
Incidence of pneumonia in lambs/kids during the preceding season (%)
Incidence of diarrhoea in lambs/kids during the preceding season (%)
Epg counts in faecal samples (epg)
Body condition score (score on scale 0–5, including half-scores)
Somatic cell counts in bulk-tank milk (cells mL^{-1})
Total bacterial counts in bulk-tank milk (cfu mL^{-1})
Isolation of staphylococci from bulk-tank milk (yes/no)
Isolation of antibiotic-resistant staphylococci from bulk-tank milk (yes/no)
Isolation of *Listeria* spp. from bulk-tank milk (yes/no)
Fat content in bulk-tank milk (%)
Protein content in bulk-tank milk (%)
Added water in bulk-tank milk (%)
Characteristics of Human Resources
Age of farmer (years)
Length of previous animal farming experience (years)
Farmer's general education (description: primary = European Qualifications Framework Levels 1 or 2/secondary or post-secondary = European Qualifications Framework Levels 3, 4 or 5/tertiary = European Qualifications Framework Level 6, 7 or 8)
Farmer's professional involvement in farming (full-time/part-time)
Daily period spent by farmer at the farm (hours)
Family tradition in farming (yes/no)
Presence of working staff in the farm (yes/no)
Occurrence of brucellosis in farmer (yes/no)

Appendix B

Table A2. Variables (n = 37) found with a significant association with professional relationship with a veterinarian in a cross-sectional study in 444 small ruminant farms in Greece.

Farms in Which There Was a Professional Relationship with a Veterinarian (n = 384)	Farms in Which There Was No Professional Relationship with a Veterinarian (n = 60)	p-Value
Management system applied in farms		
Intensive: 12.5%, Semi-intensive: 40.4%, Semi-extensive: 40.9%, Extensive: 6.3%	Intensive: 8.3%, Semi-intensive: 23.3%, Semi-extensive: 33.3%, Extensive: 35.0%	<0.0001

Table A2. *Cont.*

Farms in Which There Was a Professional Relationship with a Veterinarian (n = 384)	Farms in Which There Was No Professional Relationship with a Veterinarian (n = 60)	p-Value
Seasonal transfer of animals to other sites		
Yes: 15.9%, No: 84.1%	Yes: 28.3%, No: 81.7%	0.018
Availability of milking parlour		
Yes: 76.0%, No: 24.0%	Yes: 48.3%, No: 51.7%	<0.0001
Availability of isolation facilities for animals		
Yes: 77.1%, No: 22.9%	Yes: 55.0%, No: 45.0%	0.0003
Average age of culling females		
≤6 years: 62.2%, >6 years: 37.8%	≤6 years: 50.0%, >6 years: 50.0%	0.007
Preventive use of laboratory diagnostic examinations in samples of milk		
Yes: 23.7%, No: 76.3%	Yes: 6.7%, No: 93.3%	0.0003
Preventive use of laboratory diagnostic examinations in samples of faeces		
Yes: 13.3%, No: 86.7%	Yes: 0.0%, No: 100.0%	0.003
Number of occasions of administration of anthelmintic drugs annually		
2 (1)	1.5 (1)	0.009
Pharmaceutical form of anthelmintics administered		
Injectable solution: 60.7%	Injectable solution: 38.3%	0.001
Vaccination against contagious agalactia		
Yes: 61.2%, No: 38.8%	Yes: 26.7%, No: 73.3%	<0.0001
Vaccination against staphylococcal mastitis		
Yes: 39.1%, No: 60.9%	Yes: 16.7%, No: 83.3%	0.0007
Total number of optional vaccines administered annually		
3 (2)	2 (2)	<0.0001
Record keeping		
Yes: 66.7%, No; 33.3%	Yes: 51.7%, No: 48.3%	0.024
Routine administration of antimicrobials to newborns		
Yes: 24.5%, No: 75.5%	Yes: 10.0%, No: 90.0%	0.013
Means of calculating live bodyweight for the administration of pharmaceutical products		
Weighing: 20.6%, Estimation: 79.4%	Weighing: 33.3%, Estimation: 66.7%	0.027
Administration of flunixin in cases of clinical mastitis		
Yes: 9.9%, No: 90.1%	Yes: 1.7%, No: 98.3%	0.036
Quarantine of new animals arriving at the farm		
Yes: 63.8%, No: 36.2%	Yes: 45.0%, No: 55.0%	0.005
Presence of a fence or a wall around the farm		
Yes: 52.3%, No: 47.7%	Yes: 35.0%, No: 65.0%	0.012
Changes of rams/bucks into ewes/does during the mating period		
Yes: 28.6%, No: 71.4%	Yes:11.7%, No: 88.3%	0.005
Use of ultrasound for pregnancy diagnosis		
Yes: 33.9%, No: 66.1%	Yes: 15.0%, No: 85.0%	0.003
Grouping of pregnant females during the final stage of pregnancy		
Yes: 65.9%, No: 34.1%	Yes: 50.0%, No: 50.0%	0.017
Month of the start of the lambing/kidding season		
October	November	0.023
Administration of selenium to newborn animals		
Yes: 69.3%, No: 30.7%	Yes: 48.3%, No: 51.7%	0.001
Use of teat disinfection after milking		
Yes: 16.4%, No: 83.6%	Yes: 1.7%, No: 98.3%	0.003
Average quantity of hay provided daily to animals during the preceding season		
0.97 (1.18) kg	0.61 (1.00) kg	0.004
Provision of finished feed (concentrate) to adult animals throughout the year		
Yes: 31.9%, No: 68.1%	Yes: 53.4%, No: 46.6%	0.001
Type of finished feed (concentrate) provided to adult animals		
Pellets: 28.8%, Small pellets: 31.9%	Pellets: 51.7%, Small pellets: 15.5%	<0.01

Table A2. *Cont.*

Farms in Which There Was a Professional Relationship with a Veterinarian (n = 384)	Farms in Which There Was No Professional Relationship with a Veterinarian (n = 60)	p-Value
Average quantity of finished feed (concentrate) provided daily to animals during the preceding season		
0.74 (0.62) kg	0.53 (0.48) kg	<0.0001
Person responsible for nutritional management		
Veterinarian: 30.5%	Veterinarian: 14.0%	0.003
Average milk production per ewe/doe during the preceding milking period		
199.5 (127.5) L	129.0 (114.0) L	<0.0001
Average number of lambs/kids born per ewe/doe		
1.28 (0.20) newborns	1.20 (0.16) newborns	0.003
Incidence of clinical mastitis during the preceding season		
2.0% (4.5%)	3.0% (4.1%)	0.021
Epg counts in faecal samples		
228 ± 11 epg	320 ± 42 epg	0.011
Body condition score		
2.40 (0.22)	2.26 (0.61)	0.16
Somatic cell counts		
0.543×10^6 (0.504×10^6–0.583×10^6) cells mL^{-1}	0.680×10^6 (0.567×10^6–0.814×10^6) cells mL^{-1}	0.026
Length of previous animal farming experience		
25 (25)	30 (10)	0.010
Daily period spent by farmer at the farm		
15 (7) h	10 (7) h	0.035

References

1. Scott, P.R. The management and welfare of some common ovine obstetrical problems in the United Kingdom. *Vet. J.* **2005**, *170*, 33–40. [CrossRef] [PubMed]
2. Dwyer, C.M.; Bunger, L. Factors affecting dystocia and offspring vigour in different sheep genotypes. *Prev. Vet. Med.* **2012**, *103*, 257–264. [CrossRef] [PubMed]
3. Plant, J.W. Sheep ectoparasite control and animal welfare. *Small Rumin. Res.* **2006**, *62*, 109–112. [CrossRef]
4. Geddes, E.; Mohr, S.; Mitchell, E.S.; Robertson, S.; Brzozowska, A.M.; Burgess, S.T.G.; Busin, V. Exploiting scanning surveillance data to inform future strategies for the control of endemic diseases: The example of sheep scab. *Front. Vet. Sci.* **2021**, *8*, 647711. [CrossRef]
5. Crawford, P.E.; Hamer, K.; Lovatt, F.; Robinson, P.A. Sheep scab in Northern Ireland: Its distribution, costs and farmer knowledge about prevention and control. *Prev. Vet. Med.* **2022**, *205*, 105682. [CrossRef]
6. Windsor, P.A.; Lomax, S. Addressing welfare concerns in control of ovine cutaneous myiosis in sheep in Australia. *Small Rumin. Res.* **2013**, *110*, 165–169. [CrossRef]
7. Scott, P.R.; Sargison, N.D.; Wilson, D.J. The potential for improving welfare standards and productivity in United Kingdom sheep flocks using veterinary flock health plans. *Vet. J.* **2007**, *173*, 522–531. [CrossRef]
8. Strobel, H.; Spengler, D.; Voigt, K.; Hilke, J. Flock status—Sheep flock assessment ressource and management related welfare indicators. *Tierarztl. Prax. Ausg. Grosstiere Nutztiere* **2021**, *49*, 336–348.
9. Hosie, B.; Clark, S. Sheep flock health security. *In Pract.* **2007**, *29*, 246–254. [CrossRef]
10. Noremark, M.; Sternberg-Lewerin, S. On-farm biosecurity as perceived by professionals visiting Swedish farms. *Acta Vet. Scand.* **2014**, *56*, 28. [CrossRef]
11. Van der Heijden, M.; Dijkstra, E.; Holstege, M.; van den Brom, R.; Vellema, P. Data analysis supports monitoring and surveillance of sheep health and welfare in the Netherlands. *Small Rumin. Res.* **2022**, *216*, 106831. [CrossRef]
12. Higgins, H.M.; Green, L.E.; Green, M.J.; Kaler, J. How does reviewing the evidence change veterinary surgeons' beliefs regarding the treatment of ovine footrot? A quantitative and qualitative study. *PLoS ONE* **2013**, *8*, e64175. [CrossRef]
13. Gelasakis, A.I.; Kalogianni, A.I.; Bossis, I. Aetiology, risk factors, diagnosis and control of foot-related lameness in dairy sheep. *Animals* **2019**, *9*, 509. [CrossRef] [PubMed]
14. Windsor, P.A.; Lomax, S.; White, P. Progress in pain management to improve small ruminant farm welfare. *Small Rumin. Res.* **2016**, *142*, 55–57. [CrossRef]
15. Windsor, P.A. Role of topical anaesthesia in pain management of farm animals, a changing paradigm. *Animals* **2022**, *12*, 2459. [CrossRef] [PubMed]

16. Grandin, T. Livestock handling assessments to improve the welfare of cattle, pigs and sheep. *Anim. Prod. Sci.* **2018**, *58*, 403–407. [CrossRef]
17. Rioja-Lang, F.; Bacon, H.; Connor, M.; Dwyer, C.M. Prioritisation of animal welfare issues in the UK using expert consensus. *Vet. Rec.* **2020**, *187*, 490. [CrossRef]
18. Federation of Veterinarians in Europe. *Survey of the Veterinary Profession in Europe*; Federation of Veterinarians in Europe: Brussels, Belgium, 2019; 138p.
19. Lianou, D.T.; Chatziprodromidou, I.P.; Vasileiou, N.G.C.; Michael, C.K.; Mavrogianni, V.S.; Politis, A.P.; Kordalis, N.G.; Billinis, C.; Giannakopoulos, A.; Papadopoulos, E.; et al. A detailed questionnaire for the evaluation of health management in dairy sheep and goats. *Animals* **2020**, *10*, 1489. [CrossRef]
20. Martin, W.B.; Aitken, I.A. Appendix C. In *Diseases of Sheep*, 3rd ed.; Martin, W.B., Aitken, I.A., Eds.; Blackwell Science: Oxford, UK, 2000; p. 502.
21. Lianou, D.T. Mapping the Small Ruminant Industry in Greece: Health Management and Diseases of Animals, Preventive Veterinary Medicine and Therapeutics, Reproductive Performance, Production Outcomes, Veterinary Public Health, Socio-demographic Characteristics of the Farmers. Ph.D. Thesis, University of Thessaly, Volos, Greece, 2023.
22. Federation of Veterinarians of Europe. *Veterinary Act-European Veterinary Code of Conduct*; Federation of Veterinarians in Europe: Brussels, Belgium, 2009.
23. Hellenic Veterinary Association. *Code of Correct Veterinary Practice*; Hellenic Veterinary Association: Athens, Greece, 2011.
24. Grant, S.W.; Hickey, G.L.; Head, S.J. Statistical primer: Multivariable regression considerations and pitfalls. *Eur. J. Cardiothor. Surg.* **2018**, *55*, 179–185. [CrossRef]
25. Wiggans, G.R.; Shook, G.E. A lactation measure of somatic cell count. *J. Dairy Sci.* **1987**, *70* (Suppl. 13), 2666–2672. [CrossRef]
26. Franzoi, M.; Manuelian, C.L.; Penasa, M.; De Marchi, M. Effects of somatic cell score on milk yield and mid-infrared predicted composition and technological traits of Brown Swiss, Holstein Friesian, and Simmental cattle breeds. *J. Dairy Sci.* **2020**, *103*, 791–804. [CrossRef] [PubMed]
27. Pulina, G.; Milan, M.J.; Lavin, M.P.; Theodoridis, A.; Morin, E.; Capote, J.; Thomas, D.L.; Francesconi, A.H.D.; Caja, G. Current production trends, farm structures, and economics of the dairy sheep and goat sector. *J. Dairy Sci.* **2018**, *101*, 6715–6729. [CrossRef] [PubMed]
28. Lianou, D.T.; Fthenakis, G.C. Scientometrics approach to research in ovine mastitis from 1970 to 2019 (with a complete list of relevant literature references). *Pathogens* **2020**, *9*, 585. [CrossRef] [PubMed]
29. Lianou, D.T.; Fthenakis, G.C. Scientometrics study of research output on sheep and goats from Greece. *Animals* **2022**, *12*, 2666. [CrossRef] [PubMed]
30. Davies, P.; Remnant, J.G.; Green, M.J.; Gascoigne, E.; Gibbon, N.; Hyde, R.; Porteous, J.R.; Schubert, K.; Lovatt, F.; Corbishley, A. Quantitative analysis of antibiotic usage in British sheep flocks. *Vet. Rec.* **2017**, *181*, 511. [CrossRef] [PubMed]
31. Landfried, L.K.; Barnidge, E.K.; Pithua, P.; Lewis, R.D.; Jacoby, J.A.; King, C.C.; Baskin, C.R. Antibiotic use on goat farms: An Investigation of knowledge, attitudes, and behaviors of Missouri goat farmers. *Animals* **2018**, *8*, 198. [CrossRef]
32. Lovatt, F.; Duncan, J.; Hinde, D.; King, L. *Industry Guidance Document for Veterinary Surgeons and Farmers on Responsible Use of Antibiotics in Sheep*; Sheep Antibiotic Guardian Group, Ruminant Health & Welfare: UK, 2019; 18p.
33. Lovatt, F.; Duncan, J.; Hinde, D. Responsible use of antibiotics on sheep farms: Application at farm level. *In Pract.* **2019**, *41*, 23–33. [CrossRef]
34. Henderson, D.C. Neonatal conditions. In *Diseases of Sheep*, 3rd ed.; Martin, W.B., Aitken, I.A., Eds.; Blackwell Science: Oxford, UK, 2000; pp. 58–64.
35. Donachie, W. Pasteurellosis. In *Diseases of Sheep*, 3rd ed.; Martin, W.B., Aitken, I.A., Eds.; Blackwell Science: Oxford, UK, 2000; pp. 191–198.
36. Sargison, N. *Sheep Flock Health: A Planned Approach*; Blackwell Science: Oxford, UK, 2008; 465p.
37. Smith, M.C.; Sherman, D.M. *Goat Medicine*, 2nd ed.; Wiley-Blackwell: Ames, IW, USA, 2009; 871p.
38. Lianou, D.T.; Fthenakis, G.C. Use of antibiotics against bacterial infections on dairy sheep and goat farms: Patterns of usage and associations with health management and human resources. *Antibiotics* **2022**, *11*, 753. [CrossRef]
39. Papadopoulos, E.; Gallidis, E.; Ptochos, S. Anthelmintic resistance in sheep in Europe: A selected review. *Vet. Parasitol.* **2012**, *189*, 85–88. [CrossRef]
40. Sargison, N.D. Pharmaceutical treatments of gastrointestinal nematode infections of sheep—Future of anthelmintic drugs. *Vet. Parasitol.* **2012**, *189*, 79–84. [CrossRef]
41. Torres-Acosta, J.F.J.; Mendoza-de-Gives, P.; Aguilar-Caballero, A.J.; Cuéllar-Ordaz, J.A. Anthelmintic resistance in sheep farms: Update of the situation in the American continent. *Vet. Parasitol.* **2012**, *189*, 88–96. [CrossRef] [PubMed]
42. Arsenopoulos, K.; Minoudi, S.; Symeonidou, I.; Triantafyllidis, A.; Katsafadou, A.; Lianou, D.; Fthenakis, G.; Papadopoulos, E. Frequency of resistance to benzimidazoles of *Haemonchus contortus* helminths from dairy sheep, goats, cattle and buffaloes in Greece. *Pathogens* **2020**, *9*, 347. [CrossRef] [PubMed]
43. Petersson-Wolfe, C.S.; Leslie, K.E.; Swartz, T.H. An update on the effect of clinical mastitis on the welfare of dairy cows and potential therapies. *Vet. Clin. N. Am. Food Anim. Pract.* **2018**, *34*, 525–535. [CrossRef] [PubMed]
44. Mainau, E.; Llonch, P.; Temple, D.; Goby, L.; Manteca, X. Alteration in activity patterns of cows as a result of pain due to health conditions. *Animals* **2022**, *12*, 176. [CrossRef] [PubMed]

45. European Food Safety Authority. Scientific opinion on the welfare risks related to the farming of sheep for wool, meat and milk production. *EFSA J.* **2014**, *12*, 3933–4060.
46. Lofstedt, J.D. Gender and veterinary medicine. *Can. Vet. J.* **2003**, *44*, 533–535.
47. Maines, R. Why Are Women Crowding into Schools of Veterinary Medicine but Are not Lining up to Become Engineers? *Cornell Cronicle.* 2007. Available online: https://news.cornell.edu/stories/2007/06/why-women-become-veterinarians-not-engineers (accessed on 30 September 2023).
48. Payne, E.; Morton, E.; Lally, C.; Remnant, J. Farm animal careers and perception of 'fit' in undergraduate veterinary students: A mixed methods study. *Vet. Rec.* **2023**, *192*, e2339. [CrossRef]
49. Huxley, J. Cattle practice: Ready to adapt to a changing world? *Vet Rec.* **2016**, *179*, 377–381. [CrossRef]
50. European Board of Veterinary Specialisation. European College of Small Ruminant Health Management. Available online: https://ebvs.eu/colleges/ECSRHM (accessed on 30 September 2023).
51. Guerra-Carrillo, B.; Katovich, K.; Bunge, S.A. Does higher education hone cognitive functioning and learning efficacy? Findings from a large and diverse sample. *PLoS ONE* **2017**, *12*, e0182276. [CrossRef]
52. Greenfield, E.A.; Akincigil, A.; Moorman, S.M. Is college completion associated with better cognition in later life for people who are the least, or most, likely to obtain a bachelor's degree? *J. Gerontol. B Psychol. Sci. Soc. Sci.* **2020**, *75*, 1286–1291. [CrossRef]
53. Panousis, N.; Giadinis, N.; Karatzias, H. Selenium, vitamin E and vitamin A status in dairy sheep reared under different feeding systems in Greece. *J. Vet. Med. A* **2007**, *54*, 123–127. [CrossRef] [PubMed]
54. Giadinis, N.D.; Panousis, N.; Petridou, E.J.; Siarkou, V.I.; Lafi, S.Q.; Pourliotis, K.; Hatzopoulou, E.; Fthenakis, G.C. Selenium, vitamin E and vitamin A blood concentrations in dairy sheep flocks with increased or low clinical mastitis incidence. *Small Rumin Res.* **2011**, *95*, 193–196. [CrossRef]
55. Corner-Thomas, R.A.; Kenyon, P.R.; Morris, S.T.; Ridler, A.L.; Hickson, R.E.; Greer, A.W.; Logan, C.M.; Blair, H.T. Influence of demographic factors on the use of farm management tools by New Zealand farmers. *N. Z. J. Agric. Res.* **2015**, *58*, 412–422. [CrossRef]
56. Moore, S.J. European perspectives on efforts to reduce antimicrobial usage in food animal production. *Ir. Vet. J.* **2020**, *73*, 2. [CrossRef]

animals

MDPI

Article

Ethical Concerns of the Veterinarian in Relation to Experimental Animals and In Vivo Research

Łukasz Kiraga [1] and Andrzej Dzikowski [2,*]

[1] Division of Pharmacology and Toxicology, Department of Preclinical Sciences, Institute of Veterinary Medicine, Warsaw University of Life Sciences, 8 Ciszewski St., 02-786 Warsaw, Poland; lukasz_kiraga@sggw.edu.pl

[2] Department of Food Hygiene and Public Health Protection, Institute of Veterinary Medicine, Warsaw University of Life Sciences, 159 Nowoursynowska St., 02-776 Warsaw, Poland

* Correspondence: andrzej_dzikowski@sggw.edu.pl

Simple Summary: The veterinarian's primary responsibility is to safeguard animal health and public health, guided by the motto "Sanitas animalium pro salute homini" (the health of animals for the well-being of humans). However, there exists a distinct realm that operates separately from the core duties of veterinarians: the oversight of in vivo research. While animal studies are crucial for scientific advancement, they unfortunately involve the suffering and demise of numerous individuals. Veterinarians strive to heal animals, prevent diseases, and alleviate their pain, but in the case of animal experiments, these objectives are often unattainable. Instead of providing care, veterinarians witness the deliberate induction of various diseases, suffering, and death in animals. This situation raises ethical concerns and prompts the question of whether a veterinarian's involvement in in vivo research conflicts with their professional deontology. This article, drawing on the definitions of ethics and deontology, examining human–animal relationships across historical periods, analyzing veterinarians' codes of ethics in select European countries, and considering legal obligations concerning in vivo experiments, aims to provide insights and conclusions on this subject.

Abstract: Animal experiments, despite their controversial nature, play an indispensable role in scientific advancement and led to numerous significant discoveries. The supervision of veterinarians in the realm of in vivo research holds immense importance. However, this particular aspect of veterinary medicine, distinct from their other activities, can pose ethical challenges. Veterinarians are entrusted with the prevention of diseases, healing, and pain elimination, yet in the case of animal experiments, they witness intentional suffering and death. This article evaluates the ethical and professional deontological aspects of this issue. It explores the historical evolution of human–animal (including experimental) relationships and discusses how deontology stems from the definition of ethics. The article also examines codes of ethics for veterinarians, providing illustrative examples. It highlights that the actions of veterinarians in this domain align with their deontology and emphasises the role of veterinarians in in vivo research as viewed within current legal frameworks. In conclusion, the veterinarian's participation in animal research is both ethically and deontologically justified, and it is also a legal requirement.

Keywords: veterinarian; ethics; deontology; experimental animal; in vivo studies

1. Introduction

In vivo animal testing is undoubtely an extremely important aspect of life sciences. It is difficult to imagine the progress of biological sciences without this domain. Mankind owes many important discoveries to animal research, not the least of which we benefit from on a daily basis. For instance, smallpox was eradicated thanks to a vaccine created in research using animals [1]. One of the first in vivo studies involved penicillin. Although

Ian Flemming discovered penicillin in vitro, he, along with Florey and Chain, won the Nobel Prize for research conducted on mice showing how penicillin could be used to fight infections [2]. In vivo research helped create modern vaccines against serious, often fatal, or incurable diseases, such as against polio, tuberculosis, meningococcus, and human papilloma virus, which causes cervical cancer [3]. In general, survival rates in cancer are increasing due to the in vivo studies conducted mainly in mice. An example is the discovery of herceptin, a humanised human protein that helped increase the survival rate of breast cancer patients [4]. Another example is the animal studies conducted on Tamoxifen, which resulted in a 30% decrease in mortality in breast cancer patients in the 1990s [5]. Today, many diseases, against which medicine was once helpless, are being successfully treated. An example is AIDS; through the use of highly effective antiretroviral therapy (HAART) developed with the use of animals, it is possible to almost completely eliminate the symptoms of the disease, although the carrier of the virus remains [6]. Social unawareness that therapies for common disease entities, such as asthma and type one diabetes, are possible through animal research, can be observed.

It is worth noting that the development of novel diagnostic methods and new surgical techniques is dependent on animals. Important discoveries in transplantation, regenerative medicine, or immunology are also derived from animals. Every drug, vaccine, or diagnostic substance has to go through a phase of preclinical testing before it enters the phases of clinical trials and is registered. It is safe to say that, to a greater or lesser extent, almost everyone benefits from animal research, taking advantage of the scientific achievements we owe to them.

In vivo testing, despite the tremendous benefits it gives, is considered controversial, as evidenced by protest actions conducted in various regions of the world, or the activity of "animal rights" organisations aimed at limiting, or even stopping, in vivo research.

The problem of using animals in experiments raises considerable emotions. It is subject to legal regulations, including administrative rules and norms of professional ethics, scientific discourse, and a lively social debate. It is argued that the suffering of the animals involved makes animal research unethical. Therefore, it should not take place.

In recent decades, there was a growing interest among animal rights organisations and the broader community in the moral and ethical issues surrounding the use of animals in scientific research. Many express their opposition to such practices, arguing that the use of animals in experiments, especially primates, is ethically wrong and violates animal rights [7].

The main ethical argument put forward by animal rights organisations is the belief that animals have a right to dignity and protection from suffering. Scientists often subject animals to stressful conditions during experiments, which can cause pain and suffering. Some claim that there are other research methods that are just as effective and do not require the use of animals. According to their claims, in vitro tests, computer models, and experiments on human tissues are some of the many alternatives that provide results comparable to those obtained in animal studies [8].

Some also raise the issue of scientific efficacy. The results of animal studies do not always directly translate to humans, raising questions about the reliability and applicability of such experiments in biomedical research [9]. False or incomplete conclusions can not only lead to delays in scientific progress and generate economic costs, but also potentially affect human health [10].

Opponents of animal research also highlight the growing public disapproval of the practice. As society evolves, more and more people view the use of animals in experiments as morally unacceptable. Therefore, animal rights organisations are calling on scientists and research institutions to take a more ethical approach to conducting research [11].

However, it should be noted that the issue of animal research is not simple. There are scientists and experts who believe that in some cases animal research is necessary, provided that strict ethical standards are met and there are no alternative research methods.

This study discusses ethical issues in animal research. Research is focused on the ethical problems of those whose participation is a common element and a prerequisite for any in vivo experiment: the veterinarian. In particular, the authors intend to indicate ethical and legal factors facilitating the making of morally charged decisions by veterinarians in the case of laboratory animals [12].

This work constitutes a new scientific approach to the researched issue, as it tries to move away from the emotions that usually accompany the issue of animal testing. Moreover, the analysis is directed to veterinary surgeons, with the possibility of practical use of the research results. It would also be desirable to use the current study in veterinary education. Therefore, this article contains certain propaedeutic elements.

It is argued that the suffering of the animals involved makes animal research unethical. Therefore, it should not take place. This study will discuss ethical issues in animal research, focusing on the ethical problems of those whose participation is a common element and a prerequisite for any in vivo experiment: the veterinarian. In particular, the authors intend to indicate ethical and legal factors facilitating the making of morally charged decisions by veterinarians in the case of laboratory animals [12].

The authors decided to limit the area of the problem analysis to the European Union, as a representative example of the Western legal tradition and the Western cultural circle.

In the Western cultural circle, uniform concepts of science and ethics in science are observed, an element of which is the work ethics of veterinarians in animal testing. In the opinion of the authors, the results obtained, conclusions drawn, and observations made are of a general nature and can be applied on a global scale.

2. Ethics

In order to reliably assess the ethical aspect in the in vivo research, it is necessary to define the concept of ethics. Ethics, or moral philosophy, is a branch of philosophy concerned with moral duty: moral right vs. moral wrong. Ethics determines its detailed content: the rightness, and seeks ultimate explanations of norms, the genesis of evil, as well as the way to overcome it. In other words, ethics can be defined as an individual's personal beliefs regarding what is right and wrong or good or bad [13].

The concept of deontology is closely related to the notion of ethics. It is one of its branches. The word deontology comes from the Greek word for duty (deon) and the word for science (logos). In the modern moral philosophy, deontology is a type of normative theory regarding which choices are morally required, prohibited, or permitted [14]. The above definitions can be merged and paraphrased: deontology is the science of the ethical means to achieve the goal. The issue of deontology particularly often refers to the proper implementation of activities related to the profession—the professional ethics. According to deontology, including veterinary professional deontology, the end should not justify the means since the ethical, moral aspect of reaching the designated goal is more important, which distinguishes this concept from consequentialism.

Deontological rules in professional ethics are formulated with special attention to the moral aspect, but have legal norms as their basis. This also applies to veterinarians, who base the rules of deontology in their professional work on the veterinary codes of professional ethics.

Thus, the code of ethics enables the veterinarian to choose the right, moral, and good means to achieve the goal set [15]. Even though it is difficult to define the concepts of good and evil, since they depend on the adopted value system, the code of ethics determines the fulfilment of professional activities in a good, and therefore, *ethical* way. Nevertheless, it is impossible to say unequivocally which actions are unambiguously good and which are evil, and the authors postpone such a categorical statement.

Each state introduced its own code of ethics for veterinarians, hence, professional deontology can vary depending on which country one practices the profession in. Some codes of ethics of veterinarians describe the issue of animal testing. In spite of local minor differences in veterinary professional ethics, the work ethics of veterinarians in animal testing was found to be uniform in the Western culture. Nevertheless, those codes express common general principles, and can be regarded as the unified voice of the veterinarian community on a global scale.

Undoubtedly, all of them were formed based on the view of the currently prevailing human–animal relationship [14–19].

Therefore, it is important to demonstrate how the human–animal relationship changed throughout history in order to understand how current ethical standards for veterinarians practicing in laboratory animal medicine formed.

2.1. Human-Animal Relations throughout History as Viewed by Various Philosophical Schools

The earliest historical rationale for the relation–animal view is at least as early as Pythagoras in 4th–5th century BC [20–22]. His belief in the metempsychosis, inspired by Orphism, resulted in the promotion of vegetarianism. It is believed that he claimed that as long as men would kill animals, they would kill each other. This view can be still found today in several Far Eastern cultures and religions.

Aristotle indicated that a hierarchy of entities exists: inanimate things, plants, animals, and humans at the top. Thus, according to Aristotle, animals have a lower ontic status than humans, and help mankind achieve their own goals. He claimed that animals do not behave morally and rationally, but are capable of feeling. He justified killing animals only when it served to achieve higher goals [20,22–24].

Aristotle inspired Thomas Aquinas, who argued that less-perfect entities should serve those, who are more perfect, referring to the human–animal relationship. This view still prevails in Christian countries, and thus, Western legal tradition today. On the other hand, Francis of Assisi promoted the view that animals are perfect as an act of His creation. He encouraged the affirmation of nature; this view, however, was marginal, and did not leave much of a mark on the human–animal relationship [7,22,25].

Descartes promoted the concept of "machine" [22,26]. According to him, animals do not have vitam sensumque, which makes them incapable of feeling, including feeling pain. Animals do not suffer, while their reactions to pain are simply reflexes to damaging agents. Nevertheless, this period of such an approach to animals led to a flourishing of the animal research, most of which was conducted inhumanely and caused great suffering (e.g., vivisection).

It is known today how wrong the Cartesian theory of the time was. The Cambridge Declaration on Consciousness, for example, signed by a group of leading scientists attending the Francis Crick Memorial Conference at the University of Cambridge in the UK in July 2012, recognises that animals, including mammals, birds, and some other vertebrates, are conscious beings capable of experiencing emotions, cognitive abilities, and awareness. The declaration highlights the neuroanatomical similarities between the brains of these animals and humans, supporting the idea of consciousness. It emphasises the ethical importance of considering the welfare and treatment of animals in scientific research and human activities [27]. Moreover, there are scientists who associate still other attributes with animals. Prominent primatologist and ethologist, Frans de Waal proved through his numerous behavioural studies that mammals even demonstrate dissociate emotional and cognitive empathy [28], whereas according to famous biologist and behavioural ecologist Marc Bekoff, animals other than humans are able to exhibit moral and emotional intelligence [29].

In opposition to Descartes' claims stood John Locke. According to him, cruelty to animals negatively affects human morality. He promoted a view that animals can be used for human purposes, provided that respect is given and proper treatment guaranted [20].

Rousseau argued that all organisms (humans and animals alike) fight for their survival. In his view, animals do not behave rationally, but they are undoubtedly conscious, and similar to humans, are subject to the laws of nature. He emphasised the superiority of men over other creatures, but commanded to give them respect.

Kant created the concept of the categorical imperative, which was intended to be a set of universal ethical norms and laws applicable to every human being. Human actions should serve the general public and have no selfish motives, but only in relation to thinking beings, which, according to Kant, include only humans. He argued that man is an end in itself, and the animal is the way to an end [20,30].

Schopenhauer was of the opinion that animals have the ability to feel and behave rationally, but to a narrower degree than humans, which was close to current views [20].

The present human–animal relationship, including in the context of the in vivo research, is most likely due to Bentham's concept of utilitarianism, according to which, every action taken should be evaluated in terms of its consequences. What is useful is good. It does not mean, however, that unethical behaviour in relation to animals is acceptable [20,22,31].

According to Bentham, the determinant is not thinking, but feeling, and animals are undoubtedly capable of feeling. Thus, they can be used, provided that it serves a good purpose, and keeping in mind their ability to feel and suffer. This view shaped the modern human–animal relationship (concerning also animal testing), and still prevails today [20,24,32–34].

Contemporary philosophical, sociological, and anthropological concepts can also be mentioned [30,35,36]. Nevertheless, the authors do not intent to provide a complete anthropological or sociological theory, nor a philosophical system. Current analysis is not an anthropology of science, nor is it a sociology of science, of the in vivo research, or of the veterinary profession.

The discussed views influenced the content of the codes of professional ethics of veterinary surgeons, which directly determine the deontology of veterinarians. The actions of veterinarians, including those related to the in vivo research, must firstly comply with the applicable law, and secondly, must be ethical. Legal norms are derived from current legislation, while ethical norms are acquired from the code of ethics. Thus, the concept of ethics depends on the norms contained in the code, and its axiological basis. It is a system of connected vessels.

The following chapter will discuss ethical standards for veterinarians who deal with animal testing, according to the representative examples of the veterinary codes of ethics enforced by the European Union.

2.2. Ethical Standards for Animal Testing According to Codes of Ethics in Force in Various States

As was revealed, the performance of experiments by veterinarians is influenced by philosophical trends shaping the relationship between man and laboratory animals [31,37], as well as various types of legislation. Nevertheless, the veterinarian remains a physiscian, and a member of the profession of public trust. Therefore, he/she is obliged to observe not only their own particular system of ethics, resulting from their own philosophical or religious beliefs. Every veterinarian must comply with professional ethics and deontology, as defined in codes of professional ethics. Failure to comply with it is subject to professional liability. One may lose his/her license to practice veterinary medicine in the case of breaches of the law regarding animal experiments, the rules of the medical art, or moral standards.

In various countries and states, veterinary professional corporations and veterinary social organisations, or other representatives of the veterinary profession [14,38–40] have different approaches to the regulation of the discussed issue. Conducted analysis, however, revealed that all these differences are of secondary importance. General principles of practicing the veterinary profession, and of conducting the in vivo animal research, were found to be universal in the Western society.

Selected representative regulations of states of the European Union, and thus, Western cultural circle, were examined. These are states at a comparable level of civilisation, common ethical, and legal sources (common history, religion, and philosophy). These states are characterised by recognition of the same rules for conducting scientific research and scientific discourse [41,42].

2.2.1. Types of Regulation

A comparative ethical and legal analysis was carried out. It should be noted that the standards of professional ethics included in the form of codes are legal standards, for non-observance, of which there is a risk of liability.

The conducted research allowed us to indicate that there are three possible forms of regulation of the professional ethics of veterinarians in the scope of laboratory animal veterinary medicine:

- Tacit form;
- Mention;
- Special regulation.

In the type designated as "tacit regulation", the issues of professional ethics in animal research are not regulated separately in the code of ethics. They are rather subject to general principles, such as lege artis performance, accordance with the law, and scientific knowledge. An example of such a type is France [43–46].

In the type defined as "mention", the issues of professional ethics in animal research are regulated in the code of ethics only to a meager extent. Typical is one short provision of this scope of professional activity. An example is the German code of veterinary professional ethics [20,40,47,48], according to which veterinary surgeon must support scientific progress in all fields of medicine and life sciences. Every veterinarian ought to support the research, development, and use of alternatives to animal experimentation, an care for animal welfare.

In the type described as the "special regulation", the issues of professional ethics in animal research are regulated separately in the code of ethics, which devotes a lot of attention to them.

In the further part of the current study selected, representative regulations in this regard will be analysed.

2.2.2. Example of the Specific Regulation: Poland

The Polish code of veterinary ethics and deontology devotes Chapter IV, Articles 31–33, to the issue of laboratory activity [49]. The premises, which allow for the participation of a veterinarian in scientific animal research and in the implementation of scientific achievements, are specified. Veterinarians' activity in animal tests is acceptable only if there are reasonable grounds that it will not be harmful to humans, animals, and the environment; if experimentation using live animals is necessary for diagnostics, teaching, or for scientific research, that is expected to be of benefit to human or animal health; and if the applicable legal provisions are observed [50], there are cumulative conditions. It should be, therefore, interpreted that any activity that does not meet all of these conditions is unlawful, illegal, and most of all, unethical.

In addition, the veterinarian is burdened with an ethical obligation to watch over the entire course of the experment. He/she has, therefore, a moral and professional responsibility for all researchers [14] and for everything that happens during the experiment. The veterinarian participating in experiments on animals, or supervising their course, is obliged to ensure that unnecessary pain, suffering, and injuries are not caused to animals [32].

2.2.3. Example of the Specific Regulation: Italy

Article 39 of the Italian code of veterinary ethics is devoted to the discussed problem [51]. Veterinarians should strive for the progress of medicine and science. It is recognised as the highest goal. Other goals, such as the welfare of mankind or animal welfare, are of intermediate importance.

To ensure this, the Italian laboratory veterinarian must rely on four criteria. These are the top criteria for ensuring the quality of research and their moral justification. They are important both from the point of view of the society, veterinary profession, science, and the veterinarian him/herself.

The first criterion refers to the earlier scientific research, improvement of knowledge, and activities taken up to protect the health and welfare of animals and humans. The second criterion is the obligation to comply with legal norms. The third is the welfare of laboratory animals (the 3R principle, the development of alternative methods, and appropriate means to avoid unnecessary suffering) [52]. Finally, the fourth criterion is the possibility of using the conscientious objection.

2.2.4. Example of the Specific Regulation: Spain

Professional deontology of Spanish veterinarians in relation to the use of laboratory animals is described in Chapter XII, Article 29, of the local code of ethics [53,54].

Spanish veterinarians cannot conduct experiments on live animals without an authorising consent of the competent state authority. All animal experiments must be based on generally recognised scientific standards. Among these scientific principles, the 3R principle is directly mentioned. Minimizing the number of animals used in the experiment is also emphasised. Further regulations (Article 29, sections 5–6) concern not as much laboratory animals as experiments in the clinical phase.

2.2.5. Other Factors

The detailed examples analysed, discussed, and presented above allow us to draw conclusions of a general nature. Although these are local regulations from the area of given European states, they can be considered as an exemplification of general global rules of professional ethics that apply to all veterinarians around the world, regardless of jurisdiction.

It should be noted that in most states, the ethical standards applicable to veterinarians can be derived indirectly from the provisions of the acts on animal experimentation. There are also international regulations, such as those of the European Union, the analysis, and legal interpretation, of which will be presented in the further part of the current paper.

It should also be noted that in addition to the above sources of legal standards, a given laboratory veterinarian can be also obliged to observe scientific ethics as an employee of laboratories operating within research institutes or universities [15].

In connection with all of the above, a gap, or conflict, between the need for evidence-based medicine and ethics may occur [55]. This may give rise to serious ideological dilemmas and may practically affect the quality of the work in the laboratory or animal facility.

Moreover, a discrepancy between the morality (philosophical, religious, etc.) of a given person, a given veterinarian, or a given society and veterinary professional ethics may be observed. Discrepancy between what the law allows and what ethics indicates may be revealed.

A significant problem is the "detachment" or "abruption" from laboratory animals by the veterinary surgeon. It is difficult for him/her, and psychologically destructive, but at the same time, it serves the objectivity of research. Each veterinarian, therefore, must balance his/hers responsibilities rising from different value systems, and choose the solution that is most compliant with the law and with the ethical standards. The instrument of this choice may be the scientific knowledge acquired in the course of studies, specialisation, or courses devoted to laboratory issues.

3. European Law Regulating In Vivo Animal Testing

Professional deontology, including that of a veterinarian, is not only conditioned by ethics prevailing in a given society, but also by its religion, history, and law. The veterinary code of professional ethics cannot be in conflict with the law in force. Standards of professional ethics for veterinarians, as well as legal regulations, must be consistent in democratic countries. This is the standard of the Western cultural circle.

In addition to the regulations of individual states, more general legal provisions with an international scope exist. They firlmy affect state laws. In this paper, the authors decided not to examine the laws of individual states. Instead, the European Union regulations will be analysed as a meaningful, and as a representative example of universal significance.

Currently, the overriding legal act in the European Union member states is the Directive 2010/63/EU of the European Parliament and of the Council of 22 September 2010 on the protection of animals used for scientific purposes [56–58].

As a result of its entry into force, member states had to introduce national regulations implementing all aspects of the directive within five years. Thus, legal regulations in individual member states regarding the issue of animal testing are conditioned by various legal acts, the common element of which is the realisation of the same crucial elements arising from the directive [40].

Therefore, the provisions of the legal acts in force in individual member states are uniform because their assumptions and axiological foundations are convergent. There is no point in analysing separately the legal acts of each member state, since their assumptions coincide.

Instead of the analysis of particularities, the authors will focus on the legal role of the veterinarian in scientific research according to Directive 2010/63. This legislative act consists of 56 points that make up the preamble, 66 articles grouped into 6 chapters, and 8 annexes.

Article 25 stipulates that member states shall ensure that each breeder, supplier, and user has a designated veterinary surgeon with expertise in laboratory animal medicine, or, if it would be more appropriate, an "expert" with appropriate qualifications performing advisory duties on animal welfare and treatment.

Thus, establishment, regardless of its form of operation, must employ a veterinarian with relevant expertise in laboratory animal medicine or an "expert with relevant qualifications". It is not clear what specific qualifications, skills, knowledge, or education this "expert" should have. Nevertheless, this position is treated as an alternative to a veterinarian to perform veterinary supervision at the establishment.

The authors hereby postulate that the ambiguous position of the "expert" should be removed from the normative acts. Moreover, in states where there is an official title of a veterinary surgeon (specialist in laboratory animal medicine), this function ought to be limited to only veterinarians who can demonstrate such a national or European specialisation.

Another reference to the role of the veterinarian in the in vivo research can be indicated in Article 9 on obtaining wild animals for research. The norm states that wild animals may be obtained for research only under the condition of scientific justification, confirming that the purpose of the procedure cannot be obtained using an animal bred for use in procedures [59].

In addition, the acquisition of wild animals shall be carried out by competent persons using methods that do not cause the animals avoidable pain, suffering, distress, or permanent damage. All animals found to be injured or in poor health during or after the capture shall be examined by a veterinarian. They should then be subject to appropriate procedures to minimise suffering. Thus, the presence of a veterinarian is indispensable when acquiring wild animals for research, because if an animal is injured, it must be properly examined and treated [60]. This requirement can be derived not only from the statutory regulations, but also from the scientific veterinary knowledge, and the veterinary professional ethics.

Another role of the veterinarian is mentioned in Article 16, concerning the use of animals in an experiment once they are subjected to procedures. This is only possible if four conditions are met:

- If the severity of the previous procedures was mild or, at most, moderate (the severity classification of the procedures is referred to in Annex VIII);
- If it is shown that the animals fully recovered their general health and welfare;
- If the subsequent procedure is classified as mild, moderate, or terminal without recovery, and;
- It is in accordance with veterinary advice, taking into account the animals' life experience.

It is possible to deviate from the first condition; after the examination performed by a veterinarian, the animal can also be reused if it was subjected to a severe procedure, but not more than once. Thus, it is for the veterinarian to make the final decision whether the animal can be reused in procedures. Such a decision cannot be made without his participation. In the authors' opinion, this is a reasonable normative solution. Only a veterinary surgeon has sufficient competence, knowledge, and skills to adjudicate on the health of the animal. Not only is the knowledge of laymen (outside observer) not enough, they also perceive science differently than researchers and veterinary professionals [36].

Article 17 considers the role of the veterinarian. It regulates the fate of animals after the procedures performed on them are completed. According to paragraph 2, the veterinarian, or another competent person, makes the decision to either kill, or keep the animal alive. It is, however, not clear what competence the "other competent person" must have to perform a function equivalent to the veterinarian in this case. Such a regulation is assessed by the authors definitely negatively. This is a potential gateway to abuse.

An animal is killed if there is a probability that it will continue to feel moderate or severe pain, suffering, or distress, or that it will experience permanent damage. This means that the veterinarian, having examined the health of the animal after the procedures, decides whether the animal can be left alive or should be killed due to the suffering it is experiencing.

Article 26 describes the connection between the veterinarian and the functioning of the animal welfare advisory body. According to the statutory provisions, each establishment must set up a welfare advisory body, which must include (at least) a person or persons responsible for the animal welfare and animal care, and in the case of a user, an academician.

The animal welfare advisory body receives information from the designated veterinarian, or expert referred to in Article 25. Thus, it can be stated that the veterinarian (or the aforementioned "expert") cooperates with the welfare body without being a member of it by him/herself. His/her role is providing information on animal welfare, emphasizing the assessment of animal health.

Each establishment must employ a "designated veterinarian" with relevant expertise in laboratory animal medicine, where he or she provides extensive veterinary services.

In light of the discussed directive, the role of the veterinarian in the in vivo research concerns: deciding whether to reuse animals in procedures, determining whether to keep animals alive or kill them after procedures are completed, and cooperating with the welfare body in implementing animal welfare. These activities, for which there is a legal requirement that they are carried out specifically by a veterinarian, are hereby considered as "direct" participation of a veterinarian in the in vivo research.

An "indirect" participation can also be distinguished: when specific functions are performed by a veterinarian, even though legally they do not have to be performed by him/her. Examples include the so-called animal facility famanager and personnel of the establishment.

As for personnel of the establishment, Article 23 of the discussed European Directive distinguishes between those who perform the functions of:

- Performing procedures on animals;
- Planning procedures and projects;
- Taking care of animals; and
- Killing animals.

Persons performing these functions must be trained in the scientific discipline relevant to the work being undertaken, and should have knowledge of the species in question. The scope of mandatory training for these individuals is detailed in the Appendix V.

The animal facility manager is an informal term, not appearing in the normative text. The animal facility manager performs the functions set forth in Article 24.1, and thus is responsible for supervising the welfare and care of the animals; as well as ensures that the personnel handling the animals have access to information on the specific species housed in the facility. Moreover, he/she is responsible for ensuring that the personnel is properly educated, competent, and continuously trained, as well as supervised till the required skills are demonstrated. The establishment may have one or more persons performing this function.

Although there is no legal requirement that any of the staff or manager positions be held by a veterinarian, they are often held precisely by veterinarians because of their knowledge experience in working with animals.

There is another legal aspect tying the veterinarian to in vivo experimentation. This is alluded to in Article 34, which deals with the obligation of member states to inspect breeders, suppliers, and users.

This article provides rules for determining the frequency of such inspections. In most of the European Union member states, the veterinary inspection is involved, and the persons directly inspecting the centers are veterinary officers (and thus, veterinarians). They inspect the legality of the conduct of in vivo experiments; that is, whether they are carried out in accordance with the law currently in force (resulting from the directive), and prepare the relevant inspection documentation, which must be kept for at least five years.

The significant role of ethical committees in the process of conducting animal tests should be indicated. Such committees decide on admission to experiments, on the number of animals, or on the end of the procedure. It was found that often, but not always, a veterinary surgeon is a member of such a committee. As already indicated, according to general legal principles (including logic and axiology of the veterinary law), veterinarians are the only people who have the right to make judgments about, and to assess the health of animals. The authors hereby propose that in each ethical committee, at least one veterinary professional should be included; preferably, veterinarians experienced in animal testing and specialised in laboratory animals' health and pathology [61].

The legal provisions, however, only seem to constitute directives of conduct. The regulations themselves do not indicate to the veterinarian what ethical decisions or what choices to make [12]. Nevertheless, if, when interpreting a legal provision, he/she takes into account the ethical background and axiological grounds on which these norms are based, then making the right decision will be easier.

Furthermore, in the opinion of the authors, ethical obligations should not be created in abstracto, or metaphorically "in vitro", in isolation from the real users of ethics (veterinarians), from their limitations, or the possibility of meeting the requirements. In the authors' opinion, professional ethics and veterinary law are not ideal or idealistic theoretical concepts, but tools for practical application. Therefore, law and professional deontology must take into account the practical eventualities and limitations of the users.

4. Conclusions

In vivo animal research undeniably has a huge impact on the development of science, and these scientific achievements are of great value to humans. However, it is important to note that not all experiments involve equal animal suffering. We have four categories of the severity of procedures: non-recovery, mild, moderate, and severe [56]. At the planning stage of an experiment, we have an obligation to implement the 3Rs principle, one component of which is "refinement", according to which we must strive for the least possible animal suffering. However, there are some experiments in which, due to the type of research, we cannot avoid causing severe pain to animals, and this raises more ethical questions: does the desire to gain new knowledge and discoveries morally justify harming animals? This is still a controversial point. According to the principle of refinement, in in vivo research, we should also strive to use animals from the lower rungs of the evolutionary ladder. Nevertheless, many experiments are being conducted on primates, which are evolutionarily closest to humans. There are still conditions with unknown pathogenesis and effective treatment, such as Alzheimer's or Parkinson's disease, and mouse or rat models of these diseases do not advance our knowledge; in order to finally discover effective methods of preventing these diseases, should we conduct research on primates, which is the most sentient group of animals? This is an ethical dilemma.

The role of the veterinarian in in vivo animal research is crucial. As demonstrated, a veterinarian is the only person who has enough knowledge, skills, and legal authorisation to assess the health of laboratory animals.

Moreover, a veterinary surgeon must be involved in the scientific research because, as the legal norms state, he/she must be employed at each animal facility, must decide whether animals are to be left alive after procedures, must have a welfare advisory body cooperating with him/her, must approve the reuse of animals in procedures, and must oversee the acquisition of wild animals for research.

It is not precluded for a veterinarian to participate in the scientific research as a so-called animal facility manager (Directive 2010/63, Article 24.1), or a staff member directly involved in the conduct of an experiment. Performing any of these functions is not unethical, as it does not contradict a veterinary code of ethics. Most of such codes explicitly state that veterinarians should strive for the proper conduct in any field (including animal experiments), and ensure humane treatment of all animals (including experimental animals). Killing animals at the end of an experiment (which is at the discretion of the veterinarian) may raise moral questions, but leaving an animal suffering alive would be far less morally correct than euthanasia, and is therefore ethically correct.

The participation of veterinarians in the discussed kind of research is legal, necessary, and should not pose major ethical problems, as it does not contradict the codes of ethics of a veterinarian. Direct participation in the in vivo experiment should also not raise questions about the ethicality of such conduct, since this issue is overseen by Ethics Commissions operating in each member country [61].

Such commissions authorise only experiments in which the suffering of animals is as low as possible and morally justified; tests that may entail the acquisition of knowledge useful to humans. These provisions, therefore, justify the use of animals in scientific research according to utilitarianism.

Ethics committees do not approve badly planned or unethical experiments. Thus, taking part in a legitimate experiment, one is assured that it does not contradict ethics, nor deontology. Whether or not it is morally correct depends on the value system one adopted, and how it will balance the different responsibilities that come from different normative sources. The ethical and axiological background of the law, including the law of professional ethics, as well as scientific veterinary knowledge in the field of health and welfare of laboratory animals can be an aid and decisive instrument.

Author Contributions: Conceptualization, A.D. and Ł.K.; methodology, A.D. and Ł.K.; formal analysis, A.D. and Ł.K.; writing—original draft preparation, A.D. and Ł.K.; writing—review and editing, A.D. and Ł.K. All authors have read and agreed to the published version of the manuscript.

Funding: This research received no external funding.

Institutional Review Board Statement: Not applicable.

Informed Consent Statement: Not applicable.

Data Availability Statement: Data sharing not applicable.

Conflicts of Interest: The authors declare no conflict of interest.

References

1. Riedel, S. Edward Jenner and the History of Smallpox and Vaccination. *Bayl. Univ. Med. Cent. Proc.* **2005**, *18*, 21–25. [CrossRef]
2. Gaynes, R. The Discovery of Penicillin—New Insights After More Than 75 Years of Clinical Use. *Emerg. Infect. Dis.* **2017**, *23*, 849–853. [CrossRef]
3. Koff, W.C.; Rappuoli, R.; Plotkin, S.A. Historical Advances in Structural and Molecular Biology and How They Impacted Vaccine Development. *J. Mol. Biol.* **2023**, *435*, 168113. [CrossRef] [PubMed]
4. Slamon, D. Herceptin®: Increasing survival in metastatic breast cancer. *Eur. J. Oncol. Nurs.* **2000**, *4*, 24–29. [CrossRef] [PubMed]
5. Jordan, V.C. Proven value of translational research with appropriate animal models to advance breast cancer treatment and save lives: The tamoxifen tale. *Br. J. Clin. Pharmacol.* **2014**, *79*, 254–267. [CrossRef]
6. Gazzard, B.G. A Decade of HAART: The Development and Global Impact of Highly Active Antiretroviral Therapy. *HIV Med.* **2009**, *10*, 458. [CrossRef]
7. Gluck, J.P. *Voracious Science and Vulnerable Animals: A Primate Scientist's Ethical Journey; Animal Lives*; University of Chicago Press: Chicago, IL, USA, 2016; ISBN 978-0-226-37565-6.

8. Greek, J.S.; Greek, C.R. Replacing the Animal Model in Biomedical Research and Education. In *What Will We Do If We Don't Experiment on Animals? Medical Research for the Twenty-First Century*; Trafford Publishing: Bloomington, IN, USA, 2004; pp. 13–30, ISBN 978-1-4120-2058-9.
9. Knight, A.; Bailey, J.; Balcombe, J. Animal Carcinogenicity Studies: 2. Obstacles to Extrapolation of Data to Humans. *Altern. Lab. Anim.* **2006**, *34*, 29–38. [CrossRef]
10. Knight, A. Systematic Reviews of Animal Experiments Demonstrate Poor Human Clinical and Toxicological Utility. *Altern. Lab. Anim.* **2007**, *35*, 641–659. [CrossRef]
11. 52% of American Public Opposes the Use of Animals in Scientific Research. Available online: https://speakingofresearch.com/2018/08/30/52-of-american-public-opposes-the-use-of-animals-in-scientific-research/ (accessed on 20 July 2023).
12. Vettical, B.S. An Overview on Ethics and Ethical Decision-Making Process in Veterinary Practice. *J. Agric. Environ. Ethics* **2018**, *31*, 739–749. [CrossRef]
13. Fischer, J. Social Responsibility and Ethics: Clarifying the Concepts. *J. Bus. Ethics* **2004**, *52*, 381–390. [CrossRef]
14. Herzog, H. Ethical aspects of relationships between humans and research animals. *ILAR J.* **2002**, *43*, 27–32. [CrossRef] [PubMed]
15. Ashall, V.; Hobson-West, P. 45. The Vet in the Lab: Exploring the Position of Animal Professionals in Non-Therapeutic Roles. In *Professionals in Food Chains*; Wageningen Academic Publishers: Wageningen, The Netherlands, 2018; pp. 291–295, ISBN 978-90-8686-321-1.
16. Sturma, D. Tierversuche: Eine Ethische Perspektive. In *Natur, Ethik und Ästhetik*; Sturma, D., Ed.; Brill | Mentis: Leiden, The Netherlands, 2022; pp. 331–352, ISBN 978-3-96975-247-0.
17. Kaleta, T. Geneza dobrostanu zwierząt—Aspekty historyczne i filozoficzne. *Przegląd Hod.* **2017**, *6*, 1–3.
18. Rollin, B. Animal Ethics and the Law. *Mich. Lawe Rev. First Impr.* **2008**, *106*, 143.
19. Schmidt, K. Concepts of Animal Welfare in Relation to Positions in Animal Ethics. *Acta Biotheor.* **2011**, *59*, 153–171. [CrossRef]
20. Riether, E.; Weiss, M.N. *Tier—Mensch—Ethik*, 1st ed.; Lit: Vienna, Austria, 2012; pp. 13–72, 107–124, 141–158. (In German)
21. Krajewski, W. Filozofia Przyrody jako Pomost Między Naukami Przyrodniczymi a Filozofią. *Rocz. Filoz.* **2005**, *53*, 418–421.
22. Tyburski, W. Człowiek—Środowisko przyrodnicze w świetle wybranych stanowisk filozoficznych i ekofilozoficznych. *Paedagog. Christ.* **2011**, *28*, 41. [CrossRef]
23. Sorabji, R. *Animal Minds and Human Morals: The Origins of the Western Debate*; Cornell University Press: Ithaca, NY, USA, 1993; pp. 1–267.
24. Anderson, L.C.; Fox, J.G.; Otto, G.M.; Pritchett-Corning, K.R.; Whary, M.T. *Laboratory Animal Medicine*, 3rd ed.; Academic Press: San Diego, CA, USA, 2015; pp. 2–42, 1371–1401, 1441–1471, 1655–1659.
25. Dietl, A. Ortodoksja i herezja w relacjach ludzi i zwierząt. *SRZ* **2021**, *18*, 179–203. [CrossRef]
26. Switankowsky, I. Dualism and its importance for medicine. *Theor. Med. Bioeth.* **2000**, *21*, 567–580. [CrossRef]
27. The Cambridge Declaration on Consciousness. Available online: https://fcmconference.org/img/CambridgeDeclarationOnConsciousness.pdf (accessed on 20 July 2023).
28. De Waal, F.B.M.; Preston, S.D. Mammalian empathy: Behavioural manifestations and neural basis. *Nat. Rev. Neurosci.* **2017**, *18*, 498–509. [CrossRef]
29. Bekoff, M. *Minding Animals: Awareness, Emotions, and Heart*; Oxford University Press: New York, NY, USA, 2002; ISBN 978-0-19-515077-3.
30. Hache, E.; Latour, B. Morality or Moralism? An Exercise in Sensitization. *Common Knowl.* **2010**, *16*, 311–330. [CrossRef]
31. Yeates, J.W. Response and responsibility: An analysis of veterinary ethical conflicts. *Veter. J.* **2009**, *182*, 3–6. [CrossRef] [PubMed]
32. Carbone, L. *What Animals Want: Expertise and Advocacy in Laboratory Animal Welfare Policy*; University Press: Oxford, MS, USA, 2004; pp. 44–66, 165–185.
33. Jedynak, S. The human-animal relationship in its ecological aspect. *Probl. Sustain. Dev.* **2008**, *3*, 73–76.
34. Lemańska, A. Praktyczna Filozofia Przyrody Alternatywą klasycznej filozofii przyrody? Kryzys klasycznej filozofii przyrody w XX wieku. *Stud. Philos. Christ.* **1997**, *33*, 133–138.
35. Latour, B. Give Me a Laboratory and I Will Raise the World. In *Science Observed: Perspectives on the Social Study of Science*; Sage: London, UK; Beverly Hills, CA, USA, 1983; pp. 141–170.
36. Latour, B.; Woolgar, S. *Laboratory Life: The Construction of Scientific Facts*; Princeton University Press: Princeton, NY, USA, 1986; ISBN 978-0-691-02832-3.
37. Morgan, C.A.; McDonald, M. Ethical Dilemmas in Veterinary Medicine. *Veter.-Clin. North Am. Small Anim. Pract.* **2007**, *37*, 165–179. [CrossRef]
38. Kaliste, E. *The Welfare of Laboratory Animals*; Springer: Dordrecht, The Netherlands, 2007; pp. 1–22.
39. Pullen, S.; Gray, C. *Ethics, Law, and the Veterinary Nurse*, 1st ed.; Elsevier Butterworth Heinemann: Edinburgh, UK, 2006; pp. 11–22, 65–76, 103–116.
40. Binder, R.; Grimm, H.; Alzmann, N. *Wissenschaftliche Verantwortung im Tierversuch. Ein Handbuch für die Praxis*; Nomos: Baden-Baden, Germany, 2013; pp. 1–268. (In German)
41. Micińska-Bojarek, M. Europejski standard doświadczeń na zwierzętach. Aspekty humanitarno-prawne. *Przegląd Prawa Ochr. Sr.* **2012**, *3*, 111–127. [CrossRef]
42. Gajewska, G. O władzy ludzi nad zwierzętami w kulturze zachodniej—Perspektywa posthumanistyczna. *Stud. Eur. Gnes.* **2015**, *11*, 213–235. [CrossRef]

43. Code de Déontologie. Available online: https://www.veterinaire.fr/la-profession-veterinaire/la-reglementation-professionnelle/code-de-deontologie (accessed on 22 June 2023).
44. Sirois, M. *Laboratory Animal and Exotic Pet Medicine: Principles and Procedures*, 3rd ed.; Elsevier: Amsterdam, The Netherlands, 2022; pp. 1–15.
45. Wolfensohn, S.; Lloyd, M. *Handbook of Laboratory Animal Management and Welfare*, 3rd ed.; Blackwell: Oxford, UK, 2003; pp. 3–40.
46. Dolan, K. *Laboratory Animal Law: Legal Control of the Use of Animals in Research*, 2nd ed.; Blackwell: Oxford, UK, 2007; pp. 1–27, 90–134.
47. Ethik-Kodex Der Tierärztinnen Und Tierärzte Deutschlands. Available online: https://www.bundestieraerztekammer.de/btk/ethik/ (accessed on 22 June 2023).
48. Boscheinen, J. Buchrezension zu: Kursbuch Bioethik. *Biospektrum* **2020**, *26*, 347. [CrossRef]
49. Kodeks Etyki Lekarza Weterynarii. Available online: https://vetpol.org.pl/dmdocuments/Kodeks%20etyki%20lekarza%20weterynarii.pdf (accessed on 26 June 2023).
50. Ach, J.S. Umgang mit Tieren in der Forschung. Grundsätze des neuen Leitbilds der Universität Münster. *Z. Für Evang. Ethik* **2019**, *63*, 34–44. [CrossRef]
51. Nagasawa, T.; Kimura, Y.; Masuda, K.; Uchiyama, H. Consiglio Nazionale FNOVI. Codice Deontologico. Available online: https://www.fnovi.it/fnovi/codice-deontologico (accessed on 26 June 2023).
52. Baumgaertner, H.; Mullan, S.; Main, D.C.J.; Bsc, H.B.; Bvms, S.M.; BVetMed, D.C.J.M. Assessment of unnecessary suffering in animals by veterinary experts. *Veter. Rec.* **2016**, *179*, 307. [CrossRef]
53. Código Deontológico Para El Ejercicio de La Profesión Veterinaria. Available online: https://colegioveterinarios.net/wp-content/uploads/2018/10/BORRADOR-C%C3%93DIGO-DEONTOL%C3%93GICO-PARA-EL-EJERCICIO-DE-LA-PROFESI%C3%93N-VETERINARIA-Versi%C3%B3n-Septiembre-de-2018.pdf (accessed on 26 June 2023).
54. García, J.M.G. Laboratory medicine and the identity change of veterinary medicine in Spain at the turn of the twentieth century. *Dynamis* **2010**, *30*, 239–260. [CrossRef]
55. Vandeweerd, J.-M.; Kirschvink, N.; Clegg, P.; Vandenput, S.; Gustin, P.; Saegerman, C. Is evidence-based medicine so evident in veterinary research and practice? History, obstacles and perspectives. *Veter. J.* **2012**, *191*, 28–34. [CrossRef] [PubMed]
56. Directive 2010/63/EU of the European Parliament and the Council of 22 September 2010 on the Protection of Animals Used for Scientific Purposes. Available online: https://eur-lex.europa.eu/legal-content/EN/TXT/HTML/?uri=CELEX:32010L0063&qid=1687795274615 (accessed on 26 June 2023).
57. Olsson, I.A.S.; da Silva, S.P.; Townend, D.; Sandøe, P. Protecting Animals and Enabling Research in the European Union: An Overview of Development and Implementation of Directive 2010/63/EU. *ILAR J.* **2016**, *57*, 347–357. [CrossRef] [PubMed]
58. Chlebus, M.; Guillen, J.; Prins, J.-B. Directive 2010/63/EU: Facilitating full and correct implementation. *Lab. Anim.* **2016**, *50*, 151. [CrossRef]
59. Skorupski, J.; Budniak, M.; Śmietana, P. Etyka badań nad dzikimi zwierzętami nocnymi w kontekście oddziaływania zanieczyszczenia światłem i zanieczyszczenia hałasem. *Stud. i Mater. CEPL w Rogowie* **2016**, 73–78.
60. Tannenbaum, J. Ethics and Pain Research in Animals. *ILAR J.* **1999**, *40*, 97–110. [CrossRef]
61. Verschuere, B.; Autissier, C.; Degryse, A.D.; Gallix, P.; Gottis, B.; Laurent, J.; Leinoe, M.; Peyclit, I. Ethics committee recommendations for laboratory animals in private research in France. *Lab. Anim.* **2000**, *34*, 236–243. [CrossRef]

animals

MDPI

Communication

Training in Honey Bee Veterinary Medicine in Italy: An Observational Study and Practical Proposals to Face Professional Challenges

Carlo D'Ascenzi [1,2], Karen Power [3,4], Paola Maiolino [3,4] and Michele Mortarino [2,4,*]

[1] Department of Veterinary Sciences, University of Pisa, 56124 Pisa, Italy; carlo.dascenzi@unipi.it
[2] Department of Veterinary Medicine and Animal Sciences, University of Milan, 26900 Lodi, Italy
[3] Department of Veterinary Medicine and Animal Productions, University of Naples "Federico II", 80137 Naples, Italy; karen.power@unina.it (K.P.); maiolino@unina.it (P.M.)
[4] Veterinary Scientific Society for Beekeeping—SVETAP, 00178 Rome, Italy
* Correspondence: michele.mortarino@unimi.it; Tel.: +39-02-50334534

Simple Summary: Currently, there are not many opportunities for undergraduate students to learn about Honey Bee Veterinary Medicine (HBVM) in their regular degree programs. This is a problem because veterinarians are increasingly responsible for taking care of honey bee health and production. Additionally, there are not many options for veterinarians to specialize in HBVM after graduation. This study aimed to monitor the educational opportunities for veterinarians in Italy. The study looked at both undergraduate and postgraduate programs, including degree programs in Veterinary Medicine, Masters, and other postgraduate courses. The results show that the training available for veterinarians in beekeeping in Italy is insufficient, which is a problem in other European and non-European countries as well. Finally, this study suggests a plan for training veterinarians in beekeeping that will meet the needs of the profession in the future while also following current and future public health regulations.

Abstract: Honey bees, like other livestock, may be affected by infectious, parasitic, and abiotic diseases that need proper sanitary monitoring and control. Currently, there are limited opportunities for undergraduate students to receive education in Honey Bee Veterinary Medicine (HBVM) as part of their regular degree program, despite the professional requirements for veterinarians to carry out the increasing tasks related to honey bee health and production. Additionally, postgraduate training and specialization in HBVM is also underdeveloped. This study was an observational survey that evaluated the educational opportunities available in HBVM for current and future veterinarians in Italy. The survey analyzed both undergraduate and postgraduate programs, including Undergraduate Degree Programs in Veterinary Medicine (UDPVM), "Scuole di Specializzazione", Masters, and other postgraduate courses. The results indicate that the current training available for veterinarians in the field of apiculture, both before and after graduation, is also insufficient in Italy, as already reported in other EU- and extra-EU countries. Finally, a roadmap for veterinary training in HBVM is developed here describing objectives and teachings aimed at fulfilling the needs of the profession in the field of beekeeping, considering the existing rules and regulations governing public health and possible evolution of this legal framework in the future.

Keywords: honey bee; beekeeping; veterinary medicine; infectious; parasitic and abiotic diseases; food safety; Italian survey; undergraduate education; postgraduate education; veterinary specialization; roadmap

1. Introduction

Most pollinating insects are wild, but some species are farmed for their economic value. Among the farmed species, the most numerous are those pertaining to the genus *Apis* and of which the most common is the honey bee (*Apis mellifera* L.), the third most important livestock species in Italy (97,938 farms), after cattle (134,298 farms) and small ruminant farming (135,591 farms) [1]; 650,000 beekeepers are found throughout the European Union, managing 17.5 million hives and producing about 280,000 tons of honey annually [2]. In Italy, 71,104 beekeepers have been counted, of which 51,483 produce for self-consumption (72% of the total) with about 354,802 hives (24% of the total), and 19,621 are professional beekeepers who produce for the market (28% of the total), with over 1,127,958 hives (76% of the total) [1]. Honey bees are mainly farmed for honey production; however, many others are the hive products, which have been used since ancient times in nutrition and for human psychophysical well-being [3–5]. The beginning of the human–honey bee relationship can be dated to at least 10,000 years ago, as documented by the rock paintings discovered in the Cave of the Spider [6]. Since then, honey bees have accompanied mankind through the centuries, and signs of the use of honey bee products have been found in all the main civilizations from Babylonians to Greeks and Romans [7–9].

Honey bees, together with wild species, provide about 70 percent of the pollination of all plant species on the planet, generating significant induced economic value related to the spontaneous or controlled service of pollination [10,11]. According to the Third Report on the State of Natural Capital in Italy [12] the economic value of the pollination service of Italian agricultural areas is estimated to be around 2 billion euros per year. Bees and other pollinators, such as bumblebees, represent the core of the One Health Concept, now more than ever of great interest and sensitivity, helping to maintain the balance between "Human-Animal-Environmental" Health [13]. In the One Health approach, it is increasingly evident that the beekeeping sector needs to make use of adequately trained veterinarians, both at the level of the Public Veterinary Services of Health Authorities (control activities) and at the level of the Universities (diagnostic and research activities), as well as within the veterinary freelance profession, to face the challenges represented by the monitoring, prevention, control, and eradication of notifiable diseases, as well as assuring food safety of beekeeping products.

To date, it appears that the relationship between veterinarians and beekeepers is mainly restricted to a controller–controlled relationship aimed at evaluating the compliance to regulations. On the contrary, veterinarians should support beekeepers in the implementation of national and international regulations concerning the identification, traceability, and movement of bees, following the evolution of the regulatory sector where particular emphasis is placed on the role of veterinarians in assessing the epidemiological risk connected to beekeeping, managing the use of veterinary drugs, and protecting consumers, i.e., against fraud, managing of information systems [14–17]. Under current regulations, veterinarians are called to play a key role in guaranteeing the health of honey bee colonies and of human individuals by securing the food safety of beekeeping products [18]. In addition, veterinarians should be trained to support the diverse services that beekeeping can provide, e.g., pollination of plant crops, monitoring of environmental contaminants, apitherapy, and apitourism. Finally, veterinarians should recognize and support the socio-cultural value of beekeeping, in relation to the appreciation of the natural environment, the creation of leisure, and work opportunities [19]. However, in the past decades, this field has elicited little interest among veterinarians, leading to the impoverishment of their knowledge. In order to face the new challenges in this sector, veterinarians should acquire adequate knowledge and skills during the Undergraduate Degree Program in Veterinary Medicine (UDPVM) to carry out the clinical examination of honey bee colonies and other veterinary tasks related to Honey Bee Veterinary Medicine (HBVM).

In this context, the interest of various institutions and organizations, both nationally and internationally, in the topic of veterinarian training in beekeeping is increasing [2,20]. Recent surveys have shown that there is considerable dissimilarity regarding the level and mode of teaching of HBVM in the different curricula of Veterinary Medicine in Europe and the rest of the world. HBVM is an area of Veterinary Medicine for which few educational opportunities are made available to undergraduate students during their regular degree program, even though as veterinarians they should have the theoretical and practical knowledge and skills that have been mentioned above. A recent study of undergraduate education in Veterinary Medicine conducted at the European Union level showed that only a portion of the UDPVM provides students with knowledge and skills in HBVM, usually as elective teaching or part of other subjects [20]. According to this study, the teaching of HBVM at the undergraduate level in the EU receives less attention in the curricula compared to other areas that are less widespread and popular, such as Veterinary Medicine of Laboratory Animals and Aquatic Species. In terms of postgraduate training, specialization in HBVM is also not particularly developed. In fact, there are only a few national specialization programs, and there Is no Veterinary College recognized by the European Board of Veterinary Specialization (EBVS) capable of providing European-wide recognition for specialists in HBVM, as is the case with other disciplines [20].

The present study was an observational survey on the educational offerings in HBVM provided by Italian universities to current and future veterinarians. The survey focused on both undergraduate and postgraduate programs analyzing the UDPVM activity in Italy, together with University Masters and Postgraduate Courses open to Veterinary Medicine graduates, and describes an educational proposal, defined y objectives and teachings, aimed at filling the needs related to the practice of the profession in the field of beekeeping.

2. Materials and Methods

The study analyzed the educational offerings of the thirteen Italian universities with Veterinary Medicine, namely the following: University of Messina (UNIME), University of Bari (UNIBA), University of Naples (UNINA), University of Sassari (UNISS), University of Teramo (UNITE), University of Perugia (UNIPG), University of Camerino (UNICAM), University of Pisa (UNIPI), University of Bologna (UNIBO), University of Parma (UNIPR), University of Torino (UNITO), University of Milano (UNIMI), University of Padova (UNIPD). Initially, the survey activity focused on analyzing the educational programs of the UDPVM. Data were evaluated based on the information provided by the "Universitaly" website (https://www.universitaly.it/ accessed on 15 November 2022). Particularly, for each UDPVM, the corresponding Scheda Unica Annuale (SUA) was examined, possibly supplemented by information available on the websites of the respective universities (Supplementary Table S1). For UDPVM, the source of the study curricula consists of the corresponding Manifesto Annuale degli Studi for the 2022/23 academic year or the Regolamento Didattico, to which the SUA files refer. The Manifesto Annuale degli Studi is the document which, in accordance with the academic teaching regulations, conveys the information relating to the educational offerings for the following academic year. The Regolamento Didattico, unlike the Academic Systems, is approved exclusively at the local level and specifies the organizational and functioning aspects of the UDCVM: objectives, entry requirements, subjects and other training activities, propaedeutics, curriculum, indications relating to the exams and the final exam, any attendance obligations, and other useful information. SUA is a management tool that is functional for the planning, implementation, self-assessment, and re-planning of the educational program. The survey identified the courses, which presented in the title a clear referral to HBVM subjects and in which the relative teaching commitment was quantifiable (European Credit Transfer and Accumulation System, ECTS, or hours). Teaching activities of HBVM were then classified as a separate subject incorporated into a curriculum (monographic), as part of other subjects in a curriculum (integrated), as mandatory or elective. Among these, the Settore Scientifico Disciplinare (SSD) for the UDPVM and the ECTS have also been identified and differentiated into lectures and practical lessons. The SSD corresponds to a specific academic discipline as reported in the Decreto Ministeriale, 4 October 2000 [21], and following amendments and modifications. The methodological tool consisted of the analysis, relating to the most recent academic year for which information was found, of the study curricula, on which programmatic documents are described in the list of courses with an indication of the reference SSD and any articulation into modules, as well as other training subjects. Subsequently, the survey focused on the postgraduate programs, namely "Scuole di Specializzazione", University Masters, and "Corsi di Perfezionamento", and a search was carried out as for the UDPVM (Table 1).

Table 1. Veterinary Medicine educational programs evaluated.

University	UDPVM	Scuole di Specializzazione		Masters and Corsi di Perfezionamento
Acronym	**AY**	**Type**	**AY**	**AY**
UNIME	2022/2023	Inspection of Food of Animal Origin	2021/2022 2022/2023	2021/2022
UNIBA	2022/2023	Inspection of Food of Animal Origin; Infectious Diseases, Prophylaxis, and Animal Health Requirements	2020/2021 2021/2022 2022/2023	2021/2022
UNINA	2022/2023	Inspection of Food of Animal Origin; Infectious Diseases, Prophylaxis, and Animal Health Requirements; Animal Feeding; Applied Ethology and Animal Welfare	2020/2021 2021/2022 2022/2023	2021/2022
UNISS	2022/2023	Inspection of Food of Animal Origin; Animal Health, Livestock Husbandry, and Productions.	2020/2021 2021/2022 2022/2023	2021/2022
UNITE	2022/2023	Inspection of Food of Animal Origin; Animal Health, Livestock Husbandry, and Productions	2020/2021 2021/2022 2022/2023	2021/2022
UNIPG	2022/2023	-	2020/2021 2021/2022 2022/2023	2021/2022
UNICAM	2022/2023	Animal Health, Livestock Husbandry, and Productions	2020/2021 2021/2022 2022/2023	2021/2022
UNIPI	2022/2023	Inspection of Food of Animal Origin; Animal Health, Livestock Husbandry, and Productions	2020/2021 2021/2022 2022/2023	2021/2022
UNIBO	2022/2023	Animal Health, Livestock Husbandry, and Productions	2020/2021 2021/2022 2022/2023	2021/2022
UNIPR	2022/2023	Inspection of Food of Animal Origin; Animal Health, Livestock Husbandry, and Productions	2020/2021 2021/2022 2022/2023	2021/2022
UNITO	2022/2023	Inspection of Food of Animal Origin	2020/2021 2021/2022 2022/2023	2021/2022
UNIMI	2022/2023	Animal Health, Livestock Husbandry, and Productions; Prophylaxis and Animal Health Requirements; Animal Feeding; Applied Ethology and Animal Welfare	2020/2021 2021/2022 2022/2023	2021/2022
UNIPD	2022/2023	Inspection of Food of Animal Origin; Animal Health, Livestock Husbandry, and Productions; Infectious Diseases, Prophylaxis, and Animal Health Requirements; Animal Feeding; Applied Ethology and Animal Welfare	2020/2021 2021/2022 2022/2023	2021/2022

Acronym of University, the Academic Year (AY) of Undergraduate Degree Program in Veterinary Medicine (UDPVM), "Scuola di Specializzazione", Masters and "Corsi di Perfezionamento", and the type of "Scuola di Specializzazione" evaluated are presented.

The "Scuole di Specializzazione" are Italian educational establishments regulated by the Decreto Ministeriale, 27 January 2006, n. 146 [22]. The" Scuole di Specializzazione", which can only be accessed by graduates in Veterinary Medicine, award the title of specialist, a prerequisite for accessing professional roles in the Italian National Public Health Service. The "Corsi di Perfezionamento", regulated by Legge 341/90 [23], are provided through postgraduate training, which allows for the development and training of high-level skills and abilities for the improvement of one's professionalism. They are promoted by universities in collaboration with other public or private institutions, and unlike masters, do not issue an academic qualification, but a certificate of participation, which certifies the skills acquired during the course. Regarding the "Scuole di Specializzazione", considering that for some schools the three-year course is not always activated in the same academic year, reference was made to the last three years, i.e., from 2020/21 to 2022/23. For the Masters and "Corsi di Perfezionamento", the reference was made to the academic year 2021/22 (Table 1).

3. Results

The survey on UDPVM revealed that only 5/13 universities present HBVM courses in the educational curricula (UNIBA, UNINA, UNISS, UNIPI, UNIMI); particularly, 1/13 universities (UNISS) delivers mandatory, though incorporated, teaching in the field of HBVM, while 2/13 universities (UNIBA and UNINA) provide incorporated monothematic courses. Moreover, 3/13 universities (UNINA, UNIPI, UNIMI) offer a traineeship in HBVM as part of the 5th year final traineeship (Table 2).

Table 2. Teaching dedicated to HBVM (5 years) in Italy.

University	Year	ECTS		Teaching		SSD
		Lectures	Practical	Type	Name	
UNIBA	4th	1	1	Monographic/ Mandatory	Hygiene and Safety of the Beekeeping Industry (1)	VET/04
UNINA	5th	3	3	Monographic/ Elective	Husbandry, Pathophysiology, and Pathology of Bees	AGR/20 VET/03
	5th	-	1	Incorporated/ Elective	Traineeship in Animal Husbandry	n.a.
UNISS	4th	2	-	Incorporated/ Mandatory	Inspection of Meat, Eggs, and Honey Products (2)	VET/04
UNIPI	4th	-	1	Incorporated/ Mandatory	Traineeship in Zooculture "Breeding of Small Species"	AGR/20
UNIMI	5th	-	4	Incorporated/ Elective	Traineeship in Zootechnics "Breeding of Major and Minor Species"	AGR/17

Acronym of University, Academic Year (AY) of UDPVM in which the teaching is offered, number of the European Credit Transfer and Accumulation System (ECTS) allocated for lectures and practical teaching, type of course provided, name of the teaching and Settore Scientifico Disciplinare (SSD) are presented. (1) The module is incorporated in the course "Food Safety 1"; (2) the subject is incorporated in the course "Food Inspection, Control and Certification"; n.a.: not available.

The survey on postgraduate teaching revealed that 5/13 universities (UNINA, UNIBA, UNITE, UNIBO, UNIMI) have HBVM-dedicated teaching in the Scuole di Specializzazione, mainly as integrated courses and only 1/13 offers practical teaching (UNIMI) (Table 3).

Regarding the offering of the University Masters or "Corsi di Perfezionamento", the survey showed that only one Master and one "Corso di Perfezionamento" are available for graduated veterinarians and are provided by UNITE and UNINA, respectively. The Master in "Beekeeping: environmental and health management" provides 30 ECTSs corresponding to 300 h of lectures, 20 ECTSs corresponding to 200 h of practical activities, 5 ECTSs of elective training activities, and 5 ECTSs for the final exam. The "Corso di Perfezionamento" in "Hygienic and sanitary management of apiaries for the protection of the environment and biodiversity" provides 15 ECTSs corresponding to a total of 375 h, of which 170 h are lectures and practical activities and 205 h are self-study.

Table 3. Teaching dedicated to "Scuole di Specializzazione" (3 years) in Italy.

University	Year	ECTS		Type of Scuola di Specializzazione and Name of Teaching	SSD
		Lectures	Practical		
UNIBA				INSPECTION OF FOOD OF ANIMAL ORIGIN	
	3th	3	-	Beehive Products and Sector Legislation	VET/04
	3th	3	-	Chemical Risk Connected to Beehive Products	VET/04
UNINA				INSPECTION OF FOOD OF ANIMAL ORIGIN	
	1st	2	-	Inspection Of Honey, Eggs, and Derivatives and Relevant Legislation	VET/04
UNITE				INSPECTION OF FOOD OF ANIMAL ORIGIN	
	1st	n.a.	n.a.	Sanitary Inspection of Dairy Products, Eggs, and Honey	VET/04
UNIBO				ANIMAL HEALTH, LIVESTOCK HUSBANDRY, AND PRODUCTIONS	
	n.a	n.a.	n.a.	Livestock Registry Management—Sanitary Control in Beekeeping	VET/06
				INSPECTION OF FOOD OF ANIMAL ORIGIN	
	n.a	3	-	Beehive Products and Sector Legislation	VET/04
	n.a	3	-	Chemical Risk Connected to Beehive Products	VET/04
UNIMI				ANIMAL HEALTH, LIVESTOCK HUSBANDRY, AND PRODUCTIONS	
	2	-	1	Parasitology and Parasitic Diseases—Sanitary Management of the Apiary	VET/06

Acronym of University, Academic Year (AY) of "Scuola di Specializzazione" in which the teaching is offered, number of the European Credit Transfer and Accumulation System (ECTS) allocated for lectures and practical teaching, type of "Scuola di Specializzazione", and name of teaching and Settore Scientifico Disciplinare (SSD) are presented. n.a.: not available.

4. Discussion

Despite Italian beekeeping representing one of the largest beekeeping sectors in Europe, with a significant number of apiaries and beekeepers involved, and the role that veterinarians are called to play under current regulations, the results of our survey show that Italian universities are currently unable to provide the education required. Furthermore, the lack of an appropriate teaching and training program in UDPVM is not compensated by an adequate postgraduate offering, which could fill the gaps in HBVM knowledge, leaving the education of veterinarians to personal initiative. In such a context, it appears evident the necessity to start training future veterinarians in the University by including HBVM subjects in the Day One Competencies. Day One Competencies represent the minimum standard skills required for a newly graduated veterinarian to initiate the different roles of the veterinary profession [24]. They were established by the European Coordination Committee for Veterinary Training (ECCVT) founded in 2004 by the European Association of Establishments for Veterinary Education (EAEVE), the European Board of Veterinary Specialization (EBVS), and the Federation of Veterinarians of Europe (FVE) [24]. The general basic veterinary competence is currently established by specific EU provisions [25]. A recent graduate who has achieved Day One Competencies should be able to independently perform the entry-level tasks and duties appropriate for veterinary practice and should be self-confident enough to self-practice veterinary medicine at the primary-care level, while knowing when it is appropriate to seek guidance from more experienced colleagues. Day One Competencies in HBVM are lacking in all the Universities analyzed in the present survey, and these skills should be implemented in the educational programs of UDPVM, and the educational programs should ensure that the theoretical and practical training is organized and delivered in the appropriate manner, enabling veterinarians to perform all of his or her functions soon after graduation, preparing them to face the world of work.

At this juncture, the European System of Evaluation of Veterinary Training (ESEVT), developed by the EAEVE in collaboration with the FVE for the European accreditation of UDPVM, can represent the tool for the standardization of veterinary curricula in the EU and ensure the correct implementation HBVM teaching. The main tasks and fundamental skills that a veterinarian should acquire to be qualified to practice in the apiary include the clinical examination of honey bee colonies with adequate safety precautions; recognition of disease signs affecting the brood and adult honey bees; sampling with compilation of formal documentation for delivery to an authorized diagnostic laboratory; basic knowledge of laboratory tests; prevention, treatment, control, and eradication of honey bee infectious, parasitic, and abiotic diseases, including those reportable on the basis of the regulatory framework governing the sector at the national and international level; management of food safety guarantees for beehive products; and support to the beekeeper in providing services related to beekeeping and the environmental context. Special attention is required for training needs in health and food safety considering the current regulatory framework of public health and future training needs based on the evolution of guidelines and rules. Currently, the veterinary staff in charge of the official control needs skills in the beekeeping sector, which are addressed for the prevention and control of health problems; this field has been governed by consolidated national and/or international legislation based on the Regolamento di Polizia Veterinaria [26], with regard to Animal health, and on the National Residues Plan [27,28], with regard to food safety. Based on the progressive implementation of the recent regulations issued in the field of veterinary public health, the beekeeping sector is susceptible to growing interactions with the aims of the juridical assets of EU-member States, including the health and welfare of farmed animals, the quality and safety of the product, the protection of the natural and man-made environment, and the socio-economic field. The issuing of EU Regulation 2016/429 [15] provides the possibility of delegating functions, principally of official control, to self-employed veterinarians who hold the role of farm veterinarians. This regulatory innovation increases the need to recognize the validity of the knowledge and skills accumulated during the exercise of the profession, where the corresponding and recognized training courses are missing. Honey bee health care can be considered one of these areas, given that, as underlined by our study, the educational programs available during both the undergraduate and postgraduate period are often incomplete and fragmented. Consequently, the training of veterinarians in the beekeeping field is substantially based on the professional experience that can be acquired in the field while working alongside already expert colleagues and on attending a portfolio of training and updating events selected on an individual and autonomous basis. This experience may be susceptible to ex-post recognition and validation through the instrument of professional certification, which takes into consideration both passive learning and the professional activity carried out in various capacities. In any case, to date, there are no adequately structured and time-lined training courses, which can guarantee the acquisition of a satisfactory level of knowledge and skills in the beekeeping field for the veterinarian. Therefore, there is the need to establish an organic and suitably designed educational program, in terms of methods and times, which leads the veterinarian to acquire the knowledge and skills necessary for the performance of his/her duties in the beekeeping sector. For the purpose of adapting the professional profile of the veterinarian, it is possible to design a curriculum in HBVM that includes the definition of specific training objectives, the formulation of the related training commitment in terms of credits with assignment of the relevant scientific disciplinary fields, represented, e.g., by the SSD required by Italian legislation. Given the complexity of the knowledge and skills necessary for adequate preparation of the veterinarian in the beekeeping sector, the training objectives should be divided into two levels: first-level objectives to be achieved during undergraduate programs, and a series of second-level objectives to be achieved in the postgraduate courses for deepening and consolidating professional skills in HBVM. According to an ideal scenario, the former should be included in the study plan of the UDPVM, as dedicated and compulsory monothematic/monographic courses, to be formulated as shown in Table 4.

Table 4. List of monographic courses aimed at achieving the first-level training objectives in HBVM in the UDPVM.

Teaching	ECTS	SSD
Honey Bee Biology and Ecology	1	AGR/02-03-11
Honey Bee Breeding and Reproduction	2	AGR/11-17-18-19-20
Pathology, Diagnosis, Therapy, and Prophylaxis of Infectious, Parasitic, and Abiotic Diseases of Honey Bees	2	VET/03-05-06-07
Commercial and Hygienic Quality of Beehive Products	2	AGR/19-VET/04
Veterinary Law and Legislation, Economics, and Management of Honey Bee Breeding	1	AGR/01-VET/08

Name of teaching, European Credit Transfer and Accumulation System (ECTS) allocated to teaching, and Settore Scientifico Disciplinare (SSD) of an ideal scenario are presented.

Given the foreseeable regulatory and practical difficulty of including compulsory single-subject courses in the current teaching systems, it is possible to hypothesize a more realistic scenario, according to which the first-level learning objectives can still be achieved by including the subjects reported in Table 4 into non-single-theme courses; the teaching load of such courses should, in any case, be adjusted proportionally and according to the context. The achievement of the first-level learning objectives during the UDPVM would enable the formulation of more specific second-level objectives and guarantee adequate in-depth study of the preparation of the veterinarians for the purpose of carrying out the profession in the beekeeping sector. Second-level objectives should include the following: honey bee anatomy, physiology, and immunology; feeding and nutrition; beekeeping techniques and good beekeeping practices; apicultural services, including pollination, environmental monitoring, apitherapy, and apitourism; current legislation and administrative fulfilments relating to the beekeeping registry; honey bee disease epidemiology; honey bee general pathology and anatomo-pathology; recognition, diagnosis, and treatment of the main infectious and parasitic diseases of honey bees, and related surveillance and eradication plans; impact of environmental and anthropic risk factors for the health and well-being of honey bees; honey bee pharmacosurveillance and pharmacovigilance; qualitative characterization of hive products; quality assurance and food safety of hive products. These objectives could be achieved during postgraduate training courses required for the mandatory and continuous updating of skills (Continuing Medical Education System) and similar initiatives, without necessarily relying on a specific type of training. Taken together, the above objectives should be placed more clearly among the fundamental knowledge and skills that a veterinarian should acquire in the training path. It would be desirable for EAEVE to define criteria and procedures for the inclusion of apicultural issues among the requirements that the UDPVM should possess for the purposes of European accreditation; this should also be included in the list of compulsory subjects and corresponding indicators for EAEVE assessment [24].

5. Conclusions

As the health and sustainability of honey bee populations become more crucial to global food security and ecosystem health, it is expected that the significance of veterinary education in beekeeping will continue to increase in the upcoming years. Based on what has been reported in recent literature and on the results of this study, the training in the field of apiculture that veterinarians may have at their disposal, both before and after graduation, cannot yet be considered sufficient. Future veterinarians need to receive education on several key topics related to beekeeping, including honey bee anatomy and physiology, behavior, diseases and pests, pesticide use and exposure, nutrition and feeding, beekeeping management practices, safety of hive-derived products, sustainable beekeeping, and research skills. The quantity and variety of teaching that should cover these subjects may vary from a necessary minimum to a more exhaustive and ideal articulation. An all-encompassing education in these subject matters will equip veterinarians to manage honey bee health effectively, prioritize sustainability, and contribute to the development of innovative solutions for beekeeping challenges. To adequately prepare veterinarians, comprehensive education in beekeeping should encompass both practical and theoretical knowledge. Finally, it would be desirable to establish a body for comparison and discussion at the international level among educational institutions active in the field of veterinary apiculture, to achieve a broad consensus on the educational objectives to be pursued and the best tools to achieve them, both in the pre-degree path and in the post-degree path.

Supplementary Materials: The following supporting information can be downloaded at: https://www.mdpi.com/article/10.3390/ani13111795/s1, Table S1: Web addresses of Universities and Veterinary Departments.

Author Contributions: Conceptualization, C.D., K.P., P.M. and M.M.; methodology, C.D. and M.M.; validation, K.P. and P.M.; investigation, C.D., K.P., P.M. and M.M.; writing—original draft preparation, C.D. and P.M.; writing—review and editing, K.P. and M.M. All authors have read and agreed to the published version of the manuscript.

Funding: This research received no external funding.

Institutional Review Board Statement: Not applicable.

Informed Consent Statement: Not applicable.

Data Availability Statement: Data are available upon request to the authors.

Conflicts of Interest: The authors declare no conflict of interest.

References

1. Ministero della Salute. 2022. Sistema Informativo Veterinario. Available online: https://www.vetinfo.it/ (accessed on 15 November 2022).
2. European Commission. Report from the Commission to the European Parliament and the Council on the Implementation of Apiculture Programmes. COM/2019/635 Final. 2019. Available online: https://eur-lex.europa.eu/legal-content/en/ALL/?uri=CELEX:52019DC0635 (accessed on 19 November 2022).
3. Sforcin, J.M.; Bankova, V.; Kuropatnicki, A.K. Medical Benefits of Honeybee Products. *Evid. Based Complement Alternat. Med.* **2017**, *2017*, 2702106. [CrossRef] [PubMed]
4. El-Seedi, H.R.; Eid, N.; Abd El-Wahed, A.A.; Rateb, M.E.; Afifi, H.S.; Algethami, A.F.; Zhao, C.; Al Naggar, Y.; Alsharif, S.M.; Tahir, H.E.; et al. Honey Bee Products: Preclinical and Clinical Studies of Their Anti-inflammatory and Immunomodulatory Properties. *Front. Nutr.* **2022**, *8*, 761267. [CrossRef]
5. Alton, K.; Ratnieks, F. Can Beekeeping Improve Mental Wellbeing during Times of Crisis? *Bee World* **2022**, *99*, 40–43. [CrossRef]
6. Nayik, G.A.; Shah, T.R.; Muzaffar, K.; Wani, S.A.; Gull, A.; Majid, I.; Bhat, F.M. Honey: Its history and religious significance: A review. *Univers. J. Pharm.* **2014**, *3*, 5–8.
7. Crane, E. *The Archeology of Beekeeping*; Duckworth: London, UK, 1983; Volume 360, p. 270.
8. Crane, E. The world's beekeeping-past and present. In *The Hive and the Honey Bee*; Dadant & Sons: Hamilton, OH, USA, 1992; pp. 1–22.
9. Crane, E. *The World History of Beekeeping and Honey Hunting*; Routledge: London, UK, 1999.
10. Garibaldi, L.A.; Aizen, M.A.; Klein, A.M.; Cunningham, S.A.; Harder, L.D. Global growth and stability of agricultural yield decrease with pollinator dependence. *Proc. Natl. Acad. Sci. USA* **2011**, *108*, 5909–5914. [CrossRef] [PubMed]
11. Ollerton, J.; Winfree, R.; Tarrant, S. How many flowering plants are pollinated by animals? *Oikos* **2011**, *120*, 321–326. [CrossRef]
12. Comitato per il Capitale Naturale (Ministero per la Transizione Ecologica). 2019. Terzo Rapporto sullo Stato del Capitale Naturale in Italia. 2019. Available online: https://www.mite.gov.it/pagina/terzo-rapporto-sullo-stato-del-capitale-naturale-italia-2019 (accessed on 17 December 2022).
13. de Jongh, E.J.; Harper, S.L.; Yamamoto, S.S.; Wright, C.J.; Wilkinson, C.W.; Ghosh, S.; Otto, S.J.G. One Health, One Hive: A scoping review of honey bees, climate change, pollutants, and antimicrobial resistance. *PLoS ONE* **2022**, *17*, e0242393. [CrossRef] [PubMed]
14. Regulation (EU) 2017/625 of the European Parliament and of the Council of 15 March 2017 on Official Controls and Other Official Activities Performed to Ensure the Application of Food and Feed Law, Rules on Animal Health and Welfare, Plant Health and Plant Protection Products, Amending Regulations (EC) No 999/2001, (EC) No 396/2005, (EC) No 1069/2009, (EC) No 1107/2009, (EU) No 1151/2012, (EU) No 652/2014, (EU) 2016/429 and (EU) 2016/2031 of the European Parliament and of the Council, Council Regulations (EC) No 1/2005 and (EC) No 1099/2009 and Council Directives 98/58/EC, 1999/74/EC, 2007/43/EC, 2008/119/EC and 2008/120/EC, and Repealing Regulations (EC) No 854/2004 and (EC) No 882/2004 of the European Parliament and of the Council, Council Directives 89/608/EEC, 89/662/EEC, 90/425/EEC, 91/496/EEC, 96/23/EC, 96/93/EC and 97/78/EC and Council Decision 92/438/EEC (Official Controls Regulation). 2017. Available online: http://data.europa.eu/eli/reg/2017/625/2022-01-28 (accessed on 17 December 2022).

15. Regulation (EU) 2016/429 of the European Parliament and of the Council of 9 March 2016 on Transmissible Animal Diseases and Amending and Repealing Certain Acts in the Area of Animal Health ('Animal Health Law'). 2016. Available online: http://data.europa.eu/eli/reg/2016/429/2021-04-21 (accessed on 15 December 2022).
16. Parlamento Italiano, Decreto Legislativo 5 August 2022, n. 136. Attuazione Dell'articolo 14, Comma 2, Lettere (a), (b), (e), (f), (h), (i), (l), (n), (o) (p), Della Legge 22 Aprile 2021, n. 53 per Adeguare e Raccordare la Normativa Nazionale in Materia di Prevenzione e Controllo Delle Malattie Animali Che Sono Trasmissibili Agli Animali o All'uomo, Alle Disposizioni del Regolamento (UE) 2016/429 del Parlamento Europeo e del Consiglio, del 9 Marzo 2016. GU Serie Generale n.213 del 12-09-2022. Available online: http://www.normattiva.it/eli/id/2022/09/12/22G00144/ORIGINAL (accessed on 15 December 2022).
17. Ministero della Salute, Decreto 7 December 2017. Sistema di Reti di Epidemio-Sorveglianza, Compiti, Responsabilità E Requisiti Professionali del Veterinario Aziendale. GU Serie Generale n. 29 del 05-02-2018. Available online: www.gazzettaufficiale.it/eli/id/2018/02/05/18A00687/sg (accessed on 20 January 2023).
18. Tlak Gajger, I.; Mañes, A.M.; Formato, G.; Mortarino, M.; Toporcak, J. Veterinarians and beekeeping: What roles, expectations and future perspectives?—A review paper. *Vet. Arh.* **2021**, *91*, 437–443. [CrossRef]
19. FAO; IZSLT; Apimondia; CAAS. Good beekeeping practices for sustainable apiculture. In *FAO Animal Production and Health Guidelines No. 25*; FAO: Rome, Italy, 2021. [CrossRef]
20. Iatridou, D.; Pohl, L.; Tlak Gajger, I.; De Briyne, N.; Bravo, A.; Saunders, J. Mapping the teaching of honeybee veterinary medicine in the European Union and European Free Trade Area. *Vet. Rec. Open* **2019**, *6*, e000343. [CrossRef] [PubMed]
21. Ministero dell'Istruzione, dell'Università e della Ricerca. Decreto Ministeriale 4 October 2000. Settori Scientifico-Disciplinari. GU Serie Generale n.249 del 24-10-2000-Suppl. Ordinario n. 175. Available online: www.gazzettaufficiale.it/eli/id/2000/10/24/00A13012/sg (accessed on 10 January 2023).
22. Ministero dell'Istruzione, dell'Università e della Ricerca. Decreto Ministeriale 27 January 2006. Riassetto delle Scuole di Specializzazione di Area Veterinaria. GU Serie Generale n. 146 del 15-06-2006. Available online: www.gazzettaufficiale.it/eli/id/2006/06/15/06A05472/sg (accessed on 10 January 2022).
23. Parlamento Italiano, Legge 19 November 1990, n. 341. Riforma Degli Ordinamenti Didattici Universitari. GU n.274 del 23-11-1990. Available online: http://www.normattiva.it/eli/id/1990/11/23/090G0387/CONSOLIDATED (accessed on 15 December 2022).
24. 24. ESEVT SOP 2019, Annex 2, 30 May 2019, as Amended in September 2021 European Association of Establishments for Veterinary Education (EAEVE). 2021. European System of Evaluation of Veterinary Training (ESEVT). Manual of Standard Operating Procedure. Available online: https://www.eaeve.org/fileadmin/downloads/SOP/ESEVT_SOP_2019_As_amended_in_September_2021.pdf (accessed on 17 December 2022).
25. Directive 2005/36/EC of the European Parliament and of the Council of 7 September 2005 on the Recognition of Professional Qualifications. 2005. Available online: http://data.europa.eu/eli/dir/2005/36/2021-12-10 (accessed on 10 December 2021).
26. Il Presidente della Repubblica Italiana. Decreto del Presidente della Repubblica 8 February 1954, n. 320. Regolamento di Polizia Veterinaria. GU n. 142 del 24-06-1954. Available online: http://www.normattiva.it/eli/id/1954/06/24/054U0320/CONSOLIDATED (accessed on 10 December 2022).
27. Il Presidente della Repubblica Italiana. Decreto Legislativo 4 August 1999, n. 336. Attuazione delle direttive 96/22/CE e 96/23/CE Concernenti il Divieto di Utilizzazione di Talune Sostanze ad Azione Ormonica, Tireostatica e delle Sostanze Agoniste Nelle Produzioni di Animali e le Misure di Controllo su Talune Sostanze e sui Loro Residui Negli Animali vivi e nei Loro Prodotti. GU n.230 del 30-09-1999. Available online: http://www.normattiva.it/eli/id/1999/09/30/099G0409/CONSOLIDATED (accessed on 13 January 2023).
28. Il Presidente della Repubblica Italiana. Decreto Legislativo 16 March 2006, n. 158. Attuazione della Direttiva 2003/74/CE che Modifica la Direttiva 96/22/CE del Consiglio, del 29 Aprile 1996, Concernente il Divieto di Utilizzazione di Talune Sostanze ad Azione Ormonica, Tireostatica e delle Sostanze Beta-Agoniste nelle Produzioni Animali e della Direttiva 96/23/CE, del Consiglio, del 29 aprile 1996, Concernente le Misure di Controllo su Talune Sostanze e sui Loro Residui Negli Animali vivi e nei Loro Prodotti, Come Modificata dal Regolamento 882/2004 del Parlamento Europeo e del Consiglio, del 29 aprile 2004, Nonché Abrogazione del Decreto Legislativo 4 Agosto 1999, n. 336. GU n. 98 del 28-04-2006. Available online: http://www.normattiva.it/eli/id/2006/04/28/006G0177/CONSOLIDATED (accessed on 13 January 2023).

animals

MDPI

Article

Effects of 3D Scans on Veterinary Students' Learning Outcomes Compared to Traditional 2D Images in Anatomy Classes

Rebecca Schirone [1,*], Giuliano Mario Corte [2], Jan P. Ehlers [3], Christina Herre [1], Maximiliane Schmedding [4], Roswitha Merle [5], Joëlle Pachtmann [1] and Mahtab Bahramsoltani [1]

1 Institute of Veterinary Anatomy, School of Veterinary Medicine, Freie Universität Berlin, Koserstraße 20, 14195 Berlin, Germany
2 Institute of Veterinary Anatomy, Vetsuisse Faculty, University of Zurich (UZH), Winterthurerstrasse 260, 8057 Zurich, Switzerland
3 Didactics and Educational Research in Health Science, Faculty of Health, Witten/Herdecke University, Alfred-Herrhausen-Straße 50, 58455 Witten, Germany; jan.ehlers@uni-wh.de
4 ISME Bern and Avenches, Vetsuisse Faculty, University of Bern, Hochschulstrasse 6, 3012 Bern, Switzerland
5 Institute of Veterinary Epidemiology and Biostatistics, School of Veterinary Medicine, Freie Universität Berlin, Königsweg 67, 14163 Berlin, Germany
* Correspondence: rebecca.schirone@fu-berlin.de

Simple Summary: 3D models are increasingly popular in veterinary teaching. However, students struggle with transferring 2D textbook images to 3D anatomical structures. Therefore, this study aimed to compare the learning outcome of 3D scans and 2D images of horse and pig skulls. Furthermore, the relationship between spatial ability and learning outcome was analyzed when using the different learning materials. Second-year veterinary medicine students participated in a practical anatomy course using 3D scans or 2D images as learning material and performed a test to determine their spatial ability. Independently of the learning material, all groups displayed high learning outcomes with no significant differences between the groups. In addition, it could not be stated that 3D scans support students with lower spatial ability. Nevertheless, students preferred 3D scans, finding them more motivating, although they did not necessarily improve learning outcomes.

Abstract: Students often struggle with interpreting traditional textbook images and translating them to anatomical structures. This study aimed to compare the impact of 3D scans versus 2D images on students' learning outcomes when learning anatomical structures on skulls from horses and pigs. Furthermore, the correlation between spatial ability and learning outcomes using 3D scans or 2D images was examined. Second-year veterinary medicine students either used 3D scans or 2D images, annotated with arrows or numbers as learning material. Students' anatomical knowledge was tested before and after the learning session, and spatial ability was assessed using the mental rotation test. All groups improved significantly in the post-test. However, the differences between groups were not significant, suggesting that 3D scans do not necessarily lead to higher learning outcomes. The analysis of the correlation between spatial ability and learning outcomes did not prove that students with weaker spatial ability benefit from 3D scans. Students preferred 3D scans over 2D images despite similar outcomes, suggesting they are valuable for learning. However, results show that the introduction of novel learning materials likely amplified the impact of reduced learning time on the 3D group, as these materials necessitated additional time for effective comprehension and integration.

Keywords: veterinary didactics; veterinary education; digital 3D models; 3D scans; 2D vs. 3D

1. Introduction

Anatomy represents one of the fundamental subjects encountered by students of veterinary and human medicine at the beginning of their studies. It forms an essential building block for further medical disciplines. By gaining knowledge and learning practical skills about anatomical structures, students acquire a foundation for related subjects, e.g., surgery, pathology, and radiology [1–3]. Moreover, anatomy holds substantial importance in the educational journey of medical students, influencing their learning experience both intellectually and emotionally [4]. Furthermore, expertise in anatomy is indispensable for graduate doctors and veterinarians [5–7]. Veterinarians of small animal practice underlined the importance of the ongoing process of learning and refreshing veterinary anatomy in order to competently carry out their profession. They emphasize the importance of teaching anatomy in the veterinary medicine curriculum. Additionally, the connection between the application of anatomy in their daily routine, psychomotor abilities, and professional skills was pointed out [6]. A study that was carried out with horses and farm animals showed that a solid and fundamental understanding of clinically relevant anatomy in combination with skills of recognizing complicated anatomical details and exploring unfamiliar areas, is crucial for the profession of a clinician. Adequate knowledge of veterinary anatomy seems to be essential for effective communication, enhancing trust and confidence for the competent performance of clinical tasks [7].

For this reason, the medical and veterinarian curriculum includes practical courses, which are carried out as cadaveric dissection [8,9]. They provide hands-on experiences that complement theoretical knowledge. The courses are indispensable for understanding the three-dimensional body, developing the ability to experience physical contact, understanding the topographical position of anatomical structures and organs and ultimately being able to master and interpret images derived from imaging procedures such as X-rays, ultrasound, or computer tomography [7,9,10]. The teaching materials used to prepare and support dissection courses have been predominantly two-dimensional drawings, supplemented by photographs and, more recently, videos. Visual materials provide valuable insights [11,12].

However, it is necessary to comment on the limitations of a two-dimensional surface. In practical anatomy courses, it has been shown that the transfer of information from two-dimensional (2D) teaching materials to the three-dimensional (3D) body was considered difficult by students [13,14]. The individual's spatial ability displays a major influencing factor. Several studies explored the correlation between spatial ability and anatomy learning [15–17]. To gain a thorough knowledge of anatomy, one must understand the comprehensive structure of organs both individually and in relation to the entire body. Anatomical structures have their own functional specificity and are often shaped asymmetrically and irregularly. Mental processing and retention of 3D configurations and the understanding of their spatial relationships are essential components for performing clinical analyses and interpretations [18]. A recent study stated that students with high spatial ability skills are significantly superior to individuals with low spatial ability skills when learning with static 2D images instead of 3D animated models. Researchers suggested that people with weaker spatial imagination could learn significantly better with 3D models [19].

In the present study, the use of 3D scans compared to 2D images as learning material in anatomy classes was investigated. The following hypotheses were tested:

1. When learning the anatomical structures of the skull, students who use 3D scans as learning material have a higher learning outcome than students who use 2D images as learning material.
2. There is an interaction effect between spatial ability and the learning material used, with students with low spatial ability having a higher learning outcome with the use of 3D scans than with 2D images.

2. Participants, Materials and Methods

2.1. Participants

For the current study, data was raised during the practical comparative anatomy lesson on the skull for second-year veterinary medicine students in October 2022 (study 1) and October 2023 (study 2).

During the previous anatomy lesson, a week before, the students were informed about the objectives and procedure of the study verbally and using an information letter. The students who agreed to take part in the study gave their informed consent for inclusion before they participated in the study by filling out and signing a data protection declaration. Students were assured that their involvement was voluntary, with data collection being anonymous. Participants were given the freedom to withdraw from the study at any time point without facing consequences. In addition, the participants were requested not to prepare for the upcoming lesson on the skull. The information letter and data protection declaration are provided in Supplement S1.

2.2. Learning Materials

2.2.1. Skulls

In both study 1 and study 2, 32 horse skulls and 32 pig skulls were used in total. The used skulls belong to the anatomical collection of the Institute of Veterinary Anatomy at Freie Universität Berlin.

2.2.2. 3D Scans

3D scans of the horse and pig skulls, which were employed in this study, were generated using the handheld 3D scanner Artec Space Spider (Artec 3D, Luxembourg). It is a high-resolution scanner based on blue light technology. It is capable of capturing the geometry and texture of an object simultaneously by taking multiple pictures. To assemble and edit the finalized 3D model, the manufacturer software Artec Studio 16 (Artec 3D, Luxembourg) was used.

First, the scanned background and interfering objects that do not belong to the model were removed via the "Erase" function, before scanning was continued. As the scanner was taking more scans simultaneously, two scans at once can be merged using the "Alignment" tool. To create one 3D object from the scans, the "Global registration" task was carried out to convert all-frame surfaces to a single coordinated system. The following "Sharp fusion" task melted and solidified the frames to create the 3D body. If the 3D body displayed an incomplete surface after the initial scans, either further scans were made to obtain more raw data or AI was used to generate a complete surface with the function "Fill holes". After the 3D body was satisfactory, surface texture was provided via the "Texture" item. Raw data can be found in Supplement S5.

Once the 3D scans were finished, they were exported from Artec Studio 16 and uploaded and annotated on Sketchfab (Figure 1), a 3D modeling platform website where 3D content can be shared, viewed and annotated (www.sketchfab.com; Sketchfab, New York, NY, USA). The 3D scans can be utilized on most technical devices with internet access. Within Sketchfab, the 3D objects can be zoomed in, zoomed out, and rotated in all 3D axes. On the horse skull, 68 anatomical structures and on the pig skull 71 structures were annotated (Supplement S2). With a mouse click or tap on a specific structure of the 3D scan, the respective annotations get presented to the users.

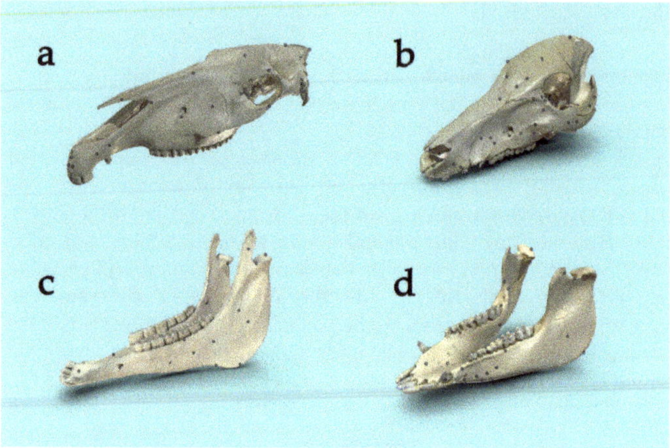

Figure 1. Annotated 3D scans of the horse's upper skull (**a**) and mandible (**c**), as well as the pig's upper skull (**b**) and mandible (**d**).

2.2.3. 2D Images

2D images of the horse and pig skulls were created using a system camera (Sony, Alpha NEX 3, Nihombashi, Tokio, Japan) and an iPhone (Apple Inc., 13. Generation, One Apple Park Way, Cupertino, CA, USA). The pictures were edited and annotated using PowerPoint (Office PowerPoint 2019, Windows). Identical structures were either portrayed using numbers (2D numbers) or arrows (2D arrows). The structures shown were exactly alike the ones annotated in the 3D scans (Figure 2). A close-up depiction of 3D and 2D annotations of selected structures can be found in Supplement S3.

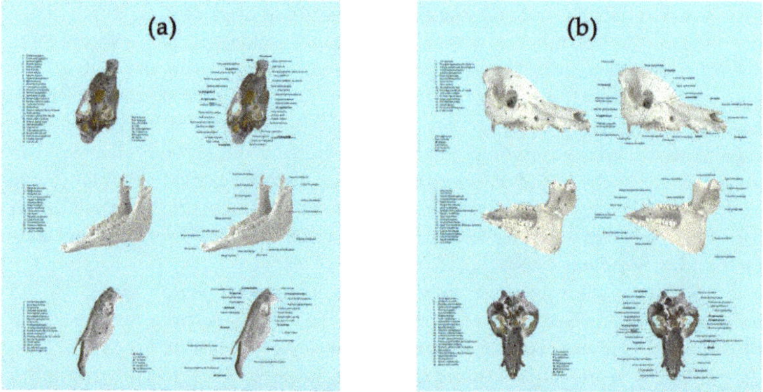

Figure 2. (**a**) 2D images of the horse skull, annotated with numbers (left) or with arrows (right), (**b**) 2D images of the pig skull, annotated with numbers (left) or with arrows (right).

2.3. *Tests*

2.3.1. Mental Rotation Test

The mental rotation test was used to assess the students' spatial ability [20]. The test had a time limit of 10 min and consisted of 18 exercises showing pictures of diverse tube figures placed in a transparent cube. Each exercise comprises two pictures of a cube, with the left one showing the cube in an initial position and the right one showing the cube from a different viewpoint. The objective of this test is to determine the position from which one observes the rotated box (right, left, up, down, behind) [20].

2.3.2. Knowledge Tests

Regarding each knowledge test, which was conducted before (pre-test) and after (post-test) the learning period, 10 structures were annotated with adhesive arrows. Each arrow was marked with a certain number and was attached to the horse and pig skulls, respectively (Figure 3). In each skull, 5 structures were identical in the pre- and post-test, while the other 5 structures were replaced by others in the post-test. During study 1, one tag got lost on pig skulls during the changeover process, resulting in one less queried structure in the post-test in comparison to the horse skull. The students' tasks in both knowledge tests consisted of writing down the anatomical terms of the annotated structures behind the corresponding numbers on the examination sheets (Supplement S4).

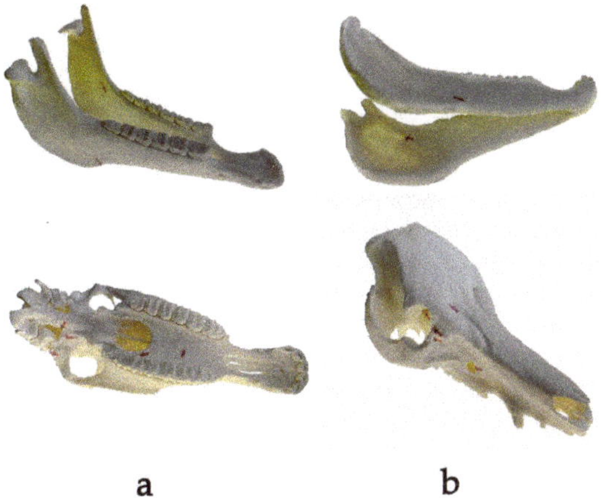

Figure 3. Annotated skulls of the horse (**a**) and of the pig (**b**) using adhesive arrows.

2.4. Student Evaluation

After performing study 1 and study 2, respectively, all students got access to all learning materials to prepare for the regular exam. After the exam, participants were requested to fill out a brief questionnaire regarding their experience of the study process. The evaluation was carried out with LimeSurvey (LimeSurvey, Version 5.6.31).

For the evaluation of the learning tools, responses for the first five questions were registered for each statement using a six-point Likert scale (1 = strongly disagree, 6 = strongly agree). Question six was a ranking, and the last three questions were noted as free-text responses. Questions and response types are listed in Table 1.

Table 1. Question and response types of the student evaluation.

	Question	Response Type
1.	By learning with the 3D scans, I felt well prepared for a practical exam on an anatomical specimen.	Likert scale
2.	By learning with the pictures with arrows, I felt well prepared for a practical exam on an anatomical specimen.	Likert scale
3.	By learning the pictures with numbers, I felt well-prepared for a practical exam on an anatomical specimen.	Likert scale
4.	The controls (turn, rotate, zoom) of the 3D scans are easy to handle.	Likert scale
5.	The controls (turn, rotate, zoom) of the 3D scans are intuitive.	Likert scale
6.	Please indicate the order of your preference for these learning materials (3D scans, 2D arrows, 2D numbers).	Ranking
7.	What positive aspects did you notice while using the visual teaching materials (3D scans, labeled specimen images)?	Free text

Table 1. *Cont.*

	Question	Response Type
8.	What negative aspects did you notice when using the visual teaching materials (3D scans, labeled specimen images)?	Free text
9.	Do you have any feedback for us regarding the course of the study?	Free text

2.5. Study Design

Study 1 and study 2 were conducted during regular anatomy lessons on the skull, in which students were regularly divided into 32 groups, each group being located at one dissection table and consisting of 5 to 6 students. Before the lesson began, 16 groups were randomly assigned to the study group 3D scans and the other 16 groups for 2D images. The study group of 2D images was further divided equally into 2D arrows and 2D numbers.

All tests were conducted by each student individually while learning time was spent in the respective groups, in which the students were allowed to interact with each other. The study began with the mental rotation test. The test started for all students at the same time. After the time had elapsed, all students stopped simultaneously. For the subsequent pre-test, annotated skulls were covered with blankets. After the students had entered their personal code and selected whether they belonged to the 3D or 2D group on their test sheet, all students began the knowledge test at the same time by removing the blankets from the skulls. At the end of the test period, the students flipped their test sheets upside down on the table. Subsequently, the students began their learning period on the non-annotated skulls of horses and pigs. In the 3D scans group, each student received the annotated 3D scans of the skulls on an iPad from Apple (Apple Inc., One Apple Park Way, Cupertino, CA, USA), of the 9th generation in study 1 and the 10th generation in study 2. In the 2D image groups, each student received a set of color-printed annotated images of the skulls.

After the learning time, the post-test proceeded identically to the pre-test, including filling out the personal code on the examination sheet again and selecting their study group (3D scans, 2D arrows, or 2D numbers). The schedule of study 1 and study 2 is shown in Table 2.

Table 2. Schedule of study 1 and study 2.

Mental rotation test	10 min (study 1 and study 2)
Knowledge test (pre-test)	15 min (study 1 and study 2)
Learning period	120 min (study 1), 40 min (study 2)
Knowledge test (post-test)	15 min (study 1 and study 2)

2.6. Statistical Analysis

Statistical and descriptive analyses and charts were carried out with IBM SPSS Statistics Version 29® (IBM, Armonk, New York, NY, USA). Only the data from people who submitted all three test forms were regarded for analysis. In order to preserve the anonymity of the participants, but to merge the three tests (pre-test, post-test, mental rotation test) of the respective person, an individual code of five letters was used, consisting of the third letter of the month of birth of their mother, the third letter of their month of birth, the second letter of their mother's first name, the second letter of their first name, and the second letter of their birthplace. In addition, the students indicated in the post-test which study group they were assigned to. In study 2, four students had to be excluded due to not submitting the three required forms and one student had to be excluded due to missing indication of the study group.

The mental rotation test was a single-choice assessment, with one point awarded for each correct answer. Incorrect or missing answers received no points. A descriptive analysis of data was conducted. Based on the random distribution of students to the study groups, no differences between the study groups were expected.

In the knowledge test, each correct term was awarded one point. No points were given for incorrect or missing terms. If terms were misspelled or incomplete, an assessment was made as to whether the term written down indicated that the correct structure had been recognized. To determine whether an individual's assessment is sufficient, the pre- and post-tests were evaluated by two researchers. Due to the minimal deviation (less than 10% in both studies), the assessment from one researcher was considered sufficient for the analysis.

The learning outcome was measured by calculating the difference of sums between post-test and pre-test. The mean score difference between the pre-test and post-test was then calculated for all study groups and compared using a paired *t*-test, followed by the analysis of variance (ANOVA) to determine the differences between study groups. Pearson's correlation was utilized to assess the correlation between spatial ability and learning outcomes of each study group of study 1 and study 2 separately.

Analysis of variance was performed to test the influence of the mental rotation test, the study groups, and study 1 and study 2 including the interaction term on the mean score difference. Levene's test revealed that the variances between the study groups in study 2 were not equal, and thus, robust parameter estimates were assessed. The normality and homoscedasticity of residuals were inspected visually. Raw data can be found in Supplement S5.

3. Results

3.1. Number of Participants

A total of 278 second-year veterinary medicine students participated in total in study 1 and study 2. They were distributed as follows: In study 1, 118 students were involved, among them 59 students joined the study group with 3D scans, 33 students with 2D numbers, and 26 students with 2D arrows. Study 2 included 160 students, 79 students joined the study group with 3D scans, 39 students with 2D numbers, and 42 students with 2D arrows.

3.2. Spatial Ability

As displayed in Figure 4, the distribution of the mental rotation test results was similar in all groups (study 1: $p = 0.195$, study 2: $p = 0.308$).

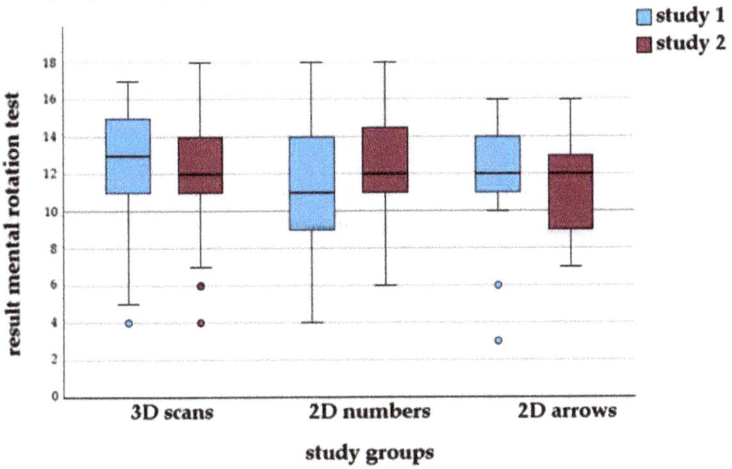

Figure 4. Boxplot of mental rotation test scores in the groups with different learning materials (annotated 3D scans, 2D images annotated with numbers or arrows) in study 1 and study 2.

3.3. Learning Outcome

Regarding the post-test, students reached significantly higher score points than in the pre-test (mean pre-test = 0.86, mean post-test = 8.3, $p < 0.001$). The post-test values were higher in study 1 (11.4 ± 4.2) than in study 2 (6.0 ± 3.1).

Analysis of variance revealed that the average learning outcome in study 1 was 5.2 score points higher than in study 2 ($p < 0.001$) and that there was an interaction between study 1 and study 2 and the study groups ($p = 0.121$, Figure 5). In study 1, the highest learning outcome was achieved by the 3D scan group, and in study 2 by the 2D numbers group (Figure 5). However, study groups did not differ significantly in their mean learning outcome ($p = 0.500$). In study 1, mean learning outcome values were 11.0 ± 3.8 for the 3D scans group and 9.97 ± 4.21 for the 2D images group ($p = 0.165$). A post hoc power analysis (conducted with G*Power 3.1.9.2) showed a medium effect (d = 0.57) and a power of 86%. Under these conditions, a significant difference between the two groups would have required a sample size of 83 students in each group. Even by comparing 2D arrows (10.0 ± 4.4) and 2D numbers (9.94 ± 4.1) to the 3D scan group, no significant difference was shown ($p = 0.383$). In study 2, mean learning outcomes were 5.0 ± 2.5 for the 3D scans group and 5.51 ± 3.32 for the 2D images group ($p = 0.292$). A post hoc power analysis revealed no effect (d = 0.00) and a power of 5%. However, when comparing 2D numbers (6.31 ± 3.6) and 2D arrows (4.76 ± 2.9) to the 3D scan group, the 2D numbers group was significantly higher ($p = 0.035$).

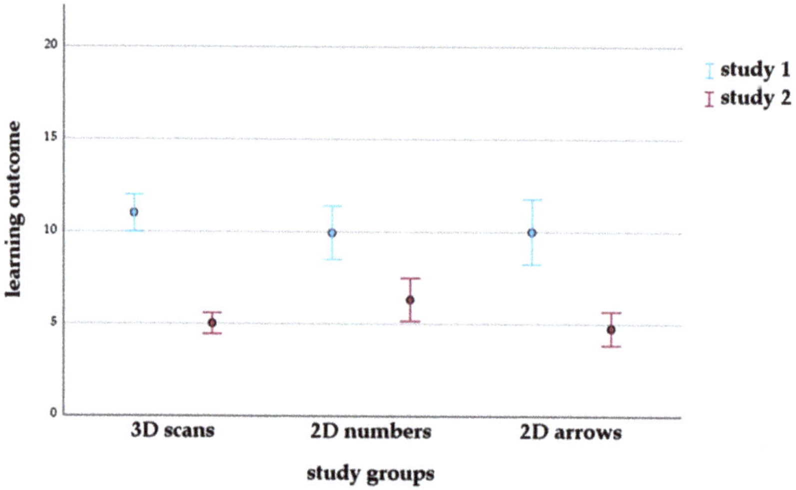

Figure 5. Estimated means and 95% confidence intervals of learning outcome in the groups with different learning materials (annotated 3D scans, 2D images annotated with numbers or arrows) in study 1 and study 2.

3.4. Correlation of Spatial Ability and Learning Outcome

The correlation between learning outcome and spatial ability, measured by the mental rotation test, was positive ($p = 0.160$) in study 1 for the study group of 3D scans with only slight differences in the correlation between study 1 (r = 0.244) and study 2 (r = 0.223). 2D numbers showed a negative correlation coefficient in study 1 (r = −0.245) (Figure 6) and a positive correlation coefficient in study 2 (r = 0.309) (Figure 7). A positive correlation was also found for 2D arrows in both studies (study 1: r = 0.400; study 2: r = 0.128).

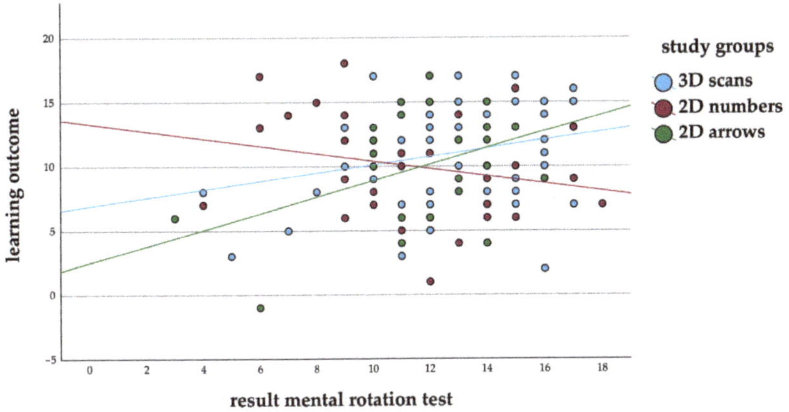

Figure 6. Correlation of learning outcome and results of the mental rotation test in the groups with different learning materials (annotated 3D scans, 2D images annotated with numbers or arrows) in study 1.

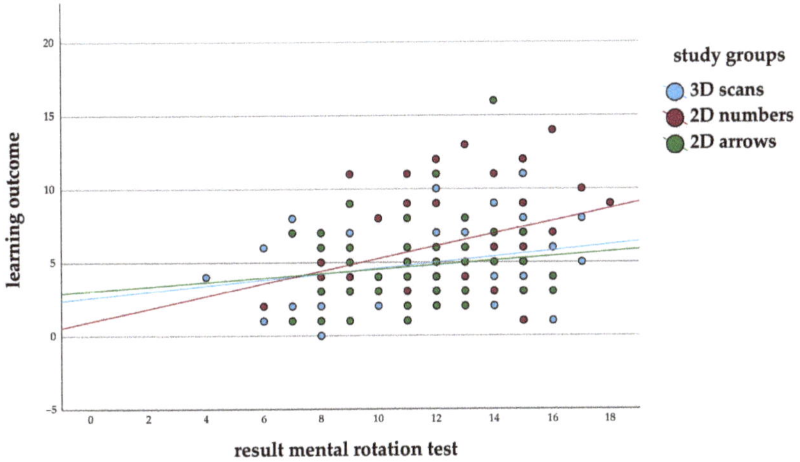

Figure 7. Correlation of learning outcome and mental rotation test in the groups with different learning materials (annotated 3D scans, 2D images annotated with numbers or arrows) in study 2.

3.5. Student Evaluation

The questionnaire to evaluate the learning tools was completed by 130 students after study 1 and 144 students after study 2. Responses were analyzed using a six-point Likert scale (1 = strongly disagree, 6 = strongly agree). Results in the range of 4 to 6 were summed up and defined as "agreeing to this statement", as well as the sums of the answers of 1 to 3 representing "disagreeing with this statement". In both studies, most of the students agreed on feeling well prepared for a practical exam by using 3D scans (74.62% in study 1, 71.09% in study 2). 58.46% in study 1 and 57.81% in study 2 agreed on feeling well prepared for an exam using pictures with arrows. By learning with pictures with numbers, 53.08% in study 1 and 46.87% in study 2 agreed on feeling well prepared for an exam. 53.84% in study 1 and 46.83% in study 2 agreed on 3D scan controls (turn, rotate, zoom) being easy to handle.

Afterward, the students were asked to indicate their order of preference for learning materials. In study 1, students most frequently chose 3D scans in first place (52.31% 3D scans, 20% 2D arrows, 13.08% 2D numbers), 2D arrows in second place (34.62% 2D arrows, 28.46% 2D numbers, 22.31% 3D scans) and 2D numbers in third place (43.08% 2D numbers, 30.77% 2D arrows, 10.77% 3D scans). In study 2, students also most frequently placed 3D scans in first place (61.06% 3D scans, 24.78% 2D arrows, 14.16% 2D numbers), 2D arrows in second place (41.44% 2D arrows, 30.63% 2D numbers, 27.93% 3D scans) and 2D numbers in third place (54.95% 2D numbers, 33.33% 2D arrows, 11.71% 3D scans).

Finally, participants were asked about the negative and positive aspects they noticed while using the visual teaching materials. A few negative aspects were mentioned, mostly referring to technical issues and difficulties in handling and orientating while using 3D scans, e.g., "slight difficulties to rotate and zoom with the 3D scans"; "The computer did not always keep up. It got hot and the pictures were slow"; and, "When you tap on an annotation, the image sometimes shifts and you are in a different place than you want to be". The mentioned positive aspects referred to a good visualization of structures, learning benefits, and availability of scans, e.g., "The visualization of the 3D scans worked well. I could visualize the skull well in my hand"; "With the 3D scans, I can memorize it faster and my attention span is greater"; and, "It is good to have the anatomical object available at home, too, which is good for learning and self-monitoring".

For 2D images, some negative comments were mentioned about the annotation with arrows being confusing, e.g., "It was not clear which structure was mentioned" and "The structures are easier to recognize in 3D scans than in 2D images". However, some positive aspects of the 2D images were referring to 2D numbers giving a good overview of the picture's structures "They were good to quiz yourself".

4. Discussion

In the presented study, the effectiveness of 3D scans versus 2D images as learning materials in veterinary anatomy classes was investigated. This research was based on the hypothesis that students using 3D scans for learning anatomical structures of skulls would achieve a higher learning outcome compared to those using 2D images. Moreover, the relation between spatial ability and the type of learning material was examined, based on the hypothesis that students with low spatial ability achieve greater success using 3D scans than 2D images.

Analysis of the data indicates that there is a significant difference between pre-test and post-test of the study groups 2D images as well as for 3D scans. This leads to the conclusion that all study groups in study 1 and study 2 were able to identify more anatomical structures correctly after the learning period. However, when comparing the study groups, no significant difference between 2D images and 3D scans was detectable. Similar findings were observed in other studies conducted to compare the effectiveness of 2D and 3D methods in anatomy education. One study tested the use of a digital 3D skull model in anatomy teaching. It was shown that the skull virtual learning resource was equally efficient as the cadaver skull and 2D atlas in teaching anatomy structures [21]. Moreover, a study by the University of Bristol evaluated a 3D computer model of the equine paranasal sinuses as a tool for veterinary anatomy education comparing it to 2D-based visualizations in a pre-test/post-test design. Also in this research, no statistically significant difference was found between 3D and 2D groups [22]. In contrast, a previous study pointed out that dynamic visualizations, including 3D models, can greatly enhance students' understanding of complex concepts in subjects such as geology, biology, and chemistry. However, the impact varied significantly between different groups of students, suggesting that factors like prior knowledge and learning styles could influence the effectiveness of these tools [23]. Thus, the hypothesis that students who use 3D scans as learning material will achieve higher learning outcomes compared to those who use 2D images could not be supported.

Moreover, time as a factor plays a crucial role in the study. In study 1, students had 120 min of learning time for both skulls. This amount seemed to be more than necessary, which was shown by students already leaving the dissection hall before time ran out. This led to the performance of study 2 which involved a shorter learning time of 40 min for learning all structures of both skulls. Since the students in study 2 had a significantly lower learning outcome, it can be assumed that this learning time was too short. Assuming that the learning time in study 1 was too long and that the average learning outcome of study 1 was, therefore, the maximum achievable, a calculated learning time of approx. 75 min would be sufficient, assuming that learning takes place in a linear fashion. In study 1, the study group 3D scans displayed the tendency of being the group with the highest learning outcome. In contrast, in study 2, which was conducted under time pressure, it was shown that 2D numbers had a significantly better learning outcome than the other groups. These findings indicate that having more time to learn a new tool makes a difference in the learning outcome, especially if it is a completely new tool that has never or occasionally been used by the participants [24–27] Students are used to learning with 2D images since school and rarely get in touch with 3D models [28]. Although students are increasingly using tablet computers as a learning tool in the dissection courses, they still mainly use them to access 2D-based visualizations, as books or their own scripts and no 3D models. It takes time to understand how to interact with the software of Sketchfab and get to know how to use the 3D scans [29]. This was mentioned by some participants as a negative aspect of the evaluation.

However, the high learning outcome for 2D numbers might be based on the regular usage of this certain type of annotation. Various veterinary anatomy book images are annotated with numbers. Therefore, veterinary medicine students are used to learning with this learning material. A former study stated that annotations, particularly numbered ones, significantly helped undergraduate students engage with scientific texts more deeply [30]. These annotations acted as frameworks, making complex information more accessible and enhancing students' comprehension and retention. Positive student feedback indicated that these annotations were especially useful for understanding graphs and interpreting scientific vocabulary, highlighting the effectiveness of numbered annotations in educational contexts [30]. Another study investigated the role of annotations in the comprehension of scientific texts, focusing on cognitive load effects. The study found that well-structured annotations, such as numbered lists, helped reduce cognitive load and improved comprehension, indicating that numbered annotations can provide clear and organized information, facilitating better understanding and learning outcomes [31].

Several findings indicate that students with low spatial ability would have a higher learning outcome using 3D scans than 2D images [16,19]. In study 1, the analysis of the correlation between learning outcome and mental rotation test showed that students on the lower scale of mental rotation test results had higher learning outcome values using 3D scans than 2D arrows. However, the same correlation was not reproduced in study 2. Therefore, the hypothesis that the 3D scans support students with weaker spatial ability could not be supported.

In the student evaluation, 3D scans were chosen as the preferred learning material, so they might enhance students' motivation. Another study showed that using 3D scans improved participants' motivation levels when compared with 2D learning materials [22,32]. Therefore, even if 3D scans do not directly result in improved learning outcomes, the element of pleasure remains crucial to the learning process [32]. It plays a significant role in motivating students, driving them to actively engage with the topic and ultimately achieve their educational goals [33]. Innovative learning methods can significantly enhance student motivation and engagement, leading to improved knowledge retention and learning outcomes [34–36]. Engaging teaching approaches can indirectly boost learning outcomes by increasing overall motivation, improving attendance, and inspiring students to adopt novel methods in their self-directed learning [37]. Additionally, the evaluation of the learning tools revealed some limitations associated with the 3D scans. These addressed issues primarily involved the use, handling, and certain technical restrictions of the 3D scans. Among the most significant challenges were the annotations created on Sketchfab. These annotations were found to be less user-friendly due to their tendency to rotate quickly and zoom in excessively, which made them difficult to navigate and interact with effectively, potentially harming the process of capturing the 3D shape. Furthermore, unlike the 2D images, Sketchfab does not provide an overview of all the annotations on the respective skull. Instead, the annotations can only be opened one at a time, which can further lead to limiting the learning process. Finding the ideal annotations for 3D models can often prove to be a challenging task [38,39]. Another limitation inherent in using 3D scans is the requirement for compatible technical devices capable of adequately processing and displaying the 3D scans. Consequently, the utilization of 3D scans necessitates the availability of suitable technology to ensure optimal viewing and utilization. The inequality of access to online technology and devices and the possibly unreliable internet makes the 3D scans not accessible to everyone anytime [40]. Interestingly, the evaluation showed that the students favored annotation by arrows over annotation by numbers for 2D images, although in study 2, under time pressure, the 2D numbers group achieved the best learning outcome. This finding confirms indications that the learning materials preferred by the students do not necessarily lead to the highest learning outcome for them [41].

One of the limitations of this study could be that the studies only had one assessment time-point, taking place during a dissection course. Additionally, these studies faced technological constraints, as they were unable to test a wide range of devices for displaying the 3D scans. This limitation has resulted in findings that are specific to the particular equipment used. Another limitation is that conclusions about the efficacy of 3D scans cannot be drawn to other anatomical structures based on the exclusive use of 3D scans of the skull.

Future research could involve conducting a comprehensive comparison among various 3D platforms, focusing particularly on their user-friendliness concerning both annotating 3D models and accessing them technically. This comparative analysis could explore interface design, ease of navigation, annotation tools, and technical requirements, aiming to provide valuable insights into optimizing the usability and accessibility of 3D platforms for educational and professional purposes. In order to eradicate the limitation of raising data solely at one assessment time-point and to analyze long-term retention of anatomical knowledge by using 3D scans, a reassessment of students' learning outcomes should be conducted involving multiple time points. To assess conclusions on other anatomical structures, similar studies could be conducted using 3D scans of different organs. Ultimately, conducting a study where students have the opportunity to familiarize themselves with the 3D surface before being introduced to the skulls would be beneficial, as it allows them to analyze learning success with the starting conditions being more aligned.

5. Conclusions

This study did not provide significant support for the hypothesis that students who use 3D scans to learn anatomical structures have a higher learning outcome compared to students who use 2D images. It was found that 3D scans do not lead to superior learning outcomes compared to 2D-based learning materials. Similarly, the hypothesis that students with low spatial ability have a higher learning outcome with the use of 3D scans than with 2D images is also not confirmed. Students with low spatial ability did not experience significantly better learning outcomes with the use of 3D scans. However, the data does provide valuable insights into the role of 3D emerging tools in veterinary anatomy education. Although practicing the handling of 3D scans appears to be time-consuming, working with 3D scans seems to enhance student motivation. The reduced learning time may have had a bigger impact on the 3D group, based on the introduction of novel learning materials, which required additional time to be understood and effectively integrated with the learning process. Similarly, the findings of this study highlight the crucial importance of allowing students adequate time to adapt to new circumstances. This need is evident not only in the specific context of the 3D skull but also more broadly in the first semester; it was noted, for example, that, expectations, relationships with professors, and the nature of examinations are significantly different than the school environment. The results of the current study provide evidence that supports the educational effectiveness of 3D scans as a complementary method to understanding anatomical structures.

Supplementary Materials: The following supporting information can be downloaded at: https://www.mdpi.com/article/10.3390/ani14152171/s1, Supplement S1: Information letter and data protection declaration, Supplement S2: List of annotated structures, Supplement S3: Close-up depiction of 3D and 2D annotations, Supplement S4: Examination sheets, Supplement S5: Raw data.

Author Contributions: Conceptualization, R.S., M.B., G.M.C. and J.P.E.; investigation, R.S., M.B., G.M.C., M.S., J.P. and C.H.; methodology, R.S., M.B., G.M.C., J.P.E. and R.M.; project administration and supervision M.B.; visualization, R.S.; writing—original draft preparation, R.S., M.B., G.M.C., C.H. and R.M.; writing—review and editing, R.S., C.H. and M.B. All authors have read and agreed to the published version of the manuscript.

Funding: This research received no external funding.

Institutional Review Board Statement: This study was conducted according to the guidelines of the Declaration of Helsinki and approved by the Ethics Committee of Freie Universität Berlin (ZEA-Nr. 2022-014, 9 June 2022).

Informed Consent Statement: Informed consent was obtained from all subjects involved in the study.

Data Availability Statement: Data are contained within the article or Supplementary Material. The data presented in this study are available in the Supplementary Material.

Acknowledgments: The authors would like to express their sincere thanks to the students involved for their brilliant participation in the studies. The authors would also like to thank Janet Weigner, Florian Grabitzky, and Harriet Wendel for their technical support during the studies as well as Martin Werner and Karsten Prühl for the photographic support.

Conflicts of Interest: The authors declare no conflicts of interest.

References

1. McLachlan, J.C.; Patten, D. Anatomy teaching: Ghosts of the past, present and future. *Med. Educ.* **2006**, *40*, 243–253. [CrossRef] [PubMed]
2. Older, J. Anatomy: Amust for teaching the next generation. *Surgeon* **2004**, *2*, 79–90. [CrossRef]
3. Sugand, K.; Abrahams, P.; Khurana, A. The anatomy of anatomy: A review for its modernization. *Anat. Sci. Educ.* **2010**, *3*, 83–93. [CrossRef] [PubMed]
4. Netterstrøm, I.; Kayser, L. Learning to be a doctor while learning anatomy! *Anat. Sci. Educ.* **2008**, *1*, 154–158. [CrossRef]
5. Cottam, W.W. Adequacy of medical school gross anatomy education as perceived by certain postgraduate residency programs and anatomy course directors. *Clin. Anat.* **1999**, *12*, 55–65. [CrossRef]
6. Wheble, R.; Channon, S.B. What Use is Anatomy in First Opinion Small Animal Veterinary Practice? A Qualitative Study. *Anat. Sci. Educ.* **2021**, *14*, 440–451. [CrossRef] [PubMed]
7. Homfray, B.; Attwood, A.; Channon, S.B. Anatomy in Practice: How Do Equine and Production Animal Veterinarians Apply Anatomy in Primary Care Settings? *J. Vet. Med. Educ.* **2022**, *50*, 643–653. [CrossRef]
8. Gummery, E.; Cobb, K.A.; Mossop, L.H.; Cobb, M.A. Student Perceptions of Veterinary Anatomy Practical Classes: A Longitudinal Study. *J. Vet. Med. Educ.* **2018**, *45*, 163–176. [CrossRef] [PubMed]
9. Böckers, A.; Jerg-Bretzke, L.; Lamp, C.; Brinkmann, A.; Traue, H.C.; Böckers, T.M. The gross anatomy course: An analysis of its importance. *Anat. Sci. Educ.* **2010**, *3*, 3–11. [CrossRef]
10. Aziz, M.A.; McKenzie, J.C.; Wilson, J.S.; Cowie, R.J.; Ayeni, S.A.; Dunn, B.K. The human cadaver in the age of biomedical informatics. *Anat. Rec.* **2002**, *269*, 20–32. [CrossRef]
11. Al-Khalili, S.M.; Coppoc, G.L. 2D and 3D stereoscopic videos used as pre-anatomy lab tools improve students' examination performance in a veterinary gross anatomy course. *J. Vet. Med. Educ.* **2014**, *41*, 68–76. [CrossRef] [PubMed]
12. Khalil, M.K.; Johnson, T.E.; Lamar, C.H. Comparison of computer-based and paper-based imagery strategies in learning anatomy. *Clin. Anat.* **2005**, *18*, 457–464. [CrossRef] [PubMed]
13. Preece, D.; Williams, S.B.; Lam, R.; Weller, R. "Let's get physical": Advantages of a physical model over 3D computer models and textbooks in learning imaging anatomy. *Anat. Sci. Educ.* **2013**, *6*, 216–224. [CrossRef] [PubMed]
14. Wainman, B.; Wolak, L.; Pukas, G.; Zheng, E.; Norman, G.R. The superiority of three-dimensional physical models to two-dimensional computer presentations in anatomy learning. *Med. Educ.* **2018**, *52*, 1138–1146. [CrossRef] [PubMed]
15. Nguyen, N.; Nelson, A.J.; Wilson, T.D. Computer visualizations: Factors that influence spatial anatomy comprehension. *Anat. Sci. Educ.* **2012**, *5*, 98–108. [CrossRef] [PubMed]

16. Berney, S.; Bétrancourt, M.; Molinari, G.; Hoyek, N. How spatial abilities and dynamic visualizations interplay when learning functional anatomy with 3D anatomical models. *Anat. Sci. Educ.* **2015**, *8*, 452–462. [CrossRef] [PubMed]
17. Garg, A.; Norman, G.; Spero, L.; Taylor, I. Learning anatomy: Do new computer models improve spatial understanding? *Med. Teach.* **1999**, *21*, 519–522. [CrossRef]
18. Dickson, J.; Gardiner, A.; Rhind, S. Veterinary Anatomy Education and Spatial Ability: Where Now and Where Next? *J. Vet. Med. Educ.* **2022**, *49*, 297–305. [CrossRef] [PubMed]
19. Höffler, T.N. Spatial Ability: Its Influence on Learning with Visualizations—A Meta-Analytic Review. *Educ. Psychol. Rev.* **2010**, *22*, 245–269. [CrossRef]
20. Mediseminar. *Trainingsbuch EMS NC Simulation "Testlauf 2"*; Band 11; Uniseminar Education AG: Trogen, Switzerland, 2023.
21. Chen, S.; Zhu, J.; Cheng, C.; Pan, Z.; Liu, L.; Du, J.; Shen, X.; Shen, Z.; Zhu, H.; Liu, J.; et al. Can virtual reality improve traditional anatomy education programmes? A mixed-methods study on the use of a 3D skull model. *BMC Med. Educ.* **2020**, *20*, 395. [CrossRef]
22. Canright, A.; Bescoby, S.; Dickson, J. Evaluation of a 3D Computer Model of the Equine Paranasal Sinuses as a Tool for Veterinary Anatomy Education. *J. Vet. Med. Educ.* **2023**, *50*, 234–242. [CrossRef] [PubMed]
23. Teplá, M.; Teplý, P.; Šmejkal, P. Influence of 3D models and animations on students in natural subjects. *Int. J. STEM Educ.* **2022**, *9*, 1–20. [CrossRef]
24. Bloom, B.S. Time and learning. *Am. Psychol.* **1974**, *29*, 682–688. [CrossRef]
25. *Time to Learn*; Program on Teaching and Learning; U.S. Department of Education, National Institute of Education: Washington, DC, USA, 1980.
26. Stoll, L. *It's About Learning (and It's About Time): What's in It for Schools?* RoutledgeFalmer: Hoboken, NJ, USA, 2002; ISBN 9780203994795.
27. Gettinger, M.; White, M.A. Which is the stronger correlate of school learning? Time to learn or measured intelligence? *J. Educ. Psychol.* **1979**, *71*, 405–412. [CrossRef]
28. Raiyn, J. The Role of Visual Learning in Improving Students' High-Order Thinking Skills. *J. Educ. Pract.* **2016**, *7*, 115–121.
29. Jacobs, H.L. SketchUp and Sketchfab: Tools for Teaching with 3D. *J. Soc. Archit. Hist.* **2022**, *81*, 256–259. [CrossRef]
30. Kararo, M.; McCartney, M. Annotated primary scientific literature: A pedagogical tool for undergraduate courses. *PLoS Biol.* **2019**, *17*, e3000103. [CrossRef] [PubMed]
31. Wallen, E.; Plass, J.L.; Brunken, R. The function of annotations in the comprehension of scientific texts: Cognitive load effects and the impact of verbal ability. *Educ. Technol. Res. Dev.* **2005**, *53*, 59–71. [CrossRef]
32. Pintrich, P.R.; Marx, R.W.; Boyle, R.A. Beyond Cold Conceptual Change: The Role of Motivational Beliefs and Classroom Contextual Factors in the Process of Conceptual Change. *Rev. Educ. Res.* **1993**, *63*, 167–199. [CrossRef]
33. Chan, L.K.; Cheng, M.M.W. An analysis of the educational value of low-fidelity anatomy models as external representations. *Anat. Sci. Educ.* **2011**, *4*, 256–263. [CrossRef]
34. Battulga, B.; Konishi, T.; Tamura, Y.; Moriguchi, H. The Effectiveness of an Interactive 3-Dimensional Computer Graphics Model for Medical Education. *Interact. J. Med. Res.* **2012**, *1*, e2. [CrossRef] [PubMed]
35. Huang, H.-M.; Rauch, U.; Liaw, S.-S. Investigating learners' attitudes toward virtual reality learning environments: Based on a constructivist approach. *Comput. Educ.* **2010**, *55*, 1171–1182. [CrossRef]
36. Shim, K.-C.; Park, J.-S.; Kim, H.-S.; Kim, J.-H.; Park, Y.-C.; Ryu, H.-I. Application of virtual reality technology in biology education. *J. Biol. Educ.* **2003**, *37*, 71–74. [CrossRef]
37. Kockro, R.A.; Amaxopoulou, C.; Killeen, T.; Wagner, W.; Reisch, R.; Schwandt, E.; Gutenberg, A.; Giese, A.; Stofft, E.; Stadie, A.T. Stereoscopic neuroanatomy lectures using a three-dimensional virtual reality environment. *Ann. Anat. Anat. Anz.* **2015**, *201*, 91–98. [CrossRef] [PubMed]
38. Ponchio, F.; Callieri, M.; Dellepiane, M.; Scopigno, R. Effective Annotations Over 3D Models. *Comput. Graph. Forum* **2020**, *39*, 89–105. [CrossRef]
39. Ohkawa, T.; Furuta, R.; Sato, Y. Efficient Annotation and Learning for 3D Hand Pose Estimation: A Survey. *Int. J. Comput. Vis.* **2023**, *131*, 3193–3206. [CrossRef]
40. Patra, A.; Asghar, A.; Chaudhary, P.; Ravi, K.S. Integration of innovative educational technologies in anatomy teaching: New normal in anatomy education. *Surg. Radiol. Anat.* **2022**, *44*, 25–32. [CrossRef] [PubMed]
41. Peterson, D.C.; Mlynarczyk, G.S.A. Analysis of traditional versus three-dimensional augmented curriculum on anatomical learning outcome measures. *Anat. Sci. Educ.* **2016**, *9*, 529–536. [CrossRef]

animals

MDPI

Article

The Impact of Low-Fidelity Three-Dimensional-Printed Models of the Equine Distal Limb and the Canine Forelimb in Teaching Veterinary Anatomy in Practical Classes

Rebecca Schirone [1,*], Maximiliane Schmedding [2], Janet Weigner [1], Martin Werner [1], Giuliano Mario Corte [3], Jan Peter Ehlers [4], Luise Grace Klass [1] and Mahtab Bahramsoltani [1]

1. Institute of Veterinary Anatomy, School of Veterinary Medicine, Freie Universität Berlin, Koserstraße 20, 14195 Berlin, Germany; janet.weigner@fu-berlin.de (J.W.); ma.werner@fu-berlin.de (M.W.); mahtab.bahramsoltani@fu-berlin.de (M.B.)
2. ISME Bern and Avenches, Vetsuisse Faculty, University of Bern, Hochschulstrasse 6, 3012 Bern, Switzerland
3. Institute of Veterinary Anatomy, Vetsuisse Faculty, University of Zurich (UZH), Winterthurerstrasse 260, 8057 Zurich, Switzerland; giuliano.corte@uzh.ch
4. Didactics and Educational Research in Health Science, Faculty of Health, Witten/Herdecke University, Alfred-Herrhausen-Straße 50, 58455 Witten, Germany; jan.ehlers@uni-wh.de

* Correspondence: rebecca.schirone@fu-berlin.de

Simple Summary: Due to limited access to animal cadavers and health concerns associated with cadavers that have been treated with formaldehyde, alternatives are needed for teaching veterinary anatomy. This study tested whether 3D-printed models with simplified representations of anatomical structures help students learn as effectively as with real specimens. In two studies, veterinary students' knowledge was tested after studying an unfamiliar anatomy topic, using either real specimens, 3D models, or a combination of both, starting with 3D models or real specimens, followed by the other. In both studies, students who used real specimens performed better on knowledge assessments. However, in the subsequent evaluation, many students stated that they prefer to start learning with 3D models followed by the real specimens, although this method had the lowest learning outcomes in the knowledge assessments. Moreover, students found 3D models helpful for learning anatomy regardless of location. They also expressed interest in having additional 3D models of other anatomical specimens. The results suggest that while 3D models cannot fully replace real specimens, they can be a useful addition to veterinary education.

Abstract: Limited cadaver availability and health risks from formaldehyde-treated cadavers have increased the need for alternative learning materials in veterinary anatomy education. Two studies were conducted to investigate whether low-fidelity 3D-printed models provide comparable learning outcomes to real specimens. In study 1, veterinary students were assigned to two groups to study the equine distal limb on a real specimen (n = 67) or a 3D model (n = 68). In study 2, students were divided into four groups to study the canine forelimb on a real specimen (n = 44), a 3D model (n = 45), a 3D model followed by a real specimen (n = 47), or the reverse combination (n = 47). Learning outcomes were measured through a knowledge assessment. Afterwards, learning materials were evaluated by students. Both studies showed significantly higher learning outcomes in the groups learning with real specimens compared to other test groups. While students preferred to start learning with 3D models before switching to real specimens, this method had the lowest learning outcomes. However, students emphasized the value of 3D models for independent learning outside the dissection hall and desired further 3D models of other anatomical specimens. Findings indicated that low-fidelity 3D-printed models cannot replace real specimens but are a useful complementary tool in veterinary anatomy education.

https://doi.org/10.3390/ani15101380

Keywords: veterinary education; experimental study; learning outcomes; student evaluation; formaldehyde-free alternatives; education sciences; musculoskeletal system

1. Introduction

Anatomy is one of the most important foundational subjects in veterinary medical education and provides an essential basis for clinical training [1]. Practical training in veterinary anatomy is usually carried out on cadavers, which creates a number of challenges. A major challenge is the limited availability of anatomical specimens for dissection [2]. These specimens are exclusively obtained from deceased or euthanized animals, which are voluntarily donated by their owners to veterinary anatomy institutes for educational purposes [1]. To extend their usability as teaching materials, formaldehyde in various concentrations is used for different fixation purposes [3]. Although the concentrations are relatively low, formaldehyde was reclassified by the European Union as a "potential carcinogen" in June 2014 [4]. Consequently, strict handling protocols are necessary to minimize potential health and environmental risks associated with formaldehyde exposure [3]. Despite preservation efforts, anatomical specimens remain subject to gradual deterioration over time, leading to structural degradation, loss of key anatomical features, and diminished educational value [5]. Therefore, there is a growing need for alternative approaches to the use of cadavers in veterinary anatomy [1].

An alternative, increasingly applied in clinical teaching, is the use of models on which clinical skills can be simulated. These models provide students with repeated opportunities to practice routine veterinary procedures in a low-pressure setting, reducing the need to use live animals [6–9]. Students who used the models reported higher confidence in procedure preparation and hand-ties compared to those who did not use them [10]. A distinction is made between low-fidelity models, which offer a simple and reduced representation of an animal's body or part of a body, and high-fidelity models, which mimic appearance, haptics, and functionality as realistically as possible. Studies show that similar learning outcomes, measured by observing students performing clinical tasks using a standardized checklist, can be achieved with low-fidelity models as with high-fidelity models when learning clinical skills [7,11]. Several 3D-printed, low-fidelity canine models for veterinary clinical skills training were used in a study, focusing on intravenous catheterization, bandaging, and anesthesia practice. Student satisfaction was assessed through a survey, revealing a positive attitude towards the use of these models as clinical simulators [9]. Therefore, low-fidelity models have become a valuable tool in human and veterinary medicine clinical training [9–16].

Low-fidelity models are also used in human anatomical teaching, albeit to a lesser extent than in clinical training [17–26]. Chan et al. described the use of various low-fidelity models from different human anatomists [17]. Among these, there was a low-fidelity model for learning midgut rotation [23], a model of the digital extensor mechanism designed to illustrate the anatomy and function of the intrinsic muscles [24], a paper model of the muscles [25], and the pipe-cleaner brachial plexus model [26]. Hindmarch et al. evaluated a low-fidelity inguinal canal model [18], while Dixit et al. developed a neuroanatomy low-fidelity model [19]. Only a few studies report the use of low-fidelity models in veterinary anatomical training [2,27,28]. A study from Kinnison et al. tested the use of a haptic simulator to teach bovine abdominal anatomy. Based on a satisfaction survey, the results demonstrate that the haptic simulator provides an effective and engaging approach for teaching bovine abdominal anatomy to large groups of students, reducing the reliance on cadavers and addressing several existing challenges in anatomy education [2]. In another study, 3D-printed models were developed for various structures, including bones, internal organs, and vascular systems, from a range of domestic and exotic animal species. These models were evaluated by comparing them to traditional teaching materials, such as fixed and plastinated specimens, through a student satisfaction survey administered after training sessions. Additionally, a general survey was conducted to gather students' opinions on traditional teaching methods. Overall, the 3D-printed models were well received by students, although acceptance varied depending on the specific model assessed [27]. The use of 3D-printed canine skulls from three different breeds was evaluated for educational purposes. Both animal science and veterinary students participated by completing a questionnaire regarding their learning experience with the 3D models. The results showed that students from both groups successfully recognized and understood the morphological differences between the skulls, suggesting that 3D-printed models are effective tools for teaching about rare skeletal specimens [28]. Very little is known about learning outcomes when using low-fidelity models in anatomy education. One study in human anatomy assessed learning outcomes using a multiple-choice test. In this study, the intervention group performed better than the control group. However, students in the intervention group received the low-fidelity model in addition to the learning materials that were also available to the control group [18]. Another study evaluated the effectiveness of an otoscopy simulator as a teaching tool to enhance knowledge of middle-ear anatomy and pathology, using a knowledge assessment questionnaire. The questionnaire was administered either at the beginning (control group) or after completion of the simulation (simulation group). Results showed that the simulation group achieved higher scores compared to the control group [21]. Moreover, another study assessed learning outcomes using a pre- and post-test design to compare virtual high-fidelity and low-fidelity liver models, and found no significant differences between the groups [22]. Given the limited research on the use of low-fidelity models in veterinary anatomy education, especially with 3D-printed models, the question arises whether such models could also be beneficial for teaching veterinary anatomy.

This study investigated the use of low-fidelity 3D-printed models compared to real anatomical specimens as learning material in veterinary anatomy classes on the musculoskeletal system. Two hypotheses regarding the effectiveness of 3D-printed low-fidelity models in anatomical education were tested. The first hypothesis proposed that students learning the anatomical structures of the equine distal limb using 3D-printed models would achieve the same learning outcomes as those using real specimens. The second hypothesis suggested that students studying the anatomical structures of the canine forelimb with 3D-printed models would achieve the same learning outcomes as those using real specimens.

2. Participants, Materials and Methods

2.1. Participants

Data for this study were collected at the Institute of Veterinary Anatomy, School of Veterinary Medicine, Freie Universität Berlin, during practical anatomy lessons on the equine distal limb for second-year veterinary students in June 2024 (study 1) and on the canine forelimb for first-year veterinary students in December 2024 (study 2). The veterinary medicine degree program consists of a total of 11 semesters, of which anatomy is taught in the first four semesters. According to the German Veterinary Licensing Regulations [29], a total of 224 teaching hours of anatomy are required. Each teaching session in anatomy consists of three teaching units, each lasting 45 min. Both present studies were conducted within the framework of one teaching session each and were integrated into the regular teaching schedule. In study 1, the topic of the teaching session was the equine distal limb, including vessels, nerves, tendons, and ligaments. In study 2, the topic of the teaching session was the canine forelimb, including muscles and nerves. One week prior to the study, students were informed about the objectives and the schedule of the study, both verbally and through an information letter. Participation was voluntary, and students provided informed consent by completing and signing a data protection declaration before taking part. They were assured that data collection was anonymous, and they could withdraw from participation at any time without consequences. Additionally, students were instructed not to prepare in advance for the lessons on the equine distal limb (study 1) and the canine forelimb (study 2). The information letter and data protection declaration are provided in Supplement S1.

2.2. Learning Materials

In accordance with ethical approval and to prevent increasing students' workload, anatomical specimens of the musculoskeletal system that are integrated into regular practical anatomy classes were selected for the studies. For study 1, which served as a pilot study, the equine distal limb was selected as a specimen with relatively few anatomical structures to be identified by students. For study 2, the canine forelimb was selected as a specimen with a larger number and complexity of anatomical structures.

2.2.1. Real Anatomical Specimens

In study 1, a total of 32 real anatomical specimens (real specimens) of the equine distal limb were used, consisting of 16 thoracic limbs and 16 pelvic limbs obtained from eight adult horses. The mean length of the equine distal limbs was 48.2 cm (±6.48), with measurements taken from the proximal point of the cannon bone to the distal aspect of the hoof wall.

Frozen equine distal limbs were defrosted cautiously at +4 °C in a cold storage room and then cleaned with a soap solution. Next, the skin was resected, and the remaining limb was fixed in a 30% ethanol–water solution (ethanol dehydrated, denatured with methyl ethyl ketone 1%) (Berkel AHK, Berlin, Germany) using immersion in boxes to preserve the natural mobility and color of the ligaments, as well as clear delineation of ligaments, vessels, and bones. Throughout the preparation, the limbs were repeatedly transferred to a new 30% ethanol solution to preserve the tissue structure and achieve gentle fixation and coloring. Between dissections, the equine distal limbs fixed in ethanol were stored in closed boxes at +4 °C. For the study, 16 distal limbs were dissected to preserve superficial structures, including the annular ligaments, superficial nerves, and vessels (superficial view). In the remaining 16 distal limbs, the palmar/plantar annular ligament and the proximal digital annular ligament were cut laterally to the flexor tendons to allow an unobstructed view of the underlying structures (deep view).

In study 2, a total of 32 real specimens of the canine forelimb were used, consisting of 16 right forelimbs and 16 left forelimbs obtained from 16 adult dogs. The mean length of the canine forelimbs was 50.4 cm (±8.27), with measurements taken from the dorsal margin of the scapula to the coronary border of the third claw.

Frozen canine forelimbs were gently thawed in a cold storage room (+4 °C) and then cleaned using a soap solution. Next, perfusion fixation of the individual limbs was performed manually via the axillary artery using a tied-in button cannula. In some cases, the fixation solution did not reach all muscle groups completely. In such cases, a targeted post-injection was necessary to ensure even and sufficient fixation of the tissue and muscle groups. The fixative solution consisted of 2% formaldehyde (Th. Geyer, Renningen, Germany), 30% ethanol, and 20% polyethylene glycol 400 (Th. Geyer, Renningen, Germany). Subsequently, the fixed limbs were stored overnight at +4 °C and then placed in a preservation bath consisting of a 2% formaldehyde solution for 8 weeks. Prior to preparation, the preserved forelimbs were soaked with preparation care solution (30% ethanol and 20% polyethylene glycol 400) and repeatedly moistened as needed during dissection. Between dissections, forelimbs were covered using cloths soaked in preparation care solution and stored in boxes at +4 °C. Dissections started by deskinning the canine forelimbs. Subsequently, muscles and nerves were dissected. To make underlying structures visible, the lateral head of the triceps brachii muscle and the superficial digital flexor muscle were cut at mid-length, angled approximately 90° to the muscle fiber orientation.

All specimens originated from animal cadavers that were obtained through the donation program of the Institute of Veterinary Anatomy of Freie Universität Berlin.

2.2.2. Low-Fidelity 3D-Printed Models

Low-fidelity 3D-printed models (3D models) of the equine distal limb and canine forelimb used in this study were modeled in the open-access software Blender 4.2.2 (Blender Foundation, Amsterdam, The Netherlands). Basic preset 3D models available within Blender were modified to represent the anatomical structures. In the sense of a low-fidelity model, the anatomical structures were displayed in a reduced form by minimizing the overall geometry of the structures, such as bones, muscles, and ligaments, while maintaining the correct positions of the structures as well as the correct origins and insertions of the muscles. Figure 1a shows an example of how the shape of the ligaments and tendons of the equine distal limb was simplified in the 3D model compared to the real specimen. Figure 1b shows a comparison of the lateral view of the canine forelimb of the real specimen and the 3D model. As part of the reduction of structures, the width and thickness of the muscles were reduced. As a result, for example, even without cutting the lateral head of the triceps brachii muscle, the other heads of this muscle, as well as other structures located below the lateral head of the triceps brachii muscle in the real specimen, are visible in the 3D model. Analogous to the real specimens, two models were made for the equine distal limb: a model representing the superficial structures (superficial view) and a model representing the deep structures (deep view). The anatomical structures of the canine forelimb were represented in one model. After the models were finalized in Blender, they were uploaded into the software GrabCAD Print 1.78 (Stratasys Ltd., Rehovot, Israel) to be prepared for 3D printing. After uploading, the software performed an automatic analysis and repaired detected issues where necessary. The models were subsequently positioned on the printing plate automatically. In GrabCAD Print, various model settings were selected for different anatomical structures, including color, shore value (degree of hardness), and surface finish (matt or glossy). Colors were defined using the RGBA (Red, Green, Blue, Alpha) color model, where values for red, green, and blue ranged from 0 to 255, and the alpha channel (A) controlled transparency on a scale from 0 (fully transparent) to 1 (fully opaque). The detailed main model settings can be found in Table 1. After selecting these model settings, the print time was automatically calculated and displayed.

For the equine distal limb, eight 3D models of the superficial view and eight 3D models of the deep view were printed. The length of the equine distal limb 3D models was 22 cm, with measurements taken from the proximal point of the cannon bone to the distal aspect of the hoof wall. Furthermore, 16 3D models of the canine forelimb were printed. The length of the 3D model of the canine forelimb was 31 cm, with measurements taken from the dorsal margin of the scapula to the coronary border of the third claw.

All models were printed using the Stratasys J55 multi-material 3D printer (Stratasys Ltd., Rehovot, Israel), which allows simultaneous printing of hard and soft materials using photopolymers. This capability enabled the production of certain parts of the model with mobility and flexibility; for example, the flexor tendons in the deep view model of the equine distal limb and the muscles in the canine forelimb model.

After printing, due to the liquid-based materials, the 3D models were completely encased in a water-soluble support material. The support material was removed by placing the printed 3D models in a water bath on a laboratory shaker (neoLab Multi Shaker Platt M, neoLab, Berlin, Germany) to facilitate the dissolution of the support material. Water was replaced periodically when it became cloudy. This process was carried out over several hours until most of the support material had dissolved. Any remaining residue of the support material was removed using a high-pressure water jet (Stratasys Ltd., Rehovot, Israel). Subsequently, the 3D models were dried and, if necessary, treated with baby or talcum powder to ensure that the material was free of any stickiness.

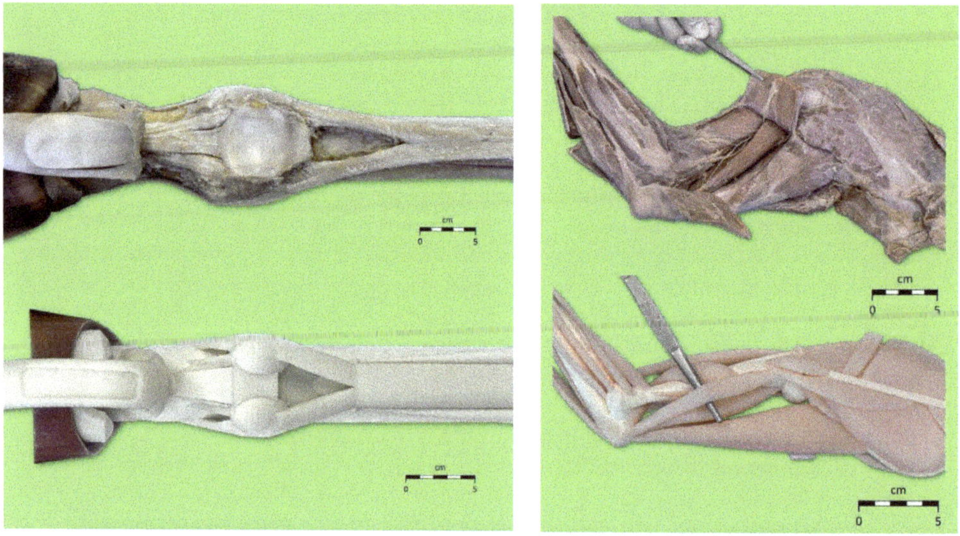

(a) (b)

Figure 1. (**a**) Example for reduction of the equine distal limb ligaments and tendons in the low-fidelity 3D model (**below**) compared to the real specimen (**above**) by simplifying the shape of these structures, shown in palmar/plantar view. (**b**) Example of the reduction of the muscles in the low-fidelity 3D model of the canine forelimb (**below**) compared to the real specimen (**above**) by reducing the width and thickness of the muscles, shown in lateral view. In the real specimen, the tweezers lift part of the sectioned lateral head of the triceps brachii muscle. In the 3D model, the tweezers are placed under the lateral head of the triceps brachii muscle.

Table 1. Main model settings in the GrabCAD Print software, including color using the RGBA color model (range 0 to 255), hardness using Shore-A (range 45 to 100) and the characteristic of the superficial surface using Surface Finish (matt/shiny).

Anatomical Structures	Color	Shore-A	Surface Finish
Bones	255(R) 253(G) 230(B) 1(A)	off	matt
Muscles	252(R) 200(G) 209(B) 0.18(A)	50	matt
Tendons	255(R) 253(G) 230(B) 0.18(A)	50	matt
Nerves	242(R) 235(G) 190(B) 0.56(A)	70	matt
Arteries	242(R) 235(G) 190(B) 0.56(A)	70	matt
Veins	108(R) 185(G) 207(B) 0.41(A)	70	matt
Hoof	107(R) 62(G) 3(B) 1 (A)	off	matt

2.2.3. Annotated Images of Real Specimens and 3D Models

Images of the real specimens and the 3D models of the equine distal limb and the canine forelimb were created using a system camera (Sony, Alpha NEX-3, Nihonbashi, Tokyo, Japan). The images were edited using Adobe Photoshop (Version 22.0) and annotated in PowerPoint (Office PowerPoint 2019, Windows) using arrows. A total of 28 structures were annotated in the images of the equine distal limb. No distinction was made between thoracic and pelvic limbs, as only structures that are morphologically similar in the thoracic and pelvic limbs were labeled. For anatomical structures that differ in their nomenclature regarding palmar/plantar, palmar was used consistently in the annotation of the images. In the images of the canine forelimb, 45 structures were annotated. To aid in the identification of different parts of muscles, unique colors were used to mark different parts of the same muscle in the images of the canine forelimb. Structures that were not visible were not labeled. The annotated images of real specimens and 3D models are shown in Figures 2 and 3.

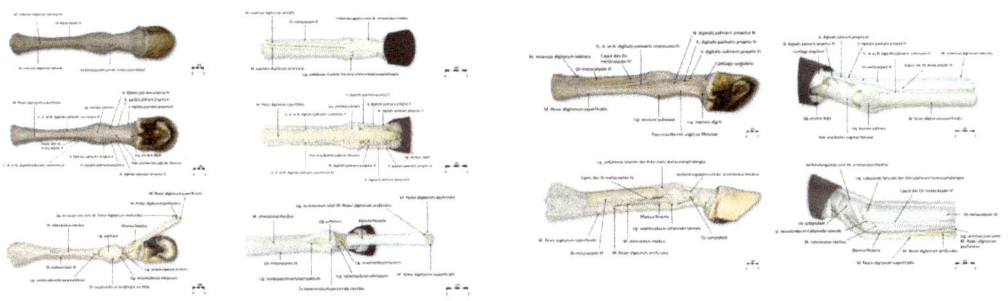

(a) (b)

Figure 2. (**a**) Annotated images of a real specimen and a 3D model of the equine distal limb, shown in dorsal and palmar/plantar views. (**b**) Annotated images of a real specimen and a 3D model of the equine distal limb, shown in lateral view.

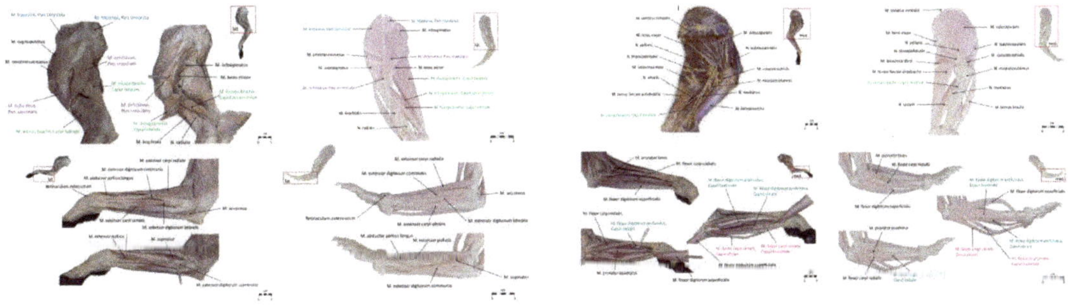

(a) (b)

Figure 3. (**a**) Annotated images of real specimens and 3D models of the canine forelimb in lateral view. (**b**) Annotated images of real specimens and 3D models of the canine forelimb in medial view.

2.3. *Knowledge Assessment*

At the end of each study, the learning outcomes were measured through a knowledge assessment in which students had to identify 20 anatomical structures on real specimens (equine distal limb in study 1, canine forelimb in study 2) and write down the corresponding anatomical terms on an examination sheet (Supplement S2). The knowledge assessment scores were defined as the learning outcomes. For the equine distal limb, both palmar and plantar were scored as correct in the knowledge assessment. In the specimens used in the knowledge assessment, anatomical structures were annotated using sewn-on beads labeled with numbers or a waterproof marker (Figure 4).

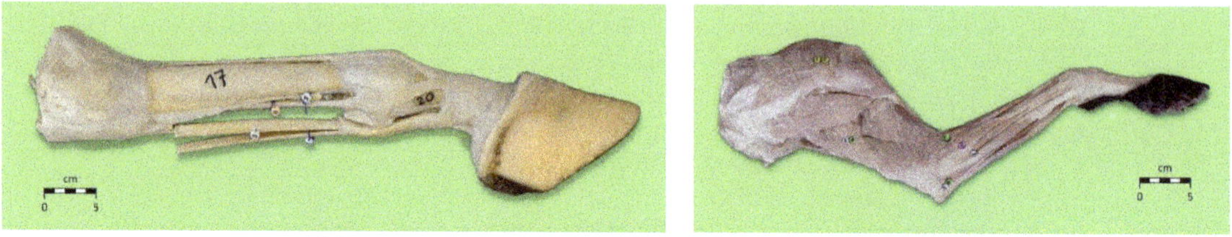

(a) (b)

Figure 4. Real specimens of the equine distal limb (**a**) and canine forelimb (**b**) used for students' knowledge assessment. Left, right, thoracic, and pelvic limbs were used as equine distal limb specimens. Both left and right forelimbs were used as canine forelimb specimens. Anatomical structures used in the knowledge assessment were labeled with numbers using sewn-on beads or a waterproof marker and are listed in Supplement S2.

2.4. *Study Design*

Both studies were carried out during regular anatomy lessons in the dissection hall, which holds 32 tables for students to study in groups. To conduct the respective knowledge assessments immediately after the learning phase, the studies were carried out in two consecutive time slots, with half of the students present in each. This way, separate tables for the learning phase and the knowledge assessment could be prepared ahead of time. Study 1 focused on the equine distal limb, while study 2 focused on the canine forelimb.

2.4.1. Study 1

All students were randomly assigned to one of two groups. One group received real specimens of the equine distal limb and the associated color-printed annotated images, while the other group learned with the 3D models of the equine distal limb and the associated color-printed annotated images. During the 10-min learning phase, students were divided into groups of 5–6 students per table and allowed to interact with each other. This phase was followed immediately by the test phase, in which students were asked to complete a knowledge assessment within 10 min. Each student completed the test individually. Before beginning the knowledge assessment, students indicated their assigned group (real specimen or 3D model) on their examination sheet. Prior to starting the knowledge assessment, the real specimens were covered with blankets. At the designated start time, all students simultaneously removed the blankets to access the annotated real specimens for the knowledge assessment. Students were asked to place their examination sheets face down on the table upon completion.

2.4.2. Study 2

For study 2, students were randomly assigned to one of four groups. The real specimen group used real specimens of the canine forelimb, while the 3D model group worked with the 3D models of the canine forelimb. Additionally, two alternating groups were introduced: the 3D model/real specimen group, which first studied with the 3D models before switching to the real specimens, and the real specimen/3D model group, which started with the real specimens and then switched to the 3D models. As in study 1, students completed the learning phase at tables of 5–6 students each and were allowed to interact with each other during this time. In this study, the learning phase lasted 30 min for each group, with the two groups that worked with both learning materials in different orders switching materials after 15 min. During the learning phase, students were provided with color-printed annotated images matching their assigned learning materials. After the learning phase, all students completed the knowledge assessment individually. The knowledge assessment was carried out in the same way as in study 1. However, in this study, students were given 15 min for the knowledge assessment, to allow extra time to find all labeled structures, since some were partially hidden by other structures.

2.5. Student Evaluation

After each of the two studies, students were given access to the entire respective learning materials, i.e., real specimens and 3D models with the corresponding annotated images, to prepare for the regular exam, which was a practical exam on real specimens. Following the exam, participants were asked to complete a brief questionnaire about their learning experiences. The evaluation was conducted via LimeSurvey (Version 5.6.31). To assess the learning materials, either a six-point Likert scale (1 = strongly disagree, 6 = strongly agree) was used, or an open-ended question was answered. A detailed overview of the questions and response types is provided in Tables 2 and 3.

Table 2. Questions and response types of the student evaluation in study 1.

	Question	Response Type
1.	By learning with the real specimen, I felt well prepared for a practical exam on an anatomical specimen.	Likert scale
2.	By learning with the low-fidelity 3D-printed model, I felt well prepared for a practical exam on an anatomical specimen.	Likert scale
3.	Do you have any feedback for us regarding the low-fidelity 3D-printed models?	Free text

Table 3. Questions and response types of the student evaluation in study 2.

Question	Response Type
1. By learning with the real specimen, I felt well prepared for a practical exam on an anatomical specimen.	Likert scale
2. By learning with the low-fidelity 3D-printed model, I felt well prepared for a practical exam on an anatomical specimen.	Likert scale
3. I think it makes sense to first learn with the low-fidelity 3D-printed model and then with the real specimen for a practical examination on an anatomical specimen.	Likert scale
4. I think it makes sense to first learn with the real specimen and then with the low-fidelity 3D-printed model for a practical examination on an anatomical specimen.	Likert scale
5. Do you have any feedback for us regarding the low-fidelity 3D-printed models?	Free text

2.6. Statistical Analysis

Statistical and descriptive analyses were performed using IBM SPSS Statistics Version 29® (IBM, Armonk, NY, USA). Graphical representations were created using BioRender (©2025 BioRender, Toronto, ON, Canada). Each correct term in the knowledge assessment was awarded one point, while no points were given for incorrect or missing responses. Misspelled or incomplete terms were evaluated to determine whether they demonstrated recognition of the correct structure. To ensure reliability, two researchers independently assessed the test results. However, due to minimal deviations (<10% in both studies; $\kappa = 0.94$), the assessment by a single researcher was deemed sufficient for analysis. Prior to further analysis, data from both studies were visually inspected for normal distribution.

Additionally, Levene's test was used to test for homogeneity of variance. The significance level was set at 5%.

In study 1, the mean knowledge assessment score was calculated for the two study groups and compared using an unpaired *t*-test. Effect sizes were calculated using Cohen's *d*. A d-value of 0.2 indicates a small effect, a d-value of 0.5 indicates a medium effect, and a d-value of 0.8 indicates a large effect [30]. In study 2, the mean knowledge assessment score was calculated for the four study groups and compared using a one-way analysis of variance (ANOVA). Bonferroni-corrected post-hoc analysis was used to verify significant differences between the study groups. Effect sizes were calculated using Cohen's *f*, whereby an f-value of 0.1 indicates a small effect, an f-value of 0.25 indicates a medium effect, and an f-value of 0.84 indicates a large effect [30]. To assess the studies' power, post-hoc power analyses were performed using G*Power 3.1.9.2.

The analysis of the Likert scale-based answers of the student evaluation was carried out for study 1 using an unpaired *t*-test (2 questions) and for study 2 using an ANOVA (4 questions). Raw data are provided in Supplement S3. A qualitative content analysis was carried out to assess the students' responses to the open-ended questions in study 1 and study 2. For this purpose, the statements were paraphrased, then abstracted in the course of generalization, and finally pooled as codes in terms of reduction [31]. Coding categories can be found in Supplement S4. To ensure reliability, the codes generated were assigned to the students' statements by a second researcher. However, given the minimal deviations (<10% in both evaluations; study 1: $\kappa = 0.9$; study 2: $\kappa = 0.95$), the assessment by a single researcher was considered adequate for the analysis.

3. Results

3.1. Number of Participants

In study 1, a total of 135 second-year veterinary students (71% of the enrolled students) participated, of whom 67 students were randomly assigned to the real specimen group and 68 were assigned to the 3D model group. In study 2, a total of 183 first-year veterinary students (88% of the enrolled students) participated. Of these, 44 students were randomly assigned to the real specimen group, 45 students to the 3D model group, 47 students to the 3D model/real specimen group, and 47 students to the real specimen/3D model group.

3.2. Learning Outcomes

Learning Outcomes in Study 1

In study 1, the unpaired *t*-test revealed a significantly higher mean knowledge assessment score in the real specimen group (8.04 ± 3.14) compared to the 3D model group (6.91 ± 2.89) ($p = 0.031$) (Figure 5). Cohen's *d* indicated a small to medium effect ($d = 0.38$). The post-hoc power analysis showed a statistical power of 0.99 (1-β err prob), which indicates sufficient power to detect the observed effect with a high degree of probability.

The structure that scored best in the knowledge assessment was the *Nervus digitalis palmaris proprius II/III* in the real specimen group (0.79 ± 0.41), while the best-scoring structure in the 3D model group was the *Musculus flexor digitorum superficialis* (0.78 ± 0.42). In both groups, the structure that scored lowest was the *Ligamentum metacarpointersesamoideum* (real specimen group: 0.13 ± 0.34; 3D model group: 0 ± 0). Raw data are provided in Supplement S3.

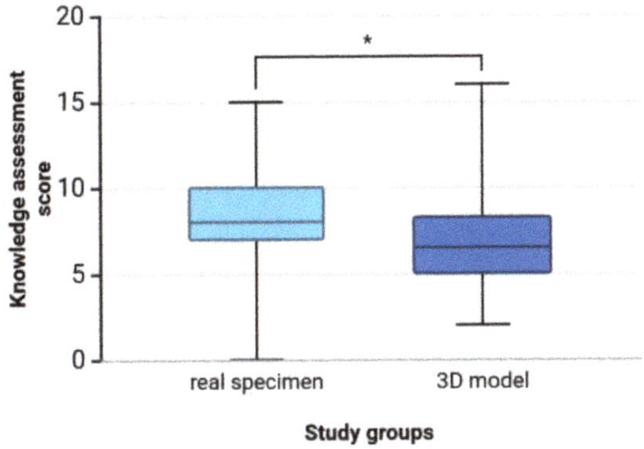

Figure 5. Study 1: Comparison of students' knowledge assessment scores between study groups after learning anatomical structures of the equine distal limb for 10 min on either a real specimen (n = 67) or a 3D model (n = 68). The knowledge assessment was based on recognition of 20 anatomical structures labeled on a real specimen of the equine distal limb. Whiskers show 10th and 90th percentiles; * $p < 0.05$.

3.3. Learning Outcomes in Study 2

The real specimen group achieved the highest mean score (6.11 ± 2.90), followed by the real specimen/3D model group (4.70 ± 2.43), the 3D model group (4.16 ± 2.90), and the 3D model/real specimen group (3.85 ± 1.93) (Figure 6). The study group had a significant influence on learning outcomes ($F(6.87)$, $p < 0.001$, $\eta p2 = 0.1$, n = 183). The effect size indicates a medium effect (f = 0.33). The post-hoc power analysis showed a statistical power of 0.97 (1-β err prob), which indicates sufficient power to detect the observed effect with a high degree of probability. Post-hoc tests with Bonferroni correction revealed that not all study groups differed significantly. However, the mean knowledge assessment score in the real specimen group was significantly higher than the scores in the 3D model group (p = 0.002) and the 3D model/real specimen group ($p < 0.001$).

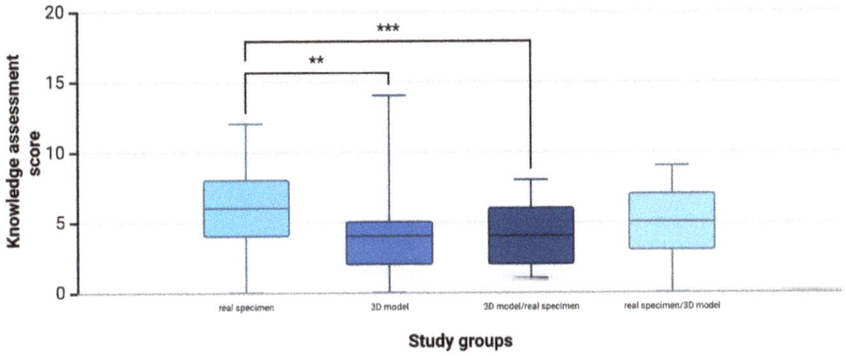

Figure 6. Study 2: Comparison of students' knowledge assessment scores between study groups after learning anatomical structures of the canine forelimb for 30 min on a real specimen (n = 44), a 3D model (n = 45), a 3D model followed by a real specimen (3D model/real specimen, n = 47), or a real specimen followed by a 3D model (real specimen/3D model, n = 47). The knowledge assessment was based on recognition of 20 anatomical structures labeled on a real specimen of the canine forelimb. Whiskers show 10th and 90th percentiles; ** $p < 0.01$, *** $p < 0.001$.

The structure that scored best in the knowledge assessment for the real specimen group (0.66 ± 0.48), the 3D model group (0.58 ± 0.50), and real specimen/3D model group (0.62 ± 0.49) was the *Musculus biceps brachii*. For the 3D model/real specimen group (0.57 ± 0.50), it was the *Musculus serratus ventralis*. Structures with the lowest scores in the knowledge assessment were the *Musculus pronator teres* in the real specimen group (0 ± 0) and the *Musculus flexor carpi radialis* in the 3D model group (0 ± 0). In the 3D model/real specimen group, the *Musculus pronator teres* (0 ± 0) and the *Musculus coracobrachialis* (0 ± 0) scored equally low. In the real specimen/3D model group, the lowest scores were observed for the *Musculus pronator teres* and the *Musculus brachialis* (both 0.02 ± 0.15). Raw data are provided in Supplement S3.

3.4. Student Evaluation

3.4.1. Student Evaluation in Study 1

Since all students had been given access to both the real specimens and the 3D models for exam preparation after study 1, 159 students took part in the evaluation of the learning materials after the exam (84% of the enrolled students). When asked which of the two learning materials students would prefer for exam preparation (assessment on a six-point Likert scale), the unpaired *t*-test revealed that students felt significantly better prepared for the practical exam by learning with the real specimens (5.17 ± 0.85) compared to the 3D models (4.76 ± 0.93) ($p < 0.001$) (Figure 7). Cohen's d showed a medium effect ($d = 0.47$). The post-hoc power analysis showed a statistical power of 0.99 (1-β err prob), which indicates sufficient power to detect the observed effect with a high degree of probability. Raw data are provided in Supplement S3.

The qualitative content analysis of the answers to the open-ended question revealed that a high number of students (19 out of 57 statements; 33.3%) preferred the 3D model when starting to learn and then moved on to the real specimen. Other statements that were made more frequently indicated that the 3D models are better suited for gaining a general basic understanding of anatomical structures (eight out of 57 statements; 14.0%) and that it is a particular advantage that the 3D models can be used for learning outside the dissection hall (eight out of 57 statements; 14.0%). In addition, several students (seven of the 57 statements; 12.3%) expressed the wish to have further 3D models of other anatomical specimens available. The list of codes is provided in Supplement S4.

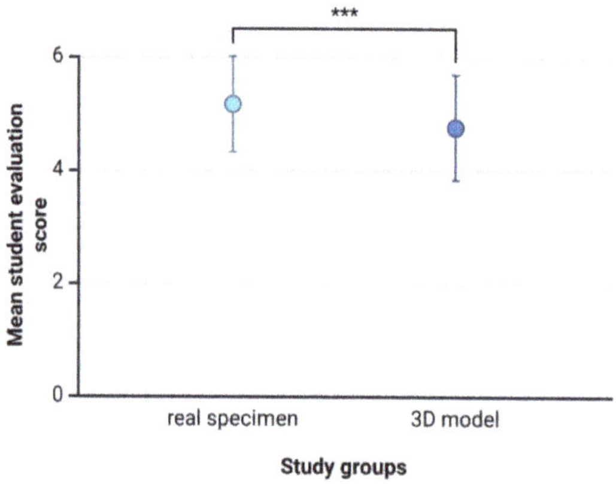

Figure 7. Study 1: Mean values and standard deviations of students' evaluations ($n = 159$) of the learning materials. Based on a six-point Likert scale, students were asked to indicate whether they felt well prepared for a practical exam on a real anatomical specimen of an equine distal limb using the respective learning materials, i.e., real specimen or 3D model; *** $p < 0.001$.

3.4.2. Student Evaluation in Study 2

The evaluation after the regular exam, after all students had been given access to real specimens and 3D models for exam preparation, included 180 students in study 2 (87% of the enrolled students). Most of the students preferred the learning method 3D model/real specimen (5.17 ± 1.24), followed by the real specimen (4.57 ± 1.03), the 3D model (4.15 ± 1.12), and real specimen/3D model (2.92 ± 1.32) (Figure 8). The results of the student evaluation revealed that the preferred learning methods differed significantly ($F(88.94)$, $p < 0.0001$, $\eta p2 = 0.33$, $n = 180$). The effect size indicates a strong effect ($f = 0.7$). The post-hoc power analysis showed a statistical power of 1.0 (1-β err prob), which indicates sufficient power to detect the observed effect with a high degree of probability. Post-hoc tests with Bonferroni correction showed that students felt significantly better prepared for the exam when using the learning materials in the order 3D model/real specimen compared to learning only with the real specimen ($p < 0.001$), only the 3D model ($p < 0.0001$), or when using the learning materials in the order real specimen/3D model ($p < 0.0001$). The differences in learning preference were also significant between real specimen and 3D model ($p = 0.021$), real specimen and real specimen/3D model ($p < 0.0001$), and 3D model and real specimen/3D model ($p < 0.0001$). The results of the evaluation show that students preferred the learning method that achieved the lowest learning outcomes in the knowledge assessment. Raw data are provided in Supplement S3.

The qualitative content analysis of students' responses to the open-ended question revealed that almost half of the statements (17 out of 40 statements; 42.5%) indicated a preference for students to start learning with the 3D model and then continue with the real specimen. Furthermore, several statements indicated that students perceived learning with the 3D models as very helpful (six out of 40 statements; 15.0%). Some students indicated that they would prefer to learn with the 3D model and real specimen simultaneously (four out of 40 statements; 10.0%). The list of codes is provided in Supplement S4.

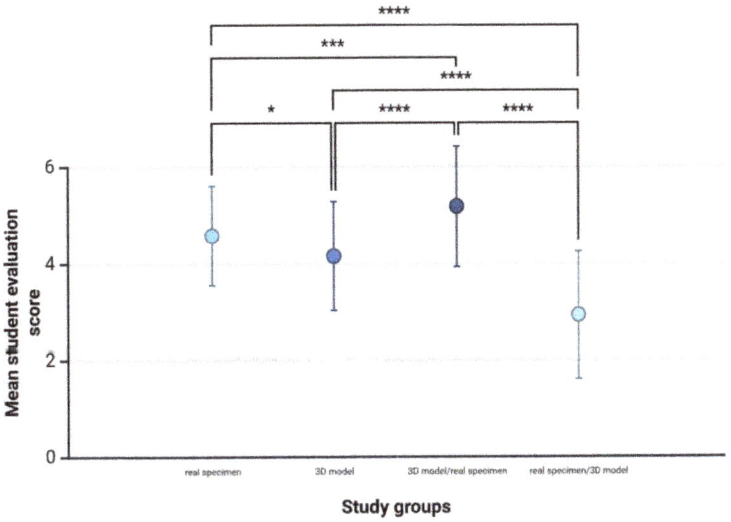

Figure 8. Study 2: Mean values and standard deviations of students' evaluations (n = 180) of the learning materials. Based on a six-point Likert scale, students were asked to indicate whether they felt well prepared for a practical exam on a real anatomical specimen of a canine forelimb using the respective learning materials, i.e., real specimen, 3D model, 3D model followed by real specimen (3D model/real specimen), or real specimen followed by 3D model (real specimen/3D model); * $p < 0.05$, *** $p < 0.001$, **** $p < 0.0001$.

4. Discussion

The presented work investigated the impact of low-fidelity 3D-printed models as learning materials in veterinary anatomy classes. The research was guided by the hypothesis that students learning the anatomical structures of the equine distal limb or the canine forelimb using low-fidelity 3D-printed models would achieve similar learning outcomes as those using the corresponding real specimens.

When students learned with either the real specimen or the 3D model, as in study 1, students who learned with the real specimen achieved significantly higher learning outcomes than students who learned with the 3D model. In addition, the evaluation of the learning materials by students after the regular anatomy exam showed that students' preference for using real specimens to prepare for the exam was significantly higher than for using the 3D model. To date, two studies on the use of 3D models as learning materials for veterinary anatomy have been published, both reporting similar findings as the present study [27,28]. A study from Japan demonstrated that 3D-printed skulls are effective as an introduction before working with real specimens [28]. Additionally, a study from Spain in the field of veterinary anatomy, which involved the creation of 3D models of various structures from various domestic and exotic species, including bone, viscera, and vascular structures, concluded that 3D-printed models are not a replacement for real specimens. Furthermore, the authors emphasized the need to improve 3D-printed models in terms of color, size, texture, and flexibility to enhance the anatomical accuracy and their potential application in surgical training [27]. It is possible that learning outcomes for 3D models differ depending on the structures and species used in the respective investigation. Since neither of those studies included the equine distal limb or the canine forelimb, comparability is limited.

Comparable results have been reported in studies on students of human medicine [32–36]. In a study carried out in human anatomy, students' preferences for anatomy learning resources and their perceived effectiveness in achieving learning outcomes were investigated. Data collection took place at the end of the spring semester, during the abdominal gross anatomy course, after medical students had completed the upper and lower limb sections, as well as the cardiovascular and respiratory system modules. The results showed that real specimens combined with clinical tutorials were rated as the preferred and most effective resource for learning anatomy, followed by dissection videos, other electronic resources, and printed materials. In contrast, the perceived usefulness of plastinated specimens and plastic models was rated lower by students [32]. Other studies in the field of human anatomy also confirm that both students and teachers rate the impact of real specimens as learning materials higher than that of 3D models [33,34]. Moreover, there is no substantial evidence that 3D models are significantly more effective in enhancing learning outcomes compared to real specimens [33,34]. In studies in which students were asked about their learning experience with 3D-printed models of human anatomical specimens compared to plastinates, students found plastinates superior to 3D models due to their more realistic nature. However, students emphasized that they would prefer 3D-printed models for learning basic anatomy [35,36]. Overall, students perceived the usefulness of 3D-printed models, particularly in gaining a general, basic understanding of anatomical structures, while real specimens or plastinates might be more likely to be used to deepen knowledge and understanding in a practical context [34,35]. In the study of Mogali et al., 3D-printed models of the thoracic limb were evaluated [35], while cardiac, head, and neck 3D-printed models were tested by Radzi et al. [36]. The student evaluations of learning materials in those studies showed similar results to the student evaluation in the present study [35,36]. Thus, in study 1, many students stated that the 3D models might be better suited than the real specimens for initially gaining a general, basic understanding of anatomical structures.

Therefore, in addition to the two test groups that used the real specimens or the 3D models for learning, two further test groups were set up in study 2, which used both learning materials, real specimens and 3D models, in different orders. However, results from study 2 show that the group that had learned with the real specimens had the highest learning outcomes, followed by the real specimen/3D model group and then the 3D model group. The group with the lowest learning outcomes was the 3D model/real specimen group, which was the group that had used the learning materials in the order that, according to the students' evaluation, should have been the most suitable. As in study 1, many students who participated in study 2 also stated in the open-ended question that they would consider it the best learning method to start with the 3D-printed models and then transition to the real specimens. The analysis of quantitative data from students' evaluations also showed that students regarded learning in the order 3D model/real specimen as most suitable, followed by learning with only the real specimen and then the 3D model only. Learning in the order real specimen/3D model was found to be least suitable by students. Students' preference for starting anatomy learning with a 3D model before transitioning to the real specimen can be explained on the basis that students often experience considerable apprehension, stress, and anxiety when encountering cadavers [37–39]. In this context, 3D models may serve as an effective introductory tool, helping students become familiar with anatomical structures, easing their discomfort, and reducing psychological barriers to working with cadavers, which remain a vital component of the anatomy curriculum [40]. In clinical training, 3D models can ease the transition to working with live animals by reducing student stress and fostering greater interest in clinical practice, for example, when they learn clinical skills such as intravenous catheterization, bandaging, or anesthesia on canine 3D-printed models [9]. The results show that students' perception of which learning method would lead to the highest learning outcomes did not match the learning method that ultimately led to the highest learning outcomes. This finding is consistent with the results of several studies that have identified a discrepancy between the learning outcomes perceived by students and the learning outcomes they actually achieved [41–43]. This could be the case because students might be more likely to perceive an increase in self-efficacy rather than measuring the actual acquisition of skills [41]. However, the lower learning outcomes when learning in the order 3D model/real specimen observed in the presented study could also arise due to students requiring more time to become familiar with the 3D models, as they were using a new and therefore unfamiliar learning tool, necessitating additional time to adapt [2,18]. In a study that evaluated a low-fidelity inguinal canal model, students explicitly expressed a desire for more hands-on time with the model [18]. Similarly, the findings of a previous study on the use of 3D scans as learning materials emphasized the vital importance of giving students sufficient time to adjust to new learning circumstances [44]. Thus, students who started learning with the 3D models may struggle to adapt and apply their knowledge effectively when switching to the real specimens. This aspect could have been underestimated by students in their evaluation. Overall, it must be considered that students' preferences are not necessarily a reliable indicator of learning efficacy, as shown in the studies presented, as well as in previous studies [32–36].

In the learning material evaluation, some students indicated that they would prefer to learn with the real specimens and the 3D models simultaneously. This way, the advantages and disadvantages of both learning materials could possibly counterbalance each other. Since dissection alone cannot meet all educational needs, combining it with innovative teaching methods offers a comprehensive approach to anatomy education, ensuring both tradition and technology work together to enhance learning [45].

An advantage of the 3D models highlighted by students' evaluations is that they can effectively support learning beyond the dissection hall. Thus, the use of 3D-printed models expands access to anatomical specimens, helping to mitigate the challenges posed by limited cadaver availability [2,28,46,47].

Not least, students expressed enthusiasm for the 3D-printed models as they perceived the 3D-printed models as highly beneficial for learning. This aligns with previous research, which has similarly reported that students find 3D-printed models to be valuable educational tools [2,9,12–14,18,19,48]. Accordingly, several students indicated that they wish to have further 3D-printed models of other anatomical specimens available. This positive commitment should be preserved, as it enhances students' motivation to engage in anatomy learning. At this point, it is important to emphasize that 3D models are tools that can be useful but are not replacements in anatomy education [27,28,35,36].

Some limitations may affect the interpretation and transferability of the results. First, the studies had only one assessment point. Further research could examine whether the same results would be obtained if there were a second assessment point with a longer time interval after the study. Second, both anatomical specimens addressed in the studies were from the musculoskeletal system. Further studies could clarify the extent to which low-fidelity 3D-printed models of specimens from other organ systems can lead to comparable learning outcomes to those of the corresponding real specimens. Third, the tests in the studies focused only on the recognition of anatomical structures on the specimen. The fact that students frequently stated that they found the 3D models helpful for initial learning could also indicate that the 3D models may be more suitable for understanding functional aspects and relationships, for example, in the muscles and ligaments. In further studies, these aspects should be considered in the tests to verify this assumption. Fourth, it is assumed that if more time were available, transitioning between different learning resources might be beneficial [45]. To examine whether a period to familiarize with the 3D model or the real specimen could reduce the differences in the learning outcomes in those groups that change the learning material during the learning period, such a period should be introduced for those test groups in subsequent studies. Lastly, this study explored the use of low-fidelity models in veterinary anatomy, and it may be possible that better learning outcomes could be achieved with high-fidelity models.

5. Conclusions

The studies did not confirm the hypothesis that the same learning outcomes can be achieved with low-fidelity 3D-printed models of the equine distal limb or the canine forelimb as with the corresponding real specimens. For both the canine forelimb and the equine distal limb, participants who studied using real specimens achieved significantly higher learning outcomes compared to those who used 3D models. In contrast, students stated in the evaluation that they would prefer to start learning with the 3D models and then switch to the real specimens. However, in the study, students achieved the lowest learning outcomes with this learning method. This discrepancy in the students' evaluation of learning materials could be, on the one hand, because the students might be more likely to measure the increase in self-efficacy than the increase in knowledge. On the other hand, it could be because familiarizing oneself with a new learning material takes some time, an aspect that was neglected in the study, which used the same learning time for all test groups, resulting in a potential disadvantage for the groups that used both learning materials in alternating order. In conclusion, equine distal limb and canine forelimb 3D models appear to be less effective for knowledge acquisition. While they may serve as useful preparatory tools, they should not be considered substitutes.

Beyond that, students were enthusiastic about the 3D models of the equine distal limb and the canine forelimb and expressed the wish to have more 3D models of further anatomical specimens, which showed that the 3D models could increase students' learning motivation. In addition, the 3D models expand opportunities for students to learn anatomy from specimens, since they can also be used outside of the dissection hall.

Supplementary Materials: The following supporting information can be downloaded at https://www.mdpi.com/article/10.3390/ani15101380/s1, Supplement S1: Information letter and data protection declaration; Supplement S2: Examination sheets; Supplement S3: Raw data; Supplement S4: List of codes for qualitative content analysis.

Author Contributions: Conceptualization, R.S., M.B., G.M.C. and J.P.E.; methodology, R.S., M.S., J.W., M.W. and M.B.; formal analysis, R.S. and M.B.; investigation, R.S., M.B. and J.W.; data curation, R.S.; writing—original draft preparation, R.S., M.B. and L.G.K.; visualization, R.S. and M.W.; supervision and project administration, M.B.; writing—review and editing, R.S., M.B., J.W. and L.G.K. All authors have read and agreed to the published version of the manuscript.

Funding: This research received no external funding. The publication of this article was funded by Freie Universität Berlin.

Institutional Review Board Statement: This study was conducted according to the guidelines of the Declaration of Helsinki and approved by the Ethics Committee of Freie Universität Berlin (ZEA-Nr. 2022-014, 9 June 2022).

Informed Consent Statement: Informed consent was obtained from all subjects involved in the study.

Data Availability Statement: Data are contained within the article or Supplementary Material. The data presented in this study are available in the Supplementary Material.

Acknowledgments: The authors would like to express their sincere thanks to the students involved for their participation in the studies. The authors would also like to thank Joëlle Pachtmann, Ioana-Alexandra Graur, Ricardo Schwarz, Lorenz Robra, and Hendrik Seipold for their brilliant support in dissecting the real specimens.

Conflicts of Interest: The authors declare no conflicts of interest.

References

1. Varner, C.; Dixon, L.; Simons, M.C. The Past, Present, and Future: A Discussion of Cadaver Use in Medical and Veterinary Education. *Front. Vet. Sci.* **2021**, *8*, 720740. [CrossRef] [PubMed]
2. Kinnison, T.; Forrest, N.D.; Frean, S.P.; Baillie, S. Teaching bovine abdominal anatomy: Use of a haptic simulator. *Anat. Sci. Educ.* **2009**, *2*, 280–285. [CrossRef]
3. Janczyk, P.; Weigner, J.; Luebke-Becker, A.; Richardson, K.C.; Plendl, J. A pilot study on ethanol-polyethylene glycol-formalin fixation of farm animal cadavers. *Berl. Munch. Tierarztl. Wochenschr.* **2011**, *124*, 225–227.
4. Office, P. European Commission. Commission Implementing Regulation (EU) No 605/2014 of 5 June 2014 Laying Down the Lists of Third Countries, Territories or Parts Thereof from Which Entry into the Union of Certain Animals and Fresh Meat is Authorized. *Off. J. Eur. Union* **2014**, *168*, 7–34. Available online: https://eur-lex.europa.eu/eli/reg/2014/605/oj/eng (accessed on 26 April 2025).
5. Peters, H.R. Erstellung von Dreidimensional Gedruckten, Anatomisch Korrekten Schädeln und Unterkiefern von Canis Familiaris für den Einsatz in der Anatomischen Lehre. Doctoral Thesis, Ludwig-Maximilians-Universität München, Munich, Germany, 2018.
6. Langebæk, R.; Toft, N.; Eriksen, T. The SimSpay-Student Perceptions of a Low-Cost Build-It-Yourself Model for Novice Training of Surgical Skills in Canine Ovariohysterectomy. *J. Vet. Med. Educ.* **2015**, *42*, 166–171. [CrossRef] [PubMed]
7. Read, E.K.; Vallevand, A.; Farrell, R.M. Evaluation of Veterinary Student Surgical Skills Preparation for Ovariohysterectomy Using Simulators: A Pilot Study. *J. Vet. Med. Educ.* **2016**, *43*, 190–213. [CrossRef]
8. Badman, M.; Höglund, K.; Höglund, O.V. Student Perceptions of the Use of a Laser Pointer for Intra-Operative Guidance in Feline Castration. *J. Vet. Med. Educ.* **2016**, *43*, 222–224. [CrossRef]
9. Hadžiomerović, N.; Šunje-Rizvan, A.; Maksimović, A.; Šatrović, L.; Tandir, F. Use of 3D printed low-cost models for veterinary clinical skills training. *Open Vet. J.* **2025**, *15*, 863–870. [CrossRef]
10. Sheats, M.K.; Burke, M.J.; Robertson, J.B.; Fiebrandt, K.E.; Fogle, C.A. Development and Formative Evaluation of a Low-Fidelity Equine Castration Model for Veterinary Education. *Front. Vet. Sci.* **2021**, *8*, 689243. [CrossRef]

11. Aulmann, M.; März, M.; Burgener, I.A.; Alef, M.; Otto, S.; Mülling, C.K.W. Development and Evaluation of Two Canine Low Fidelity Simulation Models. *J. Vet. Med. Educ.* **2015**, *42*, 151–160. [CrossRef]
12. Denadai, R.; Saad-Hossne, R.; Todelo, A.P.; Kirylko, L.; Souto, L.R.M. Low-fidelity bench models for basic surgical skills training during undergraduate medical education. *Rev. Col. Bras. Cir.* **2014**, *41*, 137–145. [CrossRef]
13. Friedman, Z.; Siddiqui, N.; Katznelson, R.; Devito, I.; Bould, M.D.; Naik, V. Clinical impact of epidural anesthesia simulation on short- and long-term learning curve: High- versus low-fidelity model training. *Reg. Anesth. Pain. Med.* **2009**, *34*, 229–232. [CrossRef] [PubMed]
14. McClelland, T.J.; Ford, K.; Dagash, H.; Lander, A.; Lakhoo, K. Low-fidelity Paediatric Surgical Simulation: Description of Models in Low-Resource Settings. *World J. Surg.* **2019**, *43*, 1193–1197. [CrossRef] [PubMed]
15. Langebæk, R.; Berendt, M.; Pedersen, L.T.; Jensen, A.L.; Eika, B. Features that contribute to the usefulness of low-fidelity models for surgical skills training. *Vet. Rec.* **2012**, *170*, 361. [CrossRef]
16. Thompson, J.-L.; MacKay, J.; Bowlt Blacklock, K. Evaluation of veterinary students' confidence and competence with surgical entrustable professional activities after repeated use of low-fidelity training models. *Vet. Rec.* **2023**, *192*, e2779. [CrossRef] [PubMed]
17. Chan, L.K.; Cheung, R.C.C. The Use of Low-Fidelity Models to Enhance the Learning of Anatomy. In *Teaching Anatomy: A Practical Guide*, 2nd ed.; Chan, L.K., Pawlina, W., Eds.; Springer International Publishing: Cham, Switzerland, 2020; pp. 325–335. ISBN 978-3-030-43283-6.
18. Hindmarch, J.; Bazzi, K.; Lahoud, J.; Malik, A.; Sinha, S. Evaluating a low-fidelity inguinal canal model. *Surg. Radiol. Anat.* **2020**, *42*, 1323–1328. [CrossRef]
19. Dixit, S.G.; Potaliya, P.; Nayeemudin, S.M.; Ghatak, S. Low fidelity model making activity by students: A novel way of learning concepts of neuroanatomy. *J. Clin. Neurosci.* **2018**, *52*, 100–104. [CrossRef]
20. Chan, L.K.; Cheng, M.M.W. An analysis of the educational value of low-fidelity anatomy models as external representations. *Anat. Sci. Educ.* **2011**, *4*, 256–263. [CrossRef]
21. Fieux, M.; Zaouche, S.; Philouze, P.; Truy, E.; Hermann, R.; Tringali, S. Low-fidelity otoscopy simulation and anatomy training: A randomized controlled trial. *Eur. Ann. Otorhinolaryngol. Head. Neck Dis.* **2021**, *138*, 231–234. [CrossRef]
22. Birbara, N.S.; Pather, N. Real Or Not Real: The Impact of the Physical Fidelity of Virtual Learning Resources on Learning Anatomy. *Anat. Sci. Educ.* **2021**, *14*, 774–787. [CrossRef]
23. Chan, L.K. Pulling my gut out--simple tools for engaging students in gross anatomy lectures. *Anat. Sci. Educ.* **2010**, *3*, 148–150. [CrossRef] [PubMed]
24. Cloud, B.A.; Youdas, J.W.; Hellyer, N.J.; Krause, D.A. A functional model of the digital extensor mechanism: Demonstrating biomechanics with hair bands. *Anat. Sci. Educ.* **2010**, *3*, 144–147. [CrossRef] [PubMed]
25. Gangata, H. An innovative approach to supplement the teaching of the spatial gross anatomy relationships of muscles to undergraduates in health sciences. *Clin. Anat.* **2008**, *21*, 339–347. [CrossRef]
26. Lefroy, H.; Burdon-Bailey, V.; Bhangu, A.; Abrahams, P. A novel technique for teaching the brachial plexus. *Clin. Teach.* **2011**, *8*, 196–199. [CrossRef] [PubMed]
27. Díaz Martínez, E.; Zarzosa, G.J.R.; Arencibia Espinosa, A.; Soler Laguía, M.; Rojo Rios, D.; Lorente, A.O.; Leotte Sánchez, M.; Ceballos-Francisco, D.; García, M.I.G.; Gil Cano, F.; et al. Veterinary Students' Assessment of 3D Anatomical Prints as New Teaching Material in Practical Veterinary Anatomy Classes. *Educ. Sci.* **2025**, *15*, 355. [CrossRef]
28. Sakaue, M.; Oishi, M.; Ozawa, A.; Tsukamoto, A.; Kayanuma, H.; Ichihara, N. Availability and issues of 3D-printed skull models for veterinary anatomy laboratories from students' perspective before and during the COVID-19 pandemic. *J. Vet. Med. Sci.* **2024**, *86*, 1081–1088. [CrossRef]
29. Verordnung zur Approbation von Tierärztinnen und Tierärzten. (TAppV). Available online: https://www.gesetze-im-internet.de/tappv/ (accessed on 26 April 2025).
30. Cohen, J. *Statistical Power Analysis for the Behavioral Sciences*; Routledge: New York, NY, USA, 2013; ISBN 9781134742707.
31. Baur, N.; Blasius, J. *Handbuch Methoden der Empirischen Sozialforschung*, 2nd ed.; Springer VS: Wiesbaden, Germany, 2019; ISBN 978-3-658-21307-7.
32. Abdullah, E.; Lone, M.; Cray, J.J.; Dvoracek, P.; Balta, J.Y. Medical Students' Opinions of Anatomy Teaching Resources and Their Role in Achieving Learning Outcomes. *Med. Sci. Educ.* **2021**, *31*, 1903–1910. [CrossRef]
33. Kerby, J.; Shukur, Z.N.; Shalhoub, J. The relationships between learning outcomes and methods of teaching anatomy as perceived by medical students. *Clin. Anat.* **2011**, *24*, 489–497. [CrossRef]
34. Azer, S.A.; Azer, S. 3D Anatomy Models and Impact on Learning: A Review of the Quality of the Literature. *Health Prof. Educ.* **2016**, *2*, 80–98. [CrossRef]
35. Mogali, S.R.; Yeong, W.Y.; Tan, H.K.J.; Tan, G.J.S.; Abrahams, P.H.; Zary, N.; Low-Beer, N.; Ferenczi, M.A. Evaluation by medical students of the educational value of multi-material and multi-colored three-dimensional printed models of the upper limb for anatomical education. *Anat. Sci. Educ.* **2018**, *11*, 54–64. [CrossRef]

36. Radzi, S.; Chandrasekaran, R.; Peh, Z.K.; Rajalingam, P.; Yeong, W.Y.; Mogali, S.R. Students' learning experiences of three-dimensional printed models and plastinated specimens: A qualitative analysis. *BMC Med. Educ.* **2022**, *22*, 695. [CrossRef] [PubMed]
37. Penney, J.C. Reactions of medical students to dissection. *Acad. Med.* **1985**, *60*, 58. [CrossRef] [PubMed]
38. Arráez-Aybar, L.-A.; Casado-Morales, M.I.; Castaño-Collado, G. Anxiety and dissection of the human cadaver: An unsolvable relationship? *Anat. Rec. B New Anat.* **2004**, *279*, 16–23. [CrossRef]
39. Boeckers, A.; Brinkmann, A.; Jerg-Bretzke, L.; Lamp, C.; Traue, H.C.; Boeckers, T.M. How can we deal with mental distress in the dissection room?-An evaluation of the need for psychological support. *Ann. Anat.* **2010**, *192*, 366–372. [CrossRef] [PubMed]
40. Lim, K.H.A.; Loo, Z.Y.; Goldie, S.J.; Adams, J.W.; McMenamin, P.G. Use of 3D printed models in medical education: A randomized control trial comparing 3D prints versus cadaveric materials for learning external cardiac anatomy. *Anat. Sci. Educ.* **2016**, *9*, 213–221. [CrossRef]
41. Persky, A.M.; Lee, E.; Schlesselman, L.S. Perception of learning versus performance as outcome measures of educational research Discussion 3D Druck. *Am. J. Pharm. Educ.* **2020**, *84*, ajpe7782. [CrossRef]
42. Deslauriers, L.; McCarty, L.S.; Miller, K.; Callaghan, K.; Kestin, G. Measuring actual learning versus feeling of learning in response to being actively engaged in the classroom. *Proc. Natl. Acad. Sci. USA* **2019**, *116*, 19251–19257. [CrossRef]
43. van Sickle, J.R. Discrepancies between Student Perception and Achievement of Learning Outcomes in a Flipped Classroom. *J. Scholarsh. Teach. Learn.* **2016**, *16*, 29–38. [CrossRef]
44. Schirone, R.; Corte, G.M.; Ehlers, J.P.; Herre, C.; Schmedding, M.; Merle, R.; Pachtmann, J.; Bahramsoltani, M. Effects of 3D Scans on Veterinary Students' Learning Outcomes Compared to Traditional 2D Images in Anatomy Classes. *Animals* **2024**, *14*, 2171. [CrossRef]
45. Ghosh, S.K. Cadaveric dissection as an educational tool for anatomical sciences in the 21st century. *Anat. Sci. Educ.* **2017**, *10*, 286–299. [CrossRef] [PubMed]
46. Patel, K.M.; Moxham, B.J. The relationships between learning outcomes and methods of teaching anatomy as perceived by professional anatomists. *Clin. Anat.* **2008**, *21*, 182–189. [CrossRef] [PubMed]
47. Dhumale, S.R.; Barraclough, T.W.; Stokes, A.; Lam, W. Producing 3D printed hand models for anatomy education using cadaveric dissection: A feasibility study. *Bulletin* **2018**, *100*, 217–222. [CrossRef]
48. Brumpt, E.; Bertin, E.; Tatu, L.; Louvrier, A. 3D printing as a pedagogical tool for teaching normal human anatomy: A systematic review. *BMC Med. Educ.* **2023**, *23*, 783. [CrossRef] [PubMed]

animals

MDPI

Article

Scientometric Analysis: An Emerging Tool in Veterinary and Animal Scientific Research

Georgia A. Vaitsi [1], Maria V. Bourganou [2], Daphne T. Lianou [1], Yiannis Kiouvrekis [2], Charalambia C. Michael [3], Dimitris A. Gougoulis [1] and George C. Fthenakis [1,*]

[1] Veterinary Faculty, University of Thessaly, 43100 Karditsa, Greece; gvaitsi@vet.uth.gr (G.A.V.); dgoug@uth.gr (D.A.G.)
[2] Faculty of Public and One Health, University of Thessaly, 43100 Karditsa, Greece; kiouvrekis.y@uth.gr (Y.K.)
[3] School of Veterinary Medicine, European University of Cyprus, Egkomi, Nicosia 2404, Cyprus
* Correspondence: gcf@vet.uth.gr

Simple Summary: Scientometrics refer to studies that quantify aspects of scholarly literature. The methodology can be a useful tool for understanding scientific trends and for mapping large relevant data. The present work has focused on the application of scientometric analysis in published research papers in the field of veterinary and animal sciences. The findings have indicated the emergence of using this analysis in works in the primary fields of scientific interest of researchers; moreover, they have provided a guide for future relevant studies.

Abstract: The present study is an evaluation of published papers in the field of scientometrics–bibliometrics in veterinary or animal studies. The objective was the quantitative evaluation of the scientific content and the bibliometric details of papers that had used scientometrics as a methodological approach to assess various topics within the broad field of veterinary or animal studies. For the search of published papers, the Web of Science database was used; the search string {ALL FIELDS = [scientometric* OR bibliometric*]} AND {ALL FIELDS = [veterinary OR animal*]} was employed. In all, 163 papers were evaluated individually. There was a progressive increase in the number of papers published annually (slope 0.314 ± 0.063) which originated from 58 countries, mostly from the United States of America (n = 24) and 306 organizations. The databases employed most frequently for record search were the Web of Science, Scopus and PubMed (in 105, 60 and 21 papers, respectively); the median timespan of the searches was 25 years (interquartile range (IQR): 31) and the median number of records was 1082.5 (IQR: 4708) (min.: 14, max.: 207,894). The papers were published in 106 journals (*Animals* (n = 21), *Scientometrics* (n = 8)), classified into 56 Web of Science categories ('veterinary sciences' (n = 26 journals)). Searches related to 88 different topics. There were 517 unique keywords in the papers, among which 'bibliometric(s)' (n = 45) occurred most often. The median number of co-authors per paper was 4 (IQR: 3) (min.: 1, max.: 17), with a total of 689 individual authors. Most papers (n = 110 (67.5%)) were published under open access. The median number of citations received per paper was 4 (IQR: 9) (max.: 68) and the h-index was 21. In multivariable analysis, the higher number of cited references in papers and the inclusion of specific animal species in the record search emerged as significant for the number of citations received per paper yearly.

Keywords: animal science; bibliometric; bibliometric analysis; health sciences; life sciences; meta-analysis; One Health; review; scientometric; veterinary science

1. Introduction

Scientometric evaluations (which include bibliometric analyses) can be useful in understanding scientific trends, in highlighting emerging topics and in mapping large amounts of relevant data [1]. That way, they can provide support to comprehend the constituents of research, the performance of journals and topics, the collaborations between researchers and thus, consequently, the further exploration of scientific research [1,2]. These studies are important parts of the development of research, as well as in its evaluation [3].

Such analyses are based on the identification of the existing scientific literature within the subject area under assessment and involve, primarily, quantitative assessment on the documents retrieved; however, analysis of qualitative traits in the content can also take place as well [3]. An advantage of scientometric analyses refers to the use of large amounts of data, which had been produced by other researchers (e.g., author groups, journals where papers were published, citations of papers), unrelated to the researchers performing the scientometric analyses [4], which leads to reliable and unbiased findings. Further, the increase in scientific output can also contribute to a risk of the traditional-style narrative reviews being potentially incomplete [5]; in this respect, it is hence notable that the availability of scientometric analyses can help people working on such reviews to provide guidance on the trends and significance of research in the topic under study.

A recent (August 2024) search into the Web of Science database by using the string [scientometric* OR bibliometric*] revealed that only 0.21% of retrieved papers were classified into the category 'veterinary sciences' and 0.17% into the category 'agriculture, dairy and animal science'. There were, however, another 33 categories in the database which included $\geq$1% of total papers retrieved in the search: these included categories in the health sciences (e.g., medicine general internal, surgery) and the life sciences (e.g., environmental sciences). The findings point out that scientometric analyses have not been used extensively in works related to veterinary and animal studies. There is, therefore, interest in further developing the approach in those areas.

The present study is an evaluation of published papers in the field of scientometrics–bibliometrics in veterinary or animal studies. The objective of the study was the quantitative evaluation of the scientific content and the bibliometric details of papers that had used scientometrics as a methodological approach to assess various topics within the broad field of veterinary or animal studies.

2. Materials and Methods

2.1. Search Procedure

The Web of Science platform (www.webofknowledge.com (accessed on 18 August 2024 and 12 September 2024); Clarivate Analytics, London, UK) was used for the search of relevant publications. For the search, we used the Web of Science Core Collection, in a search that spanned across multiple disciplines, through the inclusion of the Science Citation Index Expanded, the Emerging Sources Citation Index, the Social Sciences Citation Index, the Arts and Humanities Citation Index, the Conference Proceedings Citation Index and the Book Citation Index.

A search using the following string was performed: {ALL FIELDS = [scientometric* OR bibliometric*]} AND {ALL FIELDS = [veterinary OR animal*]} (the asterisk served as a truncation symbol to include variations of the respective terms). The search was performed on 18 August 2024 ('freeze date') and was repeated on 12 September 2024 to confirm that no additional records (i.e., delayed entries) had been added thereafter. Only records published up to 30 June 2024 were included in this study.

Thereafter, an initial document type analysis of the records obtained was performed, during which only the following types of documents were included: 'article' and 'review article'. Thus, 759 papers were retained for further assessment individually (Table S1).

2.2. Paper Evaluation

Evaluation of characteristics in the papers was performed by two persons. The evaluators worked separately and independently and compared their results after completion of their work. In case of disagreement between the two persons, the paper was evaluated by a senior author (G.C.F.) and the results returned by two of the three assessors were taken into account; this occurred with four papers in total.

During evaluation, papers not including (a) work related to veterinary or animal studies or (b) work related to scientometric or bibliometric assessment were excluded from further evaluation.

Thus, after the above, 163 papers remained and were included in the final scientometric evaluation (Table S1). In each of these papers, the following details were recorded:

1. Year of publication of paper;
2. Country and organization (university or other institution) of origin of the paper (as indicated in the affiliation(s) of the author(s));
3. Database used, timespan set and language employed for the search of records;
4. No. of records assessed in the study;
5. Journal in which the paper was published and Web of Science category(ies) into which each journal was classified;
6. Scientific topic of the scientometric assessment and keywords in the paper;
7. Number of cited references included in the relevant list;
8. Number and names of all co-authors in the paper;
9. Accessibility of paper, i.e., whether it was open access or subscription only;
10. Total number of citations received by the paper until the end of June 2024.

2.3. Data Management and Analysis

The number of papers published by 30 June 2024 on [scientometric* OR bibliometric*] only was obtained using the same procedure, in order to compare with the number of papers published on the topic of the current study.

Papers with authors affiliated with organizations of two different countries were deemed as with an international collaboration.

To assess the impact of the papers evaluated in the current study, the total number of citations received by the papers was considered. The number of citations received by the papers was normalized by calculating the average citations per year since the year of publication of each paper.

All data were systematically recorded and organized using Microsoft Excel (versions 2406-2408). Descriptive analysis was performed initially. The frequency of the various outcomes was evaluated in tables of cross-categorized frequency data using the Pearson chi-square test or the Fisher exact test, as appropriate. Comparisons between continuous data were performed using the Mann–Whitney test or the Kruskal–Wallis test. Linear regression analysis was used to establish associations with the year of publication of each paper. Spearman's rank correlation analysis was performed as indicated, and the significance of the result was evaluated according to the critical values for r.

The outcome 'citations received by a published paper yearly' was evaluated. Initially, univariable analysis was performed to assess potential associations with relevant parameters. Then, a multivariable model was developed for the above outcome, and parameters found with $p < 0.20$ in the univariable analyses previously carried out were included into this model. Progressively, parameters were removed from the model by using backward elimination. The likelihood ratio test was performed to assess the p-value of each parameter; among those found with $p > 0.20$, the one with the largest p was removed from the model. The procedure was repeated until no variable with $p > 0.20$ could be removed from the model. The parameters included in the final multivariable assessment are in Table S2. Subsequently, associations of the number of citations received by a published paper yearly and the parameters into that final multivariable assessment were evaluated by principal component analysis.

Statistical significance was defined at $p < 0.05$.

3. Results

All 163 individually assessed papers have been indexed in the Web of Science, fulfilled the search criteria and presented scientometric analysis work on veterinary or animal studies (Table S3).

3.1. Year of Publication

There was a clear progressive increase in the number of papers published (slope 0.314 ± 0.063; $p < 0.0001$) (Figure 1). The first relevant paper was published in 1988; however, most papers (66.3%) were published during the current decade (2021–today). A similar trend was observed in the entirety of published papers on scientometrics–bibliometrics internationally, where also the majority of papers was published subsequently to 2020 (60.6% of 30,702 papers) ($p = 0.14$) (Figure S1).

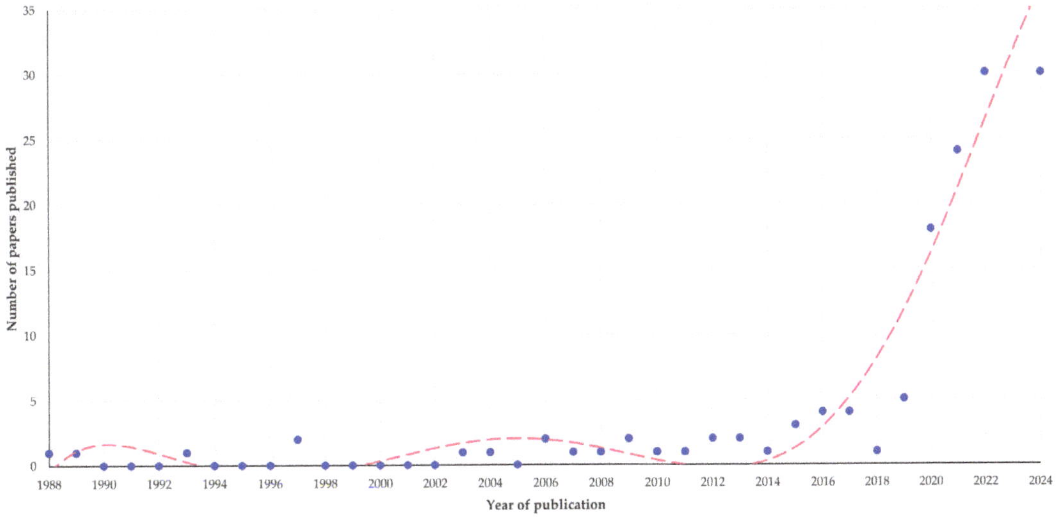

Figure 1. The number of published papers on veterinary or animal studies scientometrics according to the year of publication (the dashed line is trendline).

3.2. Origin of Published Papers

3.2.1. Countries

The papers originated from 58 countries in total. The median number of published papers per country that contributed publications was 2 (interquartile range (IQR): 4). Most papers originated from the United States of America ($n = 24$), Brazil ($n = 22$) or China ($n = 20$) (Figure 2, Table S4). Papers published up to the end of 2020 originated from 23 countries, whilst those published afterwards originated from 53 countries ($p < 0.0002$).

There were 16 countries, from which at least five published papers originated. There was a significant difference in the median year of publication of papers among these countries; France had the oldest median year of publication (2016 (IQR: 1)), whilst Egypt and Turkey had the most recent median year of publication (2023 (IQR: 1)) of relevant papers ($p = 0.020$) (Figure 3).

In 57 papers (35.0%) there was international collaboration (i.e., with affiliations from at least two countries). International collaborations were seen in 52 countries, and, in contrast, 6 countries published papers on their own only. The most frequent combination in joint papers was between Spain and the United States of America ($n = 4$) (Table S5).

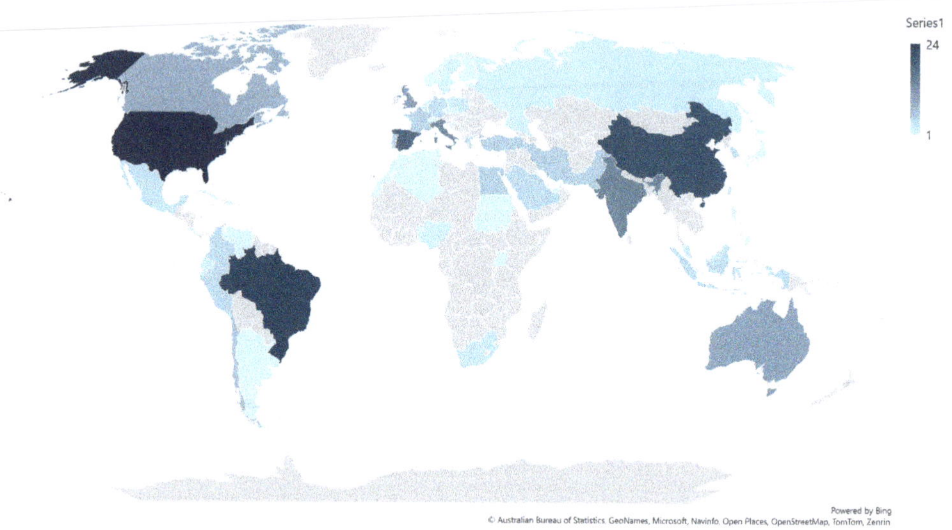

Figure 2. The countries of the world from which published papers on veterinary or animal studies scientometrics originated (blue color palette in accord with the number of papers published per country).

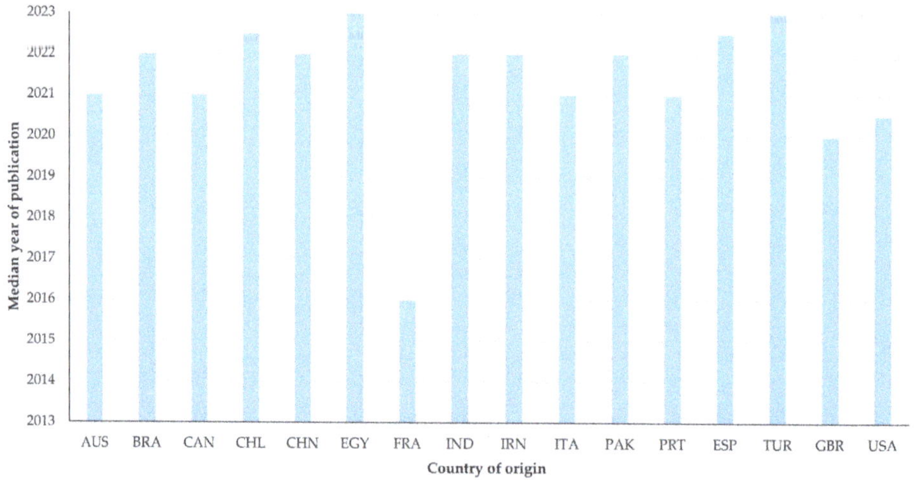

Figure 3. The median year of publication of papers on veterinary or animal studies scientometrics from the 16 countries with most papers (≥5) (the country name abbreviations are set according to International Naming Convention ISO 3166 [6]).

3.2.2. Organizations

The papers originated from 306 organizations in total. These included 240 universities and 66 organizations of other type (e.g., research institutes, government agents). The median number of published papers per organization was 1 (IQR: 0).

Most papers originated from the North Carolina State University and the São Paulo State University (n = 5) (with reference to universities), and from the Indian Council of Agricultural Research (n = 7) (Table S6). China and the United States of America were the two countries with the most organizations from which relevant papers originated (n = 28 for both). There was a clear correlation between the number of organizations in a country from which papers originated, and the number of published papers from that country ($r_{sp} = 0.882$, $p < 0.0001$) (Figure 4).

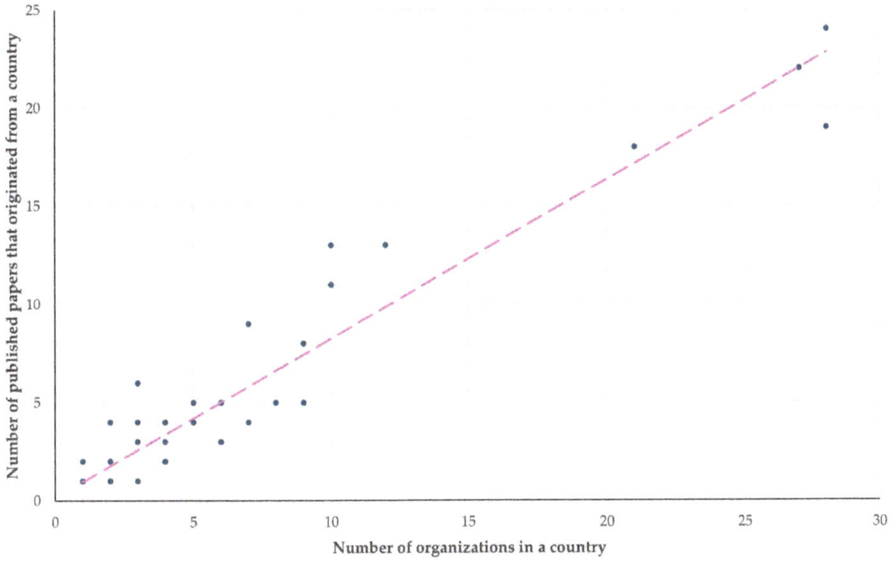

Figure 4. The number of organizations in a country, from which published papers on veterinary or animal studies scientometrics originated, and the number of published papers from that country (the dashed line is trendline).

3.3. *Search Methodologies*

3.3.1. Databases Used for Search of Records

In total, 40 different databases were employed for search of records in the studies reported in the papers (Table S7). The databases employed most frequently were the Web of Science (in 105 papers), Scopus (in 60 papers) and PubMed (in 21 papers) (Figure 5). In most papers ($n = 121$; 74.2%), use of only one database was reported for search of records, whilst in 42 papers (25.8%) use of at least two databases was reported.

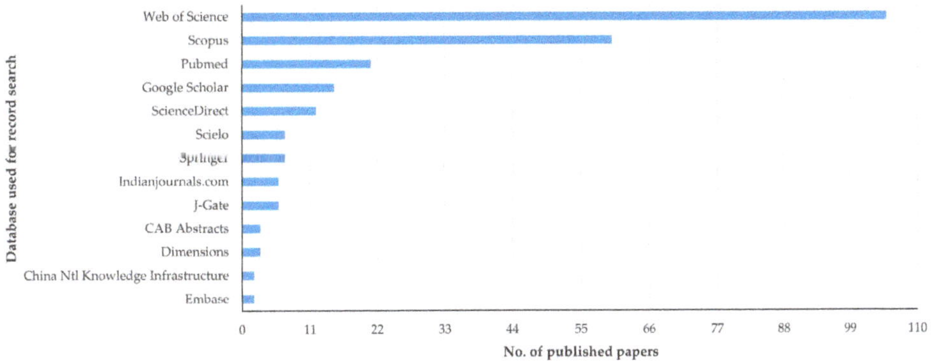

Figure 5. The databases used most frequently for record search in published papers on veterinary or animal studies scientometrics, with the number of published papers in which their use was reported (full details in Table S7).

There was no difference in the median year of publication of papers in accord with the database employed (Table S8) ($p = 0.70$). However, there was a clear difference among databases in the countries that used them ($p = 0.003$) (Table S9). Specifically, the Web of Science was employed more frequently in studies from Australia, Iran, Portugal (100%) and China (90.0%); Scopus was employed more frequently in studies from India (76.9%) and Brazil (68.2%); and PubMed in studies from India (53.8%) and USA (25.0%).

3.3.2. Timespan Set in Searches

The median timespan of searches performed in the studies reported in the various papers was 25 years (interquartile range: 31 years; minimum: 1, maximum: 223 years). There was no significant difference in the timespan of searches in accord with the database employed in the respective study ($p = 0.89$) (Figure S2).

3.3.3. Languages Employed for Search of Records

Only 15 papers reported searches performed with language limitations. Of these, in 12 papers, the language specified in the search was English only; in one paper, the language specified in the search was Spanish only; in one paper, two languages were specified in the search (English and Russian); and in another one, eight languages were specified in the search (Czech, English, Japanese, Norwegian, Polish, Russian, Slovak and Swedish).

3.3.4. Number of Records Found

The median number of records found in the various studies was 1082.5 (interquartile range: 4708; minimum: 14, maximum: 207,894). There was evidence that in studies which used the Web of Science database, significantly more records were found for use than in studies which used other databases ($p = 0.0001$) (Figure 6, Table S10). In contrast, there was no association between the number of records found in the studies and the timespan covered in these searches ($r_{sp} = 0.086$, $p = 0.09$) or the language in which searches were performed ($p = 0.22$). Finally, there was a clear inverse correlation between the number of records found in the studies and the year of publication of the paper ($r_{sp} = -0.334$, $p < 0.0001$).

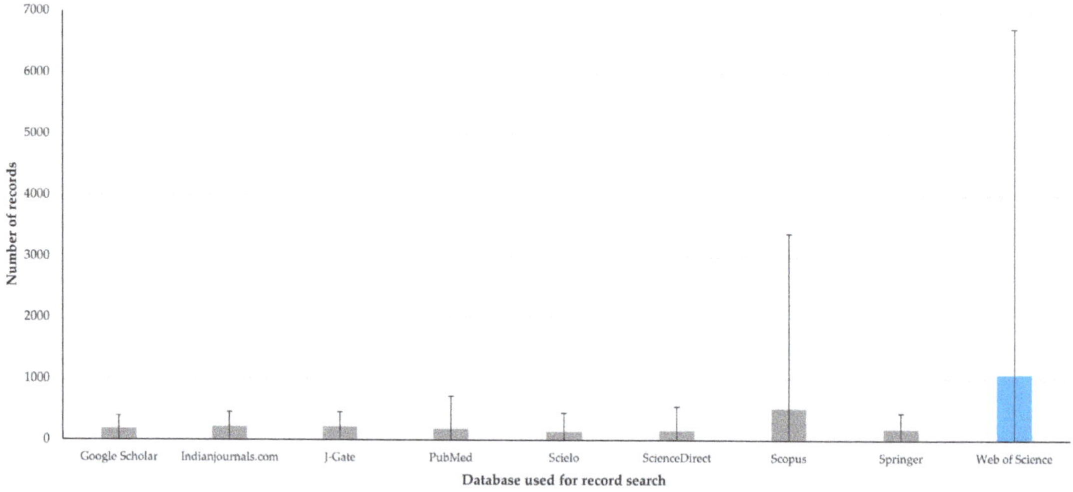

Figure 6. The number of records obtained by the most frequently used databases reported in papers on veterinary or animal studies scientometrics (bars show interquartile range).

3.4. Journals in Which Papers Were Published

The papers were published in a total of 106 journals, most frequently in *Animals* ($n = 21$ papers), *Scientometrics* ($n = 8$), *Frontiers in Veterinary Science* ($n = 7$) and *Pathogens* ($n = 4$) (Table S11). In total, 24.5% of all papers were published in these four journals, whilst 49.1% of all papers were published in the 23 journals with two or more papers in the study topic ($n = 80$ papers). Cumulatively, 65 of these papers (81.3%) originated from the 16 countries with the most papers published. There were, however, differences among these countries in the journals in which these papers were published ($p < 0.0001$) (Figure 7, Table S12).

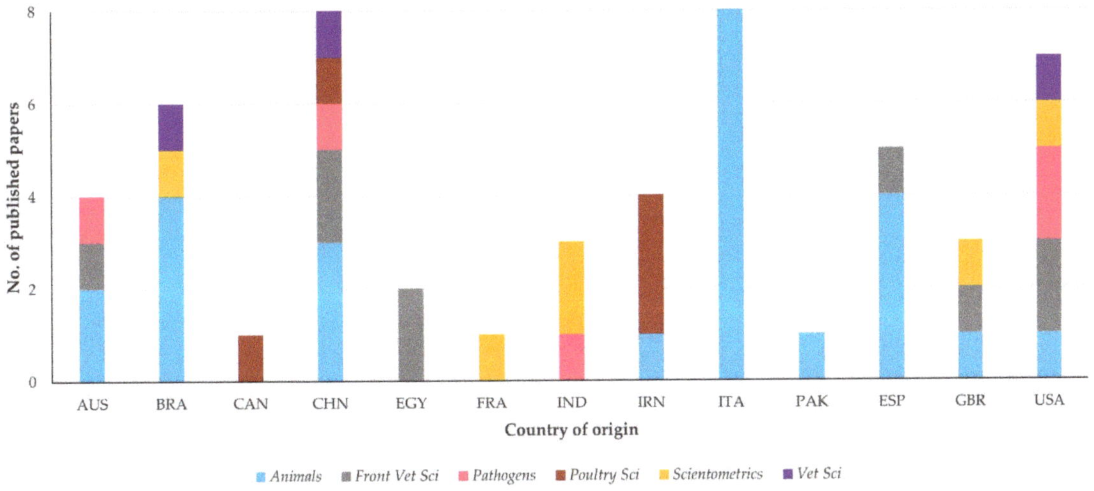

Figure 7. The number of published papers on veterinary or animal studies scientometrics, in accord with the country of origin and the journal of publication (abbreviations of country names according to International Naming Convention ISO 3166 [6]; abbreviations of journals from left to right: *Animals, Frontiers in Veterinary Science, Pathogens, Poultry Science, Scientometrics, Veterinary Sciences*).

These 106 journals were classified into 56 Web of Science categories, most frequently in 'veterinary sciences' ($n = 26$ journals, with 61 papers published in these journals), 'environmental sciences' ($n = 13$, with 16 papers published in these journals) and 'agriculture, dairy and animal science' ($n = 11$, with 36 papers published in these journals) (Table S13). The largest density of published papers per journal within a category was seen in the category 'computer science, interdisciplinary applications', with 8 papers in one journal (namely *Scientometrics*), followed by 'agriculture, dairy & animal science' (3.3 papers per journal) and 'microbiology' (2.5 papers per journal) (Table S13).

Among the categories with the most published papers in journals therein, 'parasitology' (2023 (IQR: 2)); 'environmental sciences' (2022 (IQR: 2)); and 'agriculture, dairy and animal science', 'biodiversity conservation', 'ecology' and 'veterinary sciences' (2022 (IQR: 3)) included the most recently published papers, whilst the categories 'computer science, interdisciplinary applications' (2001.5 (IQR: 23)) and 'information science and library science' (2010 (IQR: 18)) included the oldest published papers. The difference between the categories was significant ($p < 0.0001$) (Figure 8).

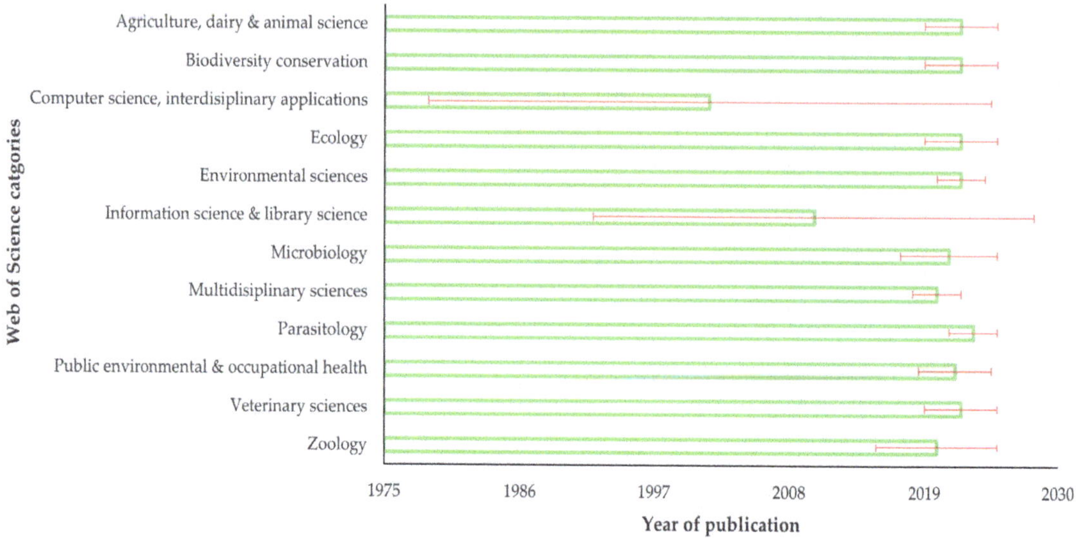

Figure 8. Median year of publication of papers on veterinary or animal studies scientometrics, in accord with Web of Science categories with the most published papers therein (bars indicate interquartile range).

3.5. Content of Papers

3.5.1. Topics of Scientometric Assessment

Searches were found to be related to 88 different topics of scientometric assessment in total. The most frequent search topics referred to country-related research (n = 16); the other frequent topics were specific journal-related research, or animal species-related research, or animal welfare (n = 10 for each). Details are in Tables 1 and S14.

Table 1. The most frequently assessed topics (n = 18) in published papers on veterinary or animal studies scientometrics and the respective number of published papers (full details in Table S14).

Topic of Assessment	Papers (n)
Country-related scientometrics [1]	16
Specific journal-related scientometrics [2]	10
Animal species-related scientometrics [3]	10
Animal welfare	10
Genetic improvement	6
Animal ethology	5
Mastitis	5
Conservation plan	4
Antibiotic resistance	3
Gastrointestinal parasitism	3
Heat stress	3
Human–animal interactions	3
Veterinary education	3
Epilepsy	2
Infections	2
Precision livestock farming	2
Tuberculosis	2
Zoo archaeology—palaeontology	2

[1] Full details in Table S15; [2] full details in Table S16; [3] full details in Table S17.

There was a significant difference in the year of publication of papers in accord with the topic of assessment (r_{sp} = 0.438, p = 0.0004). Papers on scientometrics of genetic improvement or animal ethology were the most recent (median year of publication: 2023); papers on journal-related (median year: 2011) or country-related scientometrics (median year: 2018) were the oldest (Figure 9, Table S18).

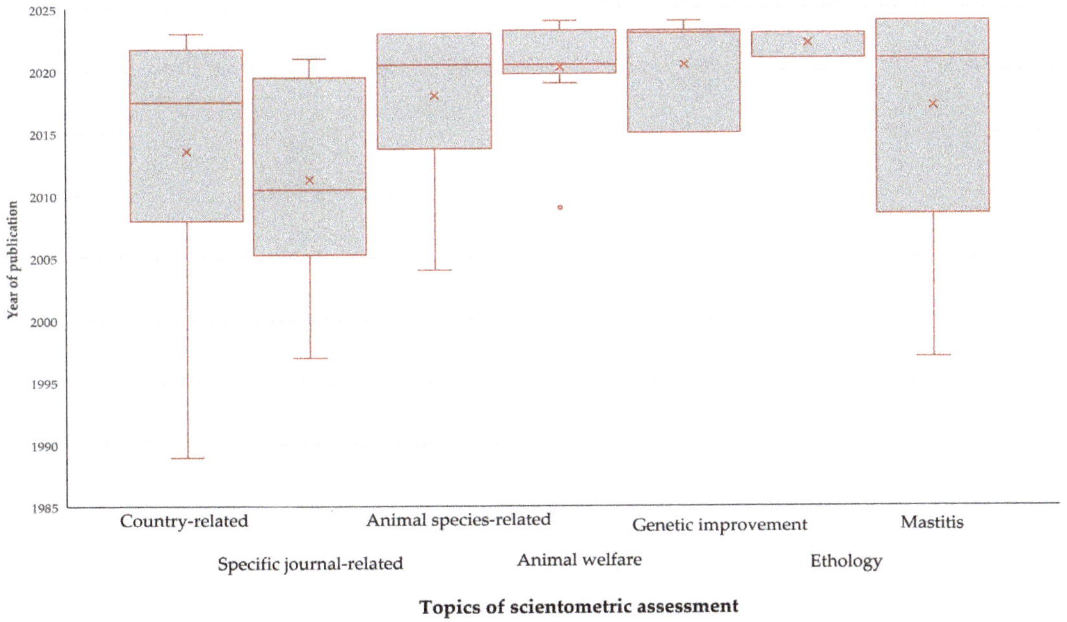

Figure 9. Box and whisker plot of the year of publication in papers on veterinary or animal studies scientometrics in accord with the topic of study and scientometric assessment (only most frequently assessed topics shown).

In contrast, no association was found between the topic of assessment and the country of origin of papers (p = 0.16). Notably, most papers on scientometrics of animal welfare originated from Australia (40.0%), on scientometrics of genetic improvement from Brazil (50.0%) and on scientometrics of mastitis from Greece (40.0%) and the United States of America (40.0%).

Also, no pattern emerged regarding the journals in which the various topics were published. It is, however, noted that most papers on scientometrics of mastitis were published in *Pathogens* (42.9%) and most papers on scientometrics of animal welfare were published in *Animals* (40.0%).

There was an association between the number of records obtained and the topic of scientometric assessment: the median number of records obtained for studies reported in papers on country-related scientometrics (6465 (IQR: 12,954)) or on animal species-related scientometrics (6362 (IQR: 5176)) were the highest, whilst the median number of records for papers on mastitis (250 (IQR: 336)) were the lowest (r_{sp} = 0.319, p = 0.015) (Figure 10, Table S19).

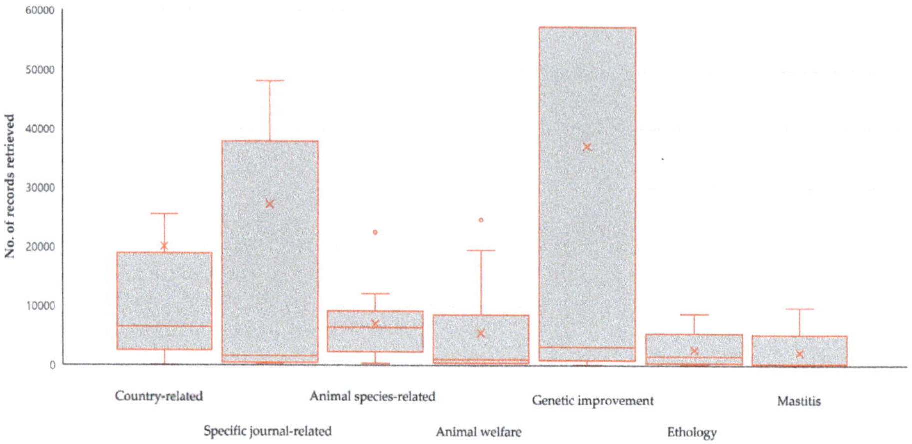

Figure 10. Box and whisker plot of the number of obtained records in papers on veterinary or animal studies scientometrics in accord with the topic of study and scientometric assessment (only most frequently assessed topics shown).

3.5.2. Animal Species Referred to in Scientometric Assessments

In total, 92 papers reported studies with reference to specific animal species in the respective searches. Animal species most frequently studied were cattle ($n = 14$ papers); poultry ($n = 12$ papers); and pigs, sheep and wildlife ($n = 9$ papers each) (Table S20).

Among these papers, there was no association between the animal species referred to and the number of records obtained ($p = 0.29$ when all animal species were taken into account, $p = 0.09$ when only the 10 animal species in most papers were taken into account) (Figure S3).

3.5.3. Keywords in Papers

In total, there were 790 keywords in the 163 papers, i.e., a median number of 5 (IQR: 2) keywords per paper. These corresponded to 517 unique keywords, among which 'bibliometric(s)' ($n = 45$), 'bibliometric analysis(es)' ($n = 32$) and 'scientometric(s)' ($n = 17$) occurred the most frequently (Figure 11, Table S21).

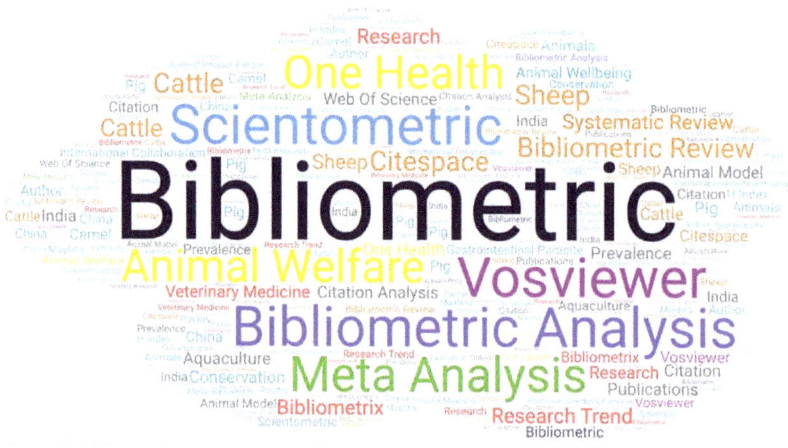

Figure 11. Word cloud of the most frequently occurring keywords in published papers on veterinary or animal studies scientometrics (full details in Table S21).

Notably, there was a clear increase in the number of keywords in a published paper in accord with the year of publication ($r_{sp} = 0.275$, $p = 0.0004$). Further, there was also a tendency for inverse correlation between the number of keywords in the published papers and the number of records obtained in the search ($r_{sp} = -0.156$, $p = 0.051$).

3.5.4. Cited References in Papers

The median number of cited references in the papers was 47 (interquartile range: 44). There was a clear positive correlation between the number of cited references therein and the year of publication of the paper ($r_{sp} = 0.462$, $p < 0.0001$), as well as an inverse correlation between the number of cited references therein and the numbers of retrieved records in the paper ($r_{sp} = -0.169$, $p = 0.034$).

3.6. Authors

Cumulatively, there were 770 co-authors; the median number of co-authors per paper was 4 (IQR: 3) (min.: 1, max.: 17). In total, there were 689 individual authors. Among them, 11 (1.6%) had published at least three papers (max.: 5). In 11 papers, there was only one author. There was a clear progressive increase in the number of co-authors per published paper throughout the years (slope: 0.117 ± 0.08) ($p = 0.0002$) (Figures 12 and S4).

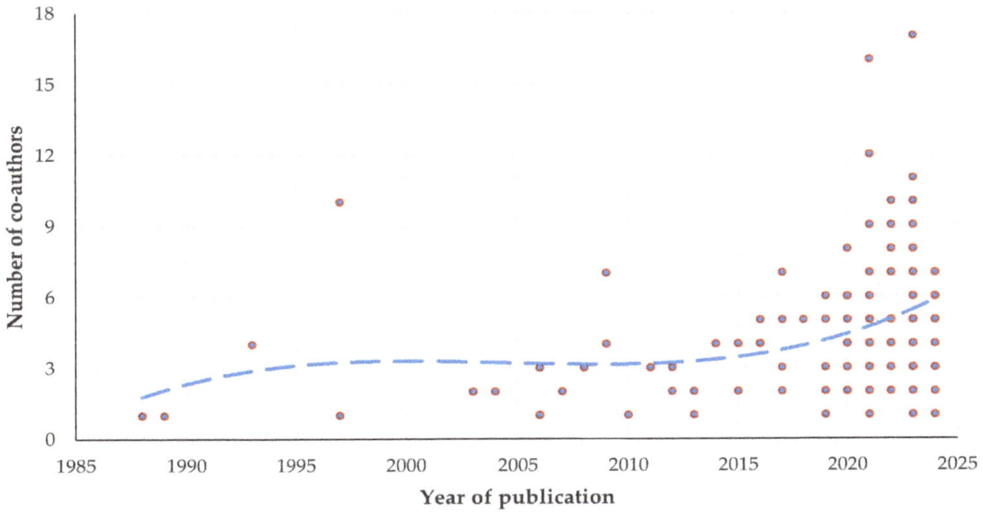

Figure 12. The number of authors per published paper in accord with the year of publication of the paper (the dashed line is trendline).

Further, there were 286 individual authors (41.5% of all), who were first or last authors in the papers. Among these, one author was first or last in four papers and 26 authors in two papers. The 11 authors with at least three papers, were, on average, first or last authors in 66.7% (25.0%) of their papers (min.: 0.0%, max.: 100.0%), whilst the 52 authors with two papers, were, on average, first or last authors in 50.0% (100.0%) of their papers.

Of the 11 authors with at least three papers as first or last, 9 were affiliated with scientific organizations in the 16 countries from which originated most published papers. Among these 11 authors, there were three clearly distinct groups of co-authors identified with joint papers, who were affiliated with the same organization in each of three different countries, specifically in India ($n = 5$ co-authors), France ($n = 2$ co-authors) and Greece ($n = 2$ co-authors).

There were no significant differences between the 16 countries with most published papers in the median number of authors per paper: papers from Canada had the smallest median number of authors, 3 (IQR: 4.5), whilst papers from Pakistan and Egypt had the highest number, 7 (IQR: 0) and 8 (IQR: 2), respectively ($p = 0.24$) (Figure S5).

The Web of Science categories of the journals of papers published by the above 11 authors, were as follows: (a) agriculture, dairy and animal science, (b) agronomy, (c) computer science, interdisciplinary applications, (d) ecology, (e) infectious diseases, (f) information science and library science, (g) microbiology, (h) parasitology, (i) public environmental and occupational health, (j) veterinary sciences and (k) zoology.

3.7. Accessibility of Papers

Most papers ($n = 110$ (67.5%)) were published under open access. The median year of publication of open access papers was significantly more recent than that of subscription access papers: 2022 (IQR: 3) versus 2021 (IQR: 12) ($p = 0.021$) (Figure 13). No differences were seen among countries in the proportion of papers published under open access ($p = 0.22$) (Figure S6).

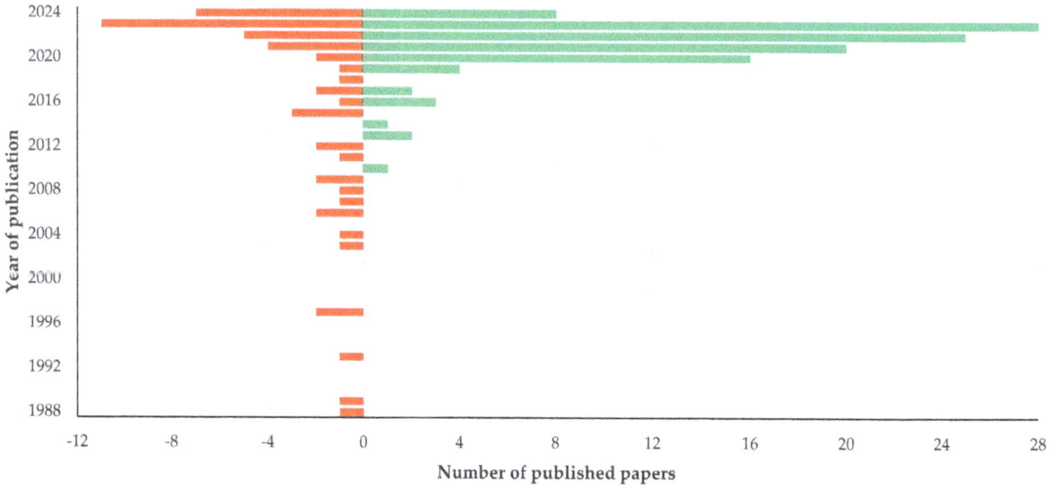

Figure 13. Frequency of published papers on veterinary or animal studies scientometrics, in accord with year of publication and accessibility of papers (red: subscription access, green: open access).

3.8. Impact of Papers

The median number of citations received per paper was 4 (IQR: 9) (max.: 68) and the *h*-index for this set of published papers was 21. The median value of yearly citations received per paper was 1.3 (IQR: 2.8) (max.: 21) and the *m*-index was 0.5.

The univariable analyses indicated the following parameters with significant association with the number of citations received per paper yearly: (a) the timespan covered in the search for records ($p = 0.002$), (b) the inclusion of specific animal species in searches ($p = 0.037$), (c) the number of cited references in papers ($p = 0.0003$) and (d) publication under open access ($p = 0.011$) (Figure 14) (Table S22). There were also differences in the number of citations received by published papers yearly among the countries with most published papers; papers from Portugal, Pakistan and China had the highest median yearly number of citations: 5.7 (IQR: 6.3), 4.7 (IQR: 1.2) and 3.5 (IQR: 3.5), respectively, whilst papers from Chile, France and India had the lowest: 0.0 (IQR: 0.7), 0.2 (IQR: 1.0) and 0.5 (IQR: 2.0) ($p = 0.018$) (Figure 15) (Table S23). In contrast, there was no difference in the number of citations received per paper yearly, in accord with the topic of assessment ($p = 0.44$ when all topics were considered, $p = 0.35$ when only the seven topics with most published papers were taken into account (Figure S7)).

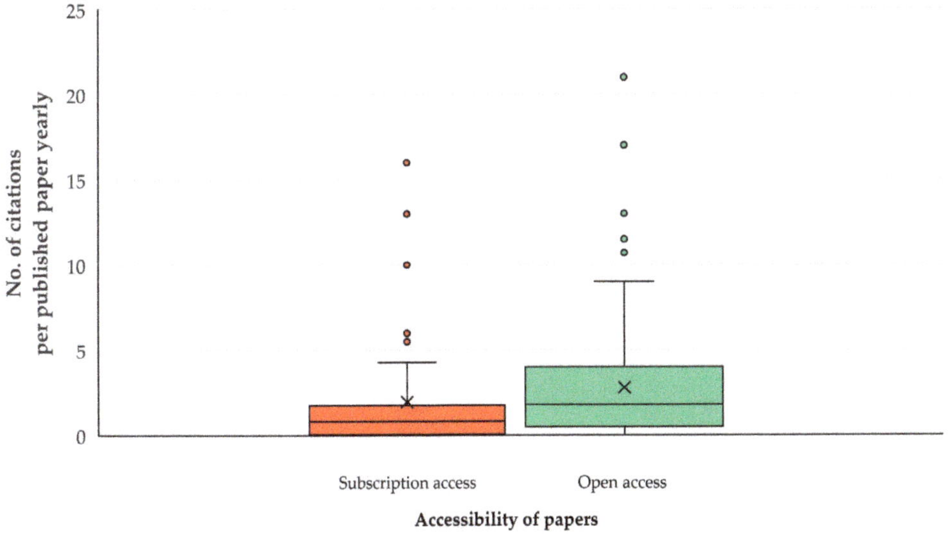

Figure 14. Box and whisker plot of the yearly citations per published paper on veterinary or animal studies scientometrics, in accord with accessibility of papers.

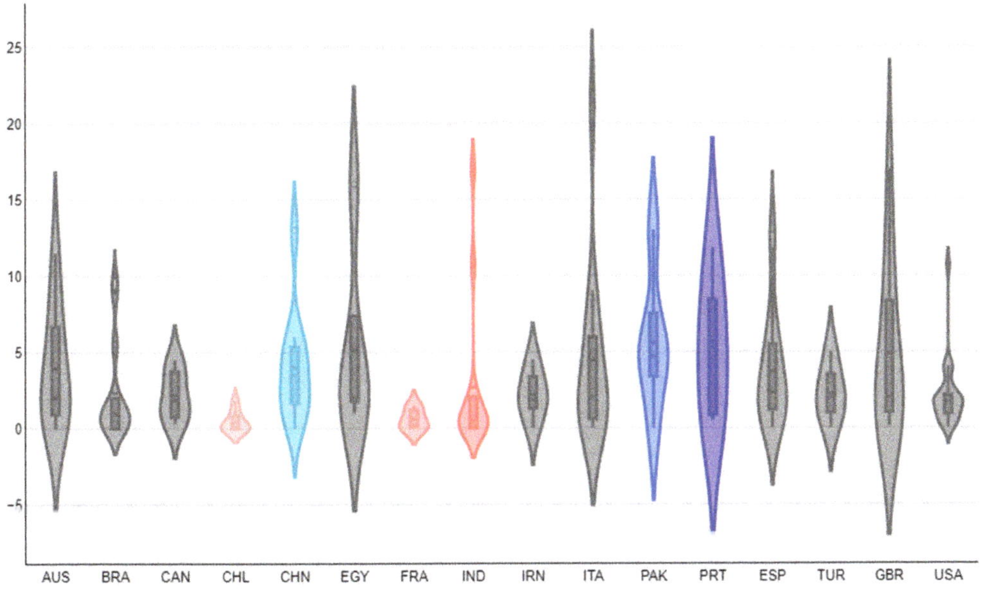

Figure 15. Violin plot of the yearly citations per published paper on veterinary or animal studies scientometrics, among the 16 countries with most relevant published papers (abbreviations of country names according to the International Naming Convention ISO 3166 [6]; pink violins: three countries with papers with lowest median citations yearly, blue-shaded violins: three countries with papers with highest median citations yearly).

In the multivariable analysis, the following parameters emerged as significant: (a) the higher number of cited references in papers ($p = 0.030$) and (b) the inclusion of specific animal species in the searches for records ($p = 0.045$) (Figure 16, Table 2). There was also a tendency for significance for the larger number of keywords included in the published paper (p = 0.07).

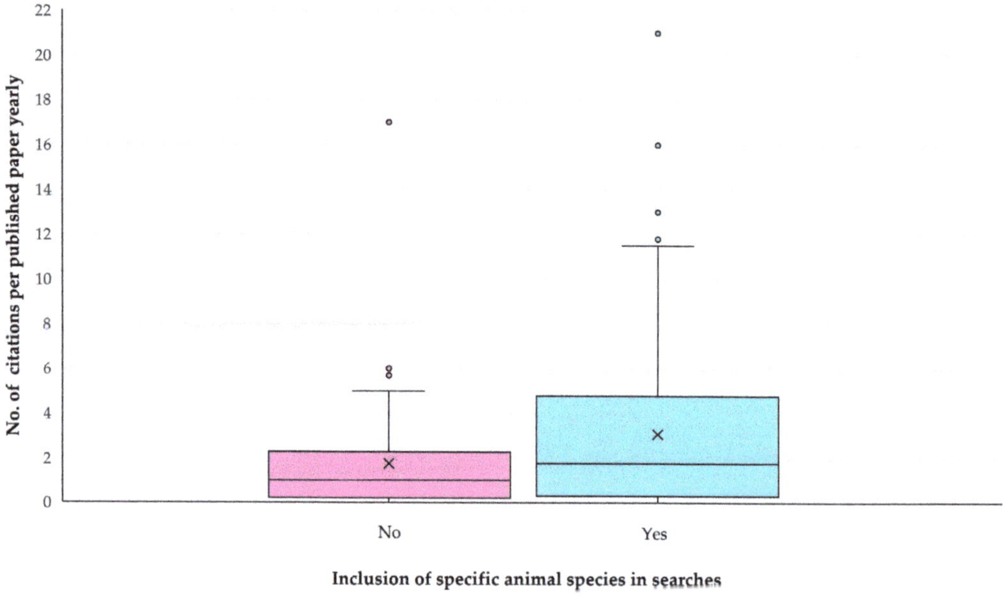

Figure 16. Number of citations per paper yearly, in papers on veterinary or animal studies scientometrics, in accord with the inclusion of specific animal species in the searches.

Table 2. Results of multivariable analysis for parameters with significant association with yearly citations of published papers on veterinary or animal studies scientometrics.

Parameters	Odds Risk (±se) [1]	p
Cited references in papers		0.030
Per unit increase	1.021 ± 1.007	0.003
Inclusion of specific animal species in searches		0.045
No (1.0 (2.0) [2])	Reference	-
Yes (1.8 (4.3))	3.738 ± 1.721	0.016

[1] se: standard error; [2] median (interquartile range) number of yearly citations.

Principal component analysis for the citations received by the published papers yearly and the four parameters included in the final multivariable assessment, revealed that the two principal components accounted for 59.9% of the variation (Figures 17 and S8, Table 3).

Table 3. Eigenvalues for principal component analysis for the citations received by the published papers yearly.

Parameter	PC_1	PC_2	PC_3	PC_4
Eigenvalue	1.34	1.06	0.84	0.76
% of Variance	33.5	26.4	21.1	19.0
Cumulative variance (%)	33.5	59.9	81.0	100.0

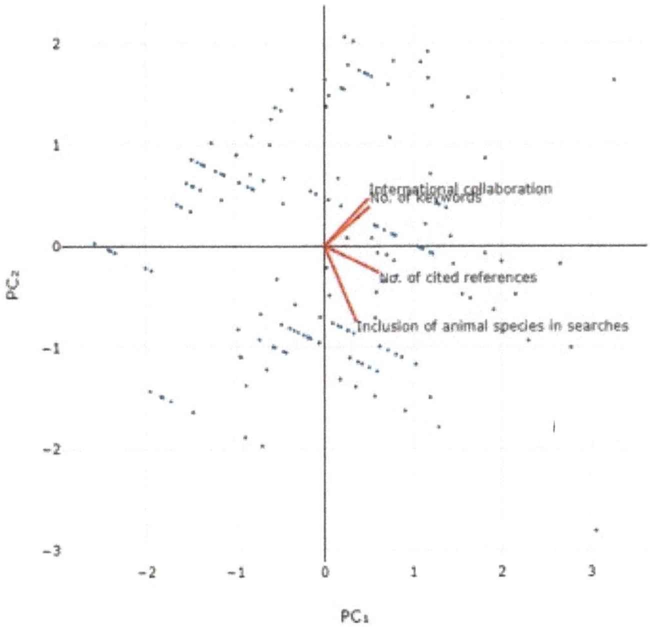

Figure 17. Bi-plot of results of principal component analysis for the yearly citations received by the published papers on veterinary or animal studies scientometrics.

4. Discussion

The idea of scientometric analyses was initiated in the 1950s and 1960s [7]. In the field of scientometrics of veterinary and animal studies, the first papers appeared in the 1980s and 1990s and were followed by sporadic publications until 2020. At that time, a massive increase in relevant publications occurred and was followed by further expansion of papers in the topic [8]. First, this increase reflects the general trend for an increased number of published papers seen across the scientific fields and the countries worldwide [9]. Moreover, we also postulate that this increase in 2020 and thereafter was triggered during the COVID-19 quarantine period, when scientists could not carry out extensive experimental or field work [10] and thus directed their interest (and energy) towards performing computational studies [11,12], as part of the general development of the information science at that period [13]. In this context, they developed and performed scientometric studies, which also answered questions pertinent to their field of research. As scientists fully appreciated the usefulness and the potential of these studies, they continued these even after all measures were lifted, leading to the continued growth of published papers.

The wide geographic expansion of the origin of published papers (the increase in author affiliations from 23 to 53 countries), the diversity of scientific organization of origin of the papers (universities, research institutes, etc.) and the proportion of papers with international collaboration lend support to our argument. Also, they point to the wide international expansion of scientometric studies.

The findings indicate that the Web of Science was the most popular database for record search, in line with the findings of Liu and He [9], who also reported that the platform was the most popular database for literature search. The Web of Science platform is a bibliometric platform unaffiliated to any publishing house, unlike other similar platforms; moreover, it applies strict quality control measures for the inclusion of journals in the database. The findings of the study have also confirmed that use of the Web of Science platform provided the largest number of records during the search. The authors of the present paper also used this database for record search in previous studies [14–17], as well as in the present one, and have found it easy to navigate and use, as well as equipped with various tools that facilitate record search and assessment.

Recently, Fassin and Rousseau [8] have reported that using the term scientometr* in an 'ALL FIELDS' search might yield unnecessary papers, in comparison to a 'TOPIC' search, due to the existence of the journal *Scientometrics*. In the present study, an 'ALL FIELDS' search wide approach was used. This contributed to eliminating the possibility of missing relevant records. Subsequent to using this search approach, all the records retrieved from the search were individually assessed to confirm that they were within the remit of our study. That way, superfluous papers returned from the search ('false positives') were eliminated during the individual assessment.

When taking into account the Web of Science categories in which journals were included, it becomes evident that there has been a shift in where papers were published. Earlier, journals related to information science were preferred for publication of relevant papers; however, in recent years, papers were published in journals concurring with the topic under assessment. This corroborates, at least to some extent, the hypothesis that scientists started included scientometric studies in the methodological approaches used in the study of their primary field of interest.

A variety of topics have been studied by means of scientometric methodologies. Most of them are directly related to veterinary science (e.g., mastitis, gastrointestinal parasitism, veterinary education); several include studies within the One Health approach (e.g., antibiotic resistance, heat stress), which is also a topic of significant veterinary involvement; and others deal with the use of animals as models for human disorders (e.g., epilepsy, tuberculosis) and also fields of veterinary work [18]. Although others have focused more on animal science (e.g., genetic improvement, precision livestock farming), it was deemed useful to include them, in order to encompass the full literature on animal-related scientometric studies.

Such, more specific, studies were found to proliferate in more recent years, in distinction to more generalized topics which had been addressed in earlier scientometric studies (country-related, specific journal-related and animal species-related studies), potentially indicating that researchers have started to include scientometric methodologies in the study of their particular fields of interest. The decrease in the number of retrieved records in correlation with the year of publication is in accord with the performance of more specific and focused scientometric studies in recent years, in more narrow topics. Consequently, the number of keywords in the published papers increased, as researchers had to include more terms of reference to describe better the topic of assessment.

In this context, the progressive increase in the number of authors in recent papers may possibly reflect the situation hypothesized above, i.e., larger groups working in various scientific topics have started scientometric analyses in their primary fields of scientific interest. Moreover, the weak connections seen between author groups confirm that the authors of the papers have focused on topics of different disciplines, which reduces the possibilities for cross-disciplinary studies on scientometrics.

The recent increase in papers published as open access papers is in line with the international trend for open science, transparency in research and availability to the public of scientific results, particularly when derived from public funds [19]. This also reflects the public requirements for expansion of open access publishing, which further promotes dissemination of scientific findings and knowledge to the academic community and the general public [20].

An increased number of citations indicates a useful study ('reference paper') or, alternatively, an article that has attracted attention and reference to it (in a good or bad context) [21]. Thus, high citation numbers reflect impact, but not necessarily quality [22,23]. In the same way, low citations numbers do not automatically indicate a low-quality paper, but may possibly mirror a more narrow field of study [21].

The increased number of citations found to be associated with a high number of cited references within a paper likely reflects a variety of issues dealt with in the paper and a diversity of ideas presented therein, which make it citable more easily, as the result of including more information and more hypotheses. Similar results have been reported previously by other researchers [24–28], as well as by our group [16]. Further, it has been suggested that such papers may become more 'visible' in online searches [28]. This aligns with the increased number of keywords, which reflects the diversity of ideas in the manuscript, and has been found with a tendency for association with the number of citations. Furthermore, the association of increased citations with the inclusion of specific animal species (Table S20) in the search for records aligns with a focused approach in the paper, thus making the paper visible in searches which include species-related strings.

5. Conclusions

The work refers to a study of 'scientometrics of scientometrics' focusing on the field of veterinary and animal studies. The Web of Science database was found to be the database employed most often, and also the one through which the highest number of records for analysis was obtained. The findings confirmed a clear increase in relevant papers during recent years. It is suggested that the results show a trend of including scientometrics analysis as part of the work in the primary fields of scientific interest of researchers.

There are advantages in the use of this methodological approach in veterinary and animal scientific research. Through this approach, researchers can assess large amounts of data, which have been produced independently (i.e., by other researchers) and which can provide insights in the development of a scientific field of work or a topic of research; they can also identify potential collaborators for future joint work. Thus, in all, scientometrics would be a useful tool or practice for understanding the situation in a specific research field or topic.

Supplementary Materials: The following supporting information can be downloaded at: https://www.mdpi.com/article/10.3390/ani14213132/s1, Table S1: PRISMA flow diagram for the identification and exclusion of records from Web of Science database; Table S2: Details of a multivariable model employed for evaluation of predictors for yearly citations of papers on veterinary or animal studies scientometrics; Table S3: Details of 163 papers published until 30 June 2024 on veterinary or animal studies scientometrics and listed in the Web of Science platform; Figure S1: Proportions of published papers (a) up to 2020 and (b) from 2021 up to July 2024 among all published papers on scientometrics and among published papers on veterinary or animal studies scientometrics; Table S4: The countries of origin of published papers on veterinary or animal studies scientometrics and the respective number of published papers; Table S5: The combinations of countries of origin of published papers on veterinary or animal studies scientometrics and the respective number of published papers; Table S6: The organization of origin of published papers on veterinary or animal studies scientometrics and the respective number of published papers; Table S7: The databases used for record search in published papers on veterinary or animal studies scientometrics and the respective number of published papers, in which their use was reported; Table S8: The databases used most frequently for record search in published papers on veterinary or animal studies scientometrics and the year of publication of respective papers that reported use of database; Table S9: Frequency of published papers on veterinary or animal studies scientometrics, in accord with the country of origin of the papers and the database used for record search; Figure S2: The databases used most frequently for record search for published papers on veterinary or animal studies scientometrics and the timespan of searches in respective published papers; Table S10: The databases used most frequently for record search in published papers on veterinary or animal studies scientometrics and the number of records in respective studies; Table S11: The journals in which papers on veterinary or animal studies scientometrics were published, and the respective number of published papers; Table S12: Frequency of published papers on veterinary or animal studies scientometrics, in accord with the country of origin of the papers and the journal in which they were published; Table S13: The Web of Science categories in which journals with published papers on veterinary or animal studies scientometrics were classified, and the respective number of journals and of published papers in these journals; Table S14: The topics assessed in published papers on veterinary or animal studies scientometrics and the respective number of published papers; Table S15: The countries referred to in work reported in published papers on veterinary or animal studies scientometrics in the topic of assessment of country-related scientometrics and the respective number of published papers; Table S16: The journals referred to in work reported in published papers on veterinary or animal studies scientometrics in the topic of assessment of specific journal-related scientometrics and the respective number of published papers; Table S17: The animal species referred to in work reported in published papers on veterinary or animal studies scientometrics in the topic of assessment of specific animal species-related scientometrics and the respective number of published papers; Table S18: The topics assessed most frequently in published papers on veterinary or animal studies scientometrics and the year of publication of respective papers; Table S19: The topics assessed most frequently in published papers on veterinary or animal studies scientometrics and the number of records in respective papers; Table S20: The specific animal species referred to in papers on veterinary or animal studies scientometrics and the respective number of published papers; Figure S3: Box and whisker plot of number of records in papers on veterinary or animal studies scientometrics, in accord with the most frequently referred to specific animal species; Table S21: The keywords in papers on veterinary or animal studies scientometrics and the respective number of occurrences in the papers; Figure S4: Trendline of the progressive change of the median number of co-authors in papers on veterinary or animal studies scientometrics published yearly; Figure S5: Box and whisker plot of number of co-authors in papers on veterinary or animal studies scientometrics, among the countries with most published papers; Figure S6: Histogram of the proportion of papers published under open access among the countries with most published papers on veterinary or animal studies scientometrics; Table S22: Results of univariable analysis for associations with the number of citations received per paper on veterinary or animal studies scientometrics yearly; Table S23: The median number of yearly citations per published paper on veterinary or animal studies scientometrics from the 16 countries with most papers; Figure S7: Box and whisker plot of the yearly citations per published paper on veterinary or animal studies scientometrics in accord with the topic of study and scientometric assessment; Figure S8: Scree-plot of results of principal components analysis for the yearly citations received by the published papers on veterinary or animal studies scientometrics.

Author Contributions: Conceptualization, G.A.V. and G.C.F.; methodology, G.A.V. and G.C.F.; formal analysis, G.A.V., D.T.L. and G.C.F.; investigation, G.A.V., M.V.B., D.T.L., C.C.M. and G.C.F.; data curation, G.A.V.; writing—original draft preparation, G.A.V., M.V.B. and G.C.F.; writing—review and editing, G.A.V., M.V.B., D.T.L., Y.K., C.C.M., D.A.G. and G.C.F.; visualization, G.A.V. and G.C.F.; supervision, G.C.F. All authors have read and agreed to the published version of the manuscript.

Funding: This research received no external funding.

Institutional Review Board Statement: Not applicable.

Informed Consent Statement: Not applicable.

Data Availability Statement: All data are available in the Web of Science platform and in the Supplementary Materials.

Conflicts of Interest: The authors declare no conflicts of interest.

References

1. Donthu, N.; Kumar, S.; Mukherjee, D.; Pandey, N.; Lim, W.M. How to conduct a bibliometric analysis: An overview and guidelines. *J. Bus. Res.* **2021**, *133*, 285–296. [CrossRef]
2. Verma, S.; Gustafsson, A. Investigating the emerging COVID-19 research trends in the field of business and management: A bibliometric analysis approach. *J. Bus. Res.* **2020**, *118*, 253–261. [CrossRef] [PubMed]
3. Ellegaard, O.; Wallin, J.A. The bibliometric analysis of scholarly production: How great is the impact? *Scientometrics* **2015**, *105*, 1809–1831. [CrossRef]
4. Donthu, N.; Kumar, S.; Pandey, N.; Lim, W.M. Research constituents, intellectual structure, and collaboration patterns in journal of international marketing: An analytical retrospective. *J. Int. Market.* **2021**, *29*, 1–25. [CrossRef]
5. Ramos-Rodrígue, A.R.; Ruíz-Navarro, J. Changes in the intellectual structure of strategic management research: A bibliometric study of the Strategic Management Journal, 1980–2000. *Strat. Manag. J.* **2004**, *25*, 981–1004. [CrossRef]
6. *ISO 3166-1:2020(en)*; Codes for the Representation of Names of Countries and Their Subdivisions—Part 1: Country Code. International Organization for Standardization: Geneva, Switzerland, 2020. Available online: https://www.iso.org/obp/ui/en/#iso:std:iso:3166:-1:ed-4:v1:en (accessed on 15 August 2024).

7. Wallin, J.A. Bibliometric methods: Pitfalls and possibilities. *Bas. Clin. Pharmacol. Toxicol.* **2005**, *97*, 261–275. [CrossRef] [PubMed]
8. Fassin, Y.; Rousseau, R. Use of bibliometrics-related terms, their evolution, and the growth of metrics in science. *J. Scientometr. Res.* **2023**, *12*, 509–519. [CrossRef]
9. Liu, Y.; He, H. Scientometrics of scientometrics based on web of science core collection data between 1992 and 2020. *Information* **2023**, *14*, 637. [CrossRef]
10. Heo, S.; Chan, A.Y.; Diaz Peralta, P.; Jin, L.; Ribeiro Pereira Nunes, C.; Bell, M.L. Impacts of the COVID-19 pandemic on scientists' productivity in science, technology, engineering, mathematics (STEM), and medicine fields. *Human. Soc. Sci. Comm.* **2022**, *9*, 434. [CrossRef]
11. Stachan, A.L. The Impact of COVID-19 on Research Methods and Approaches. Covid Collective 2021. Available online: https://opendocs.ids.ac.uk/articles/report/The_Impact_of_Covid-19_on_Research_Methods_and_Approaches/26430931?file=48080689 (accessed on 15 July 2024).
12. Volpe, M.; Ralli, M.; Isidori, A. The impact of the COVID-19 pandemic on research activities: A survey of the largest Italian academic community. *PLoS ONE* **2024**, *19*, e0304078. [CrossRef]
13. Dwivedi, Y.K.; Hughes, D.L.; Coombs, C.; Constantiou, I.; Duan, Y.; Edwards, J.S.; Gupta, B.; Lal, B.; Misrah, S.; Prashant, P.; et al. Impact of COVID-19 pandemic on information management research and practice: Transforming education, work and life. *Int. J. Inform. Manag.* **2020**, *55*, 102211. [CrossRef]
14. Lianou, D.T.; Fthenakis, G.C. Scientometrics study of research output on sheep and goats from Greece. *Animals* **2022**, *12*, 2666. [CrossRef]
15. Lianou, D.T.; Fthenakis, G.C. Scientometrics approach to research in ovine mastitis from 1970 to 2019 (with a complete list of relevant literature references). *Pathogens* **2020**, *9*, 585. [CrossRef] [PubMed]
16. Bourganou, M.V.; Chatzopoulos, D.C.; Lianou, D.T.; Tsangaris, G.T.; Fthenakis, G.C.; Katsafadou, A.I. Scientometrics evaluation of published scientific papers on the use of proteomics technologies in mastitis research in ruminants. *Pathogens* **2024**, *13*, 324. [CrossRef] [PubMed]
17. Bourganou, M.V.; Kiouvrekis, Y.; Chatzopoulos, D.C.; Zikas, S.; Katsafadou, A.I.; Liagka, D.V.; Vasileiou, N.G.C.; Fthenakis, G.C.; Lianou, D.T. Assessment of published papers on the use of machine learning in diagnosis and treatment of mastitis. *Information* **2024**, *15*, 428. [CrossRef]
18. Lerner, H.; Berg, C. The concept of health in One Health and some practical implications for research and education: What is One Health. *Ecol. Epidemiol.* **2015**, *5*, 25300. [CrossRef]
19. European Commission. Open Access. 2022. Available online: https://research-and-innovation.ec.europa.eu/strategy/strategy-2020-2024/our-digital-future/open-science/open-access_en (accessed on 20 February 2024).
20. Pampel, H. Promoting open access in research-performing organizations: Spheres of activity, challenges, and future action areas. *Publications* **2023**, *11*, 44. [CrossRef]
21. Chew, F.S.; Relyea-Chew, A. How research becomes knowledge in radiology: An analysis of citations to published papers. *Am. J. Roentgenol.* **1988**, *150*, 31–37. [CrossRef]
22. Moed, H.F.; Burger, W.J.M.; Frankfort, J.G.; Van Raan, A.F.J. The use of bibliometric data for the measurement of university research performance. *Res. Policy* **1985**, *14*, 131–149. [CrossRef]
23. Van Raan, A.F.J.; Van Leeuwen, T.N. Assessment of the scientific basis of interdisciplinary, applied research—Application of bibliometric methods in nutrition and food research. *Res. Policy* **2002**, *31*, 611–632. [CrossRef]
24. Evans, J.A. Electronic publication and the narrowing of science and scholarship. *Science* **2008**, *321*, 395. [CrossRef] [PubMed]
25. Onodera, N.; Yoshikane, F. Factors affecting citation rates of research articles. large-scale study based on Web of Science data. *J. Assoc. Inform. Sci. Technol.* **2015**, *66*, 739–764. [CrossRef]
26. Fox, C.W.; Paine, C.E.T.; Sauterey, B. Citations increase with manuscript length, author number, and references cited in ecology journals. *Ecol. Evol.* **2016**, *6*, 7717–7726. [CrossRef]
27. Ahlgren, P.; Colliander, C.; Sjögårde, P. Exploring the relation between referencing practices and citation impact: A large-scale study based on Web of Science data. *J. Assoc. Inform. Sci. Technol.* **2018**, *69*, 728–743. [CrossRef]
28. Mammola, S.; Fontaneto, D.; Martínez, A.; Chichorro, F. Impact of the reference list features on the number of citations. *Scientometrics* **2021**, *126*, 785–799. [CrossRef]

MDPI AG
Grosspeteranlage 5
4052 Basel
Switzerland
Tel.: +41 61 683 77 34

Animals Editorial Office
E-mail: animals@mdpi.com
www.mdpi.com/journal/animals

www.ingramcontent.com/pod-product-compliance
Lightning Source LLC
LaVergne TN
LVHW070451061126
851858LV00011B/208
9783725882519